Encyclopedia of Drug Discovery and Development: Essential Topics in Drug Discovery

Volume VI

Encyclopedia of Drug Discovery and Development: Essential Topics in Drug Discovery Volume VI

Edited by **Ned Burnett**

FOSTER
A C A D E M I C S

New Jersey

Published by Foster Academics,
61 Van Reypen Street,
Jersey City, NJ 07306, USA
www.fosteracademics.com

Encyclopedia of Drug Discovery and Development:
Essential Topics in Drug Discovery
Volume VI
Edited by Ned Burnett

International Standard Book Number: 978-1-63242-141-8 (Hardback)

Contents

Preface

The purpose of the book is to provide a glimpse into the dynamics and to present opinions and studies of some of the scientists engaged in the development of new ideas in the field from very different standpoints. This book will prove useful to students and researchers owing to its high content quality.

Natural products are a consistent source of potentially effective compounds for the treatment of several disorders. It is believed that the tropical and Middle East regions have the most abundant supplies of natural products across the globe. Secondary metabolites obtained from plants have been employed by humans to treat health disorders, acute infections and chronic illness for a large number of years. Natural products have been greatly replaced by synthetic drugs in the past 100 years. Estimates of 200,000 natural products in plant species have been revised upward as mass spectrometry methodologies have advanced. For advancing countries the recognition and use of endogenous medicinal plants as cures for cancers have become appealing. This book presents essential topics in drug discovery covering an introduction to biochemical pharmacology, anticancer drug discovery, drug interactions, molecule screens to identity inhibitors of infectious disease, oxidative stress in human infectious disease, etc.

At the end, I would like to appreciate all the efforts made by the authors in completing their chapters professionally. I express my deepest gratitude to all of them for contributing to this book by sharing their valuable works. A special thanks to my family and friends for their constant support in this journey.

Editor

Introduction to
Biochemical Pharmacology and Drug Discovery

Gabriel Magoma

Additional information is available at the end of the chapter

1. Introduction

This chapter introduces biochemical pharmacology and highlights drug absorption and drug transformation reactions and a general introduction to pharmacology, drug discovery and clinical trials for new drug candidates. It also introduces the concept of individualization of drug therapies. After studying this chapter, one is expected to demonstrate understanding the following: (i) Linkage between the various pharmacological processes (ii) Routes of drug administration, (iii) Mechanisms of drug absorption (iv) The kinetics of drug disposition and concepts, such as volume of distribution, initial dose and half-life, (v) The biotransformation and excretion of drugs.(vi) The role of biochemical knowledge in the discovery and development of candidate drug compounds into useful drugs (vii) Basic design of clinical trials of new drugs and the drug approval process.(viii) The linkage between genetic variations and varied drug responses in different individuals (ix) The various adverse drug reactions in different patients (x) How different dosage regimens are calculated with respect to the prevailing health status of individuals and how adjustments are carried out in old patients or geriatrics.

2. Pharmacology

Pharmacology is the science that deals with drugs, their properties, actions and fate in the body. It embraces the sciences of pharmaceutics (preparation of drugs), therapeutics (treatment of diseases by use of drugs) and toxicosis or adverse side-effects that arise from the therapeutic interventions. Pharmacology can be divided into the following processes:-

i.   The pharmaceutical process of drugs; deals with chemical synthesis, formulation and distribution of drugs.

ii.   Pharmacokinetic process; deals with the time course of drug concentration in the body.This process can be further subdivided into; absorption, distribution, biotransformation and excretion of the drug.

iii.   The pharmacodynamic process; deals with the mechanism of drug action: that is interaction of drugs with the molecular structures in the body.

iv.   The therapeutic process; deals with the clinical response arising from the pharmacodynamic process.

v.   Toxicologic process; deals with adverse effects of drugs arising from either over dosage or interference of biochemical pathways unrelated to the intended drug target. The five processes are related as exemplified in Figure1.

3. Biochemical pharmacology

Biochemical pharmacology is concerned with the effects of drugs on biochemical pathways underlying the pharmacokinetic and pharmacodynamic processes and the subsequent therapeutic and the toxicological processes. The pharmaceutical process is, however, outside the realms of biochemical pharmacology.

4. Routes of drug administration and systemic availability

This depends on the actual biochemical characteristics of the drug and the interaction of drug molecules with body fluids and tissues. The main routes of drug administration are the topical application, parenteral, and enteral routes.

The route of drug application determines how quickly the drug reaches its site of action. The choice of the route of administration of a drug, therefore, depends on the therapeutic objectives of the treatment. For instance, intravenous injection or inhalation may be selected to produce intense, but rather short-lived effects, whereas oral dosing may be better and more convenient for long lasting effects and even intensity. The various types of drug administration include;

4.1. Topical application

This is the most direct and easiest mode of drug administration. It involves local application of a drug to the site of action e.g. eye drop solutions, sprays and lotions for oral, rectal, vaginal and urethral use. These drugs are absorbed through the cell membranes. Absorption of drugs through the skin is proportional to their lipid solubility since the epidermis behaves like a hydrophilic barrier. Lipid insoluble drugs are therefore suspended in oily vehicles to enhance solubility and hence absorption.

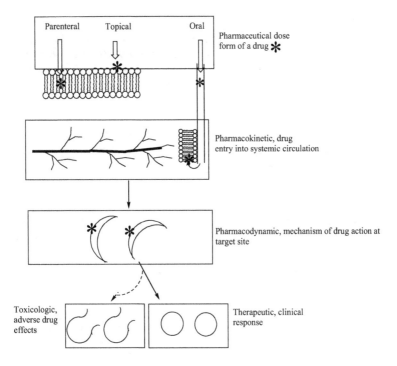

Figure 1. Relationships between the five pharmacological processes starting with the entry of the drug and ending with the clinical response and/or the toxic effects

4.2. Oral administration

The drugs administered orally are absorbed at different sites along the gastrointestinal tract (GIT):

4.2.1. Oral mucosal or sublingual

Drug absorption is generally rapid because of the rich vascular supply to the mucosa and the absence of a stratum corneum. Drugs delivered using this route are not exposed to gastric and intestinal digestive juices and are not subjected to immediate passage through the liver. Therefore there is no prior biotransformation or first-effect before the drugs enter the systemic circulation.

4.2.2. Stomach and intestine

Absorption depends on different factors such as pH, gastric emptying, intestinal motility and solubility of solid drugs. The rapidity with which a drug reaches the small intestine is enhanced when a drug is taken with water and when the stomach is relatively empty. However drugs absorbed in the stomach and intestine are subjected to first-pass effect.

4.3. Rectal administration

This is the preferred route when the oral route is unsuitable because of nausea or if the drugs have objectionable taste or odor. This route also protects susceptible drugs from the biotransformation reactions in the liver. However, absorption by this route is often irregular and incomplete. Formulations such as suppositories or enemas are applied via rectal route.

4.4. Parenteral administration

This mode of administration is also known as injection. It is generally more rapid and enables more accurate dose selection and predictable absorption. Parenteral routes include;

4.4.1. Subcutaneous injection

This mode of administration is mainly used for non-irritating drugs. It provides even and slows absorption producing sustained drug effects. Vasoconstrictor agents such as epinephrine can be added to the drug solution to decrease the rate of absorption.

Large volumes of drugs may, however, be painful because of tissue distention.

4.4.2. Intramuscular injection

This method of drug delivery ensures rapid absorption of the drug in aqueous solutions. Slow and even absorption is possible when drugs are suspended in oily vehicles.

4.4.3. Intravenous administration

This route ensures rapid delivery of the desired blood concentration of the drug to be obtained accurately and immediately and is the preferred route of delivery in emergency situations. Irritating drugs are delivered intravenously because the veins have low sensitivity to pain. This mode of delivery is also preferred for drug such as the barbiturates and phenytoin, anti-seizure drugs which dissolve only in rather strong alkaline solution and therefore need the blood to buffer the pH of the drug solution for better solubility. Drugs such as ethylene di-amine tetra acetic acid (EDTA) for treatment of heavy-metal poisoning are given by intravenous injection or through an infusion because they are poorly absorbed in the gut. The other advantage of this mode of delivery is the avoidance of the hepatic and pulmonary first-pass effect. Generally, the properties of the drug may determine the route that must be used for reasonable efficacy.

5. Mechanisms of drug absorption across membranes

In order for drugs to elicit their pharmacological effects, they have to cross the biological membranes into systemic circulation and reach the site of action. Therefore an insight into the structure and function of the membrane leads to a better understanding of drug absorption.

Membranes are phospholipid bi-layers with interspersed integral and peripheral proteins which behave either as molecular 'gates' or 'pumps'. Molecular gates are non-specific. The intake of molecules into the cell depends on the charged groups in the pore and the size of molecule to be transported across the membrane. Molecular pumps, however, are highly specific and require energy for molecular transport. There are several mechanisms by which drugs traverse membranes to reach their intended target site and they include the following:

5.1. Simple diffusion

This involves is the passage of polar but uncharged substances across water filled channels in response to the concentration gradient. Simple diffusion is the mechanism of choice for water soluble drugs and those with low molecular weight such as the an aesthetic nitrous oxide (44kD) and ethanol (46 KDa). The majority of lipid-soluble drugs permeate cell membranes by passive diffusion between the lipid molecules of the membrane. The permeation rate of a lipid soluble drug depends on the concentration of the drug, its lipid/water partition coefficient concentration of protons and the surface area of the absorbing membrane. The lipid/water partition coefficient of a drug is the principal factor determining its absorption.

The higher the value of lipid/water partition coefficient of a drug, the more rapidly it will be absorbed and vice versa. The chemical force that causes lipid-soluble drugs to move readily across membranes is termed the hydrophobic force since water molecules repels the lipid-soluble drugs. In most cases, drug absorption can be enhanced by absorption enhancers, such as fatty acids, phospholipids and muco-adhesive polymers. These compounds disrupt the lipid bilayer making it more permeable and also increase the solubility of insoluble drugs.

5.2. Facilitated diffusion

This type of diffusion is achieved by carrier molecules which combine with the drug in question to form complexes that can diffuse more rapidly across the membrane than free-drug could do alone. An example is the transport of nucleotide antimetabolites used in viral or cancer chemotherapy.

5.3. Active transport of drugs

This is the transport which is linked to a source of energy. Examples of specific active transport systems are the sodium pump, which maintains high potassium and low sodium ions inside the cell relative to the external medium and the calcium pump that maintains a high concentration of calcium inside the sarcoplasmic reticulum and a low concentration around the myofibrils. Active transport of drugs across membranes have been discovered and an example is the uptake of pentazocine (a narcotic antagonist) by leukocytes which is dependent upon energy supply (glucose) and can be inhibited by cyclazocine, which competes for the same transport mechanism.

5.4. Pinocytosis and phagocytosis of drugs

Proteins, bacterial toxins and drugs with high molecular weights, (1000 KDa or more) enter cells by means of pinocytosis and endocytosis. These substances finally enter the lysosomal system.

6. Factors affecting absorption of drugs

6.1. Surface area

For any substance that can penetrate the GIT in measurable amounts, the small intestine represents the greatest area of absorption. For instance, ethanol can be absorbed by the stomach, but it is absorbed eight times faster from the small intestine because of the large surface area provided by the villi. The rate at which the stomach empties its contents into the small intestine also markedly affects the overall rate at which drugs reach general circulation after oral administration. For this reason many agents are administered on an empty stomach with sufficient water to ensure their rapid passage to the small intestine.

6.2. Tissue pH

Drugs can be classified either as organic amines or organic acids and therefore their absorption is markedly affected by pH. Tertiary amines are not charged at high pH and have a high lipid/water partition coefficient and hence readily penetrate membranes.

At low pH, the tertiary amine is protonated and has low lipid/water partition coefficient thus lower rate of permeation.

Stomach	Small intestines
Low pH	High pH
(protonated form)	(unprotonated form)
Lower absorption	Higher absorption.

In case of an organic acid, the same general principle applies. The unprotonated organic acid at low pH permeates the tissues more readily as compared to the charged form of the drug at high pH.

Low pH   High pH

$R\text{-}COOH \rightleftharpoons R\text{-}COO^- + H^+$

Stomach   Intestine

Therefore organic acids such as barbiturates and acetyl salicylic acid (aspirin) have a higher absorption rate in the stomach.

The degree of ionization of the drug when in the GIT or other body fluids is the main determinant of the amount of the drug found in an uncharged form and this depends upon the relation between pH of the fluid and the pKa of the drug:

Acidic drugs:

$$RCOOH \overset{Ka}{\rightleftharpoons} RCOO^- + H^+$$

Basic drugs:

$$R -^+NH_3 \overset{Ka}{\rightleftharpoons} RNH_2 + H^+$$

If the pH of the fluid is low, the ionization of acidic drugs is less while the ionization of basic drugs will be high.When the pKa of a drug is equal to the pH of the surrounding fluid, there is 50% ionization.

7. Types of tissue barriers to drugs

Most of these barriers are typically the same systems that animals use for defense against invasion by foreign agents. These barriers include the skin, the GIT membranes, blood-brain barrier and placenta.

7.1. Skin

The superficial layer of the skin, stratum corneum is particularly impermeable to most drugs. The skin permeability for the drugs is enhanced by using a co-solvent system such as ethanol/water which increases drug partition into the skin. The lipid domains of the buccal and nasal mucosa also restrict drug entry and the drugs which permeate are able to do so through passive diffusion using the hydrophilic trans-cellular spaces and direct permeation through the membrane.

7.2. Tight junctions

The gap junctions between cells in different cell types within a tissue can form channels for the passage of drugs between epithelial, endothelial, and mesothelial cells of the same tissue. These channels comprise of a group of proteins known as connexin. Cells in different tissues are however connected by tight junctions and these can impair transport between cells in different tissues. The tight junctions are dynamic structures, which normally regulate the trafficking of nutrients, medium sized compounds between cells, and form a regulated barrier in spaces between cells. There is need therefore to use drug absorption enhancers such as bile salts and long chain acyl-carnitines which act as Ca^{2+}chelatorsand disrupt the tight junctions thereby improving transport across the junctions. Tight junctions are shown in Figure 2.

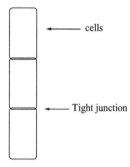

Figure 2. Arrangement of epithelial cells with tight junctions

7.3. Cerebrospinal fluid barrier (CSF)

Epithelial cells which are in contact with the brain ventricular spaces form a barrier to the movement of drugs. These epithelial cells are connected by occluding zonulae (blood- brain barrier) as shown in Figure 3. The zonulae severely restrict the passage of most molecules between the bloodstream and the parenchyma of the central nervous system. Drug entry across this barrier is through either passive diffusion or carrier mediated transport. Only the lipid soluble drugs cross into the CSF from blood.

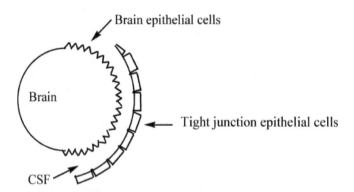

Figure 3. Epithelial cells with tight junctions as part of the blood brain barrier

Epithelial cells that separate the CSF from the brain are connected with tight junctions and are characterized by marked scarcity of pinocytic vesicles. However, the epithelial cells that lines the brain are not connected by occluding zonulae and therefore, there is unrestricted passage of drug molecules from CSF to the brain. Drugs like penicillin which are not much lipid-soluble and required in high concentrations for the treatment of brain abscesses are administered through intrathecal injections directly into the CFS.

7.4. Placental barrier

The placental membrane limits the amount of maternal blood following through the placenta to the foetus and passive diffusion is the main mechanism of drug entry from the maternal blood to the foetus. The shortest time required for equilibration of a drug between mother and foetus is about ten minutes and this delay is useful as it can allow a mother to be anaesthetized during final stages of labour.

8. Systemic availability of drugs

A drug will reach systemic arterial circulation only if it is absorbed from the GIT and if it escapes metabolism in the gut, liver, and lungs. When the concentration of the drug in plasma is measured at specified time intervals, it is possible to construct concentration versus time graph and hence be able to determine the extent of drug availability as shown in Figure 4.

The availability depends on both the extent of absorption and the extent of presystemic metabolism and comprises three aspects; Peak concentration (C_{max}), Time taken to reach the peak (T_{max}) and area under the curve (AUC)as shown in Figure 4. The C_{max} and T_{max} are measures of the rate of availability while AUC is a measure of the extent of availability (i.e. proportion of the administered drug which reaches systemic circulation intact). For the three curves shown for the formulations a, b, and c; the AUC is the same, but the rate of availability is different in each case; a, has the lowest rate of availability followed by b, while c has the highest rate of availability.

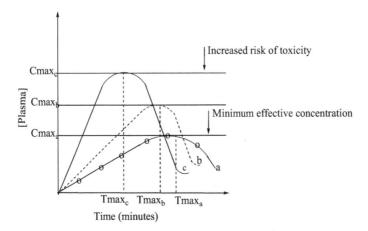

Figure 4. Plasma concentration versus time curves for different drug formulations

The speed at which a particular drug is needed to reach the site of action will determine the type of formulation to use. Drugs with the same relative bioavailability and can be used to treat the same condition using either the same routes or dosages are known as bioequivalent drugs.

9. Dosage and effect

A particular dose of an administered drug is subject to the biochemical processes in the body as shown in Figure 5. The desired effect of a drug is proportional to the concentration of the drug at its site of action which is described by the following kinetic parameters: (i) The apparent volume of distribution (V_d) which is the volume of the hydrophilic and hydrophobic spaces in the body that the drug is distributed in. It is obtained by dividing the injected dose (D_o) by the initial concentration (C_o) in blood plasma. Drugs that bind to tissues extensively exhibit low concentrations in the plasma and therefore, have higher a V_d compared to those that are mainly bound by blood plasma proteins. An average 70kg person has a total body water volume of ~ 50L of which ~ 10L occupy extra-cellular space.

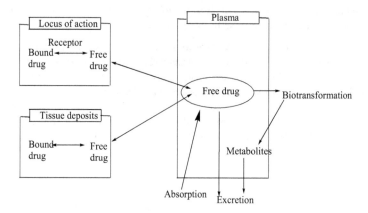

Figure 5. Drug disposition routes from absorption to excretion

The apparent volume of distribution cannot tell us where in the body the drug really is. The (C_{tox}) is the maximum drug concentration beyond which there would be toxic effects in the body, while the (C_{ther}) is the plasma concentration of a drug that would achieve a therapeutic effect or effective clinical response. The steady state concentration (C_{ss}) is that concentration that should be maintained between any two drug administration intervals. These pharmacokinetic data are important in that they characterize the fate of drugs in the body and are required by pharmacologists to calculate doses and frequencies of drug administration. However, in some clinical responses, the intensity of pharmacological action correlates better with the concentration of free drug in plasma, while in other responses there is no direct relationship between drug concentration and clinical response. The main variations of the drug response effects include;

i.   Drugs which combine with their receptors as quickly as they dissociate from them; for this category of drugs, the pharmacological effect increases or reduces in tandem with the plasma drug concentration.

ii.   Drugs which do not readily dissociate from their receptors. In this case the pharma-cological effect persists despite the falling plasma concentration.

iii.   Drugs which combine with receptors and irrespective of their rates of association/ dissociation sets in motion a cascade of events which runs on despite falling plasma concentrations.

10. Kinetics of drug disposition process

Drug disposition process most of the times follows the 1st order kinetics in which disposition is proportional to the concentration of the drug at any given time. Therefore, the concentration of a drug in plasma will decrease at a rate that is proportional at all times to the concentration itself. Therefore;

$$\frac{-d[C]}{dt} = K[C]$$

$$\int \frac{-d[C]}{[C]} = \int K dt$$

$$\left[\ln[C] \right]_{c_0}^{ct} = Kt$$

$$\ln[C]_t - \ln[C]_o = Kt \text{ or } \ln C = \ln C_o - Kt$$

$$e^{\ln} \frac{[C]_t}{[C]_o} = e^{-Kt}$$

$$[C_t] = [C_o] e^{-Kt}$$

A more convenient form of this equation is obtained by taking $\log_{10}$

Since

$$\ln x = 2.303 \log_{10} x \qquad\qquad (1)$$

It follows that;

$$2.303 \log_{10} C = 2.30.3 \log_{10} C_0 - Kt$$

and $\log_{10} C = \log_{10} C_0 - \frac{Kt}{2.303}$

A linear relationship is obtained when the logarithm of concentrations ($\log_{10} C$) is plotted against (t), times of observation (Figure 6).

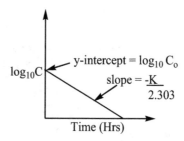

Figure 6. Logarithmic time course of drug concentration

Half-life ($t_{1/2}$) of a drug: this is the time period during which the concentration decreases to one- half of its previous value. $T_{1/2}$ can be evaluated from the elimination rate constant.

When $t = t_{1/2}$, $C_t = \frac{C_0}{2}$

therefore,

$$\frac{C_0}{2} = C_0 e^{-K t_{1/2}}$$

$$\frac{1}{2} = e^{-K t_{1/2}} \quad \text{but,} \quad K t_{1/2} = \log_e 2$$

$$t_{1/2} = \log_e \frac{2}{K} = \frac{0.693}{K}$$

11. Drug biotransformation reactions

Drugs and other foreign substances (xenobiotics) undergo series of biotransformation reactions in the body. The biotransformation reactions act as first line defense strategy against these xenobiotics. It is armed with a battery of enzymes which convert the lipid-soluble xenobiotics into more water-soluble metabolites to allow more efficient excretion of the drugs in a limited volume of water in urine or bile.

The enzymes involved in the biotransformation of endogenous chemicals are the same ones that are used in the biotransformation of xenobiotics. There is, therefore, a close relationship between drug biotransformation and fundamental homeostatic processes.

The drug biotransformation reaction may result in the following potential effects with respect to pharmacological activity:

11.1. Activation

An inactive precursor may be converted into a pharmacologically active drug. For instance, the nucleoside analogue used as an anti-HIV drug, have to undergo *in vivo* phosphorylation to form the active triphosphates which functions to inhibit the enzyme reverse transcriptase, while L– dopa (inactive), which is used in the treatment of parkinsons disease, is converted into dopamine (active) in the basal ganglia. Futamide, a drug used in the treatment of prostate cancer, undergoes hydroxylation at the alkyl side chain to form hydroxyflutamide, a metabolite that is more active and has a longer duration of action compared to the parent drug.

11.2. Maintenance of activity

An active drug is converted into another form which is also active, for instance diazepam, a sedative hypnotic, is metabolized to an equally active metabolite, oxazepam.

11.3. Inactivation

An active drug is converted to inactive products, for example, pentobarbital is hydroxylated to forminactive metabolites.

11.4. Phase I reactions

These include oxidation, reduction and hydrolytic reactions and such reactions generally introduce or unmask a functional group (hydroxyl, amine, sulfhydryl etc) that make the drug more polar.

11.5. Phase II reactions

Consist of synthetic/conjugation reactions in which an endogenous substance such as glucuronic acid or glutathione combines with the functional group derived from phase I reactions to produce a highly polar drug conjugate. All tissues have some ability to carry out drug biotransformation reactions but the most important organs of biotransformation include; the liver, GIT, lungs, skin, and kidneys in that order and most phase II reactions result in a decrease in the pharmacological activity of the drug. The fact that the GIT and liver are the major sites of drug biotransformation means that drugs which are administered orally will be extensively bio-transformed before they eventually reach systemic circulation. This first-pass effect can severely limit the oral bio- availability of some drugs. In addition, intestinal micro-organisms are capable of catalyzing drug biotransformation reactions e.g. a glucuronide conjugate of a drug may be excreted through the intestine via the bile where gut bacteria may convert the conjugate back into free drug. The free drug is then reabsorbed and re-enters the liver via the portal vein where the conjugation process is repeated. This leads to a phenomenon known as entero-hepaticcirculation.

At sub-cellular level, enzymes of drug biotransformation are located in the endoplasmic reticulum, mitochondria, cytosol and lysosome. The major site of drug biotransformation within the hepatocytes and other cells is the membrane of the smooth endoplasmic reticulum. The smooth endoplasmic reticulum constitutes the microsome fraction during differential centrifugation of whole blood. The microsome fraction can be used to carry out many drug biotransformation reactions *in vitro*.

11.6. Mechanisms of phase I reactions

11.6.1. Oxidation

Is the most important category of the microsomal drug oxidizing systems and requires participation of two distinct proteins in endoplasmic reticulum; cytochromes P_{450} (which functions as a terminal oxidase) and cytochrome P_{450} reductase. The name Cyt_{450} is derived from the fact that the reduced form of this hemoprotein complexes with carbon monoxide to form a complex that has a unique absorption spectrum with a maximum at 450nm. Cytochrome P_{450} reductase serves to transfer reducing equivalent from NADPH to the cytochrome P_{450} oxidase:

$$DrugRH + O_2 + NADPH + H^+ \rightarrow DrugROH \text{ (hydroxylated product)} + H_2O + NADP^+$$

The sequence of reactions that transform a drug to its hydroxylated product is shown below (Figure 7).

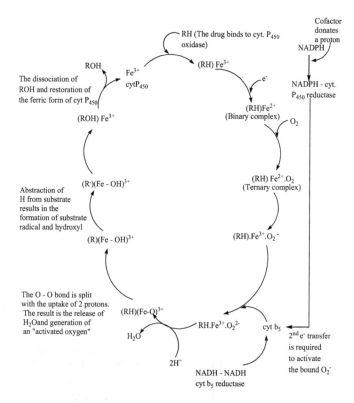

Figure 7. Phase 1 drug biotransformation reactions in the liver microsomal fraction in which the drug is converted to a more polar form.

The phospholipids of the endoplasmic reticulum are required for substrate binding, electron transfer, and facilitating the interaction between $CytP_{450}$ and its reductase. However, cytochrome P_{450} does not catalyze all Oxidation reactions. The microsomal flavin– containing monooxygenases (FMOs) catalyze NADPH – dependent oxygenation of nucleophilic phosphorous, nitrogen and sulfur atoms. These atoms are present in a wide variety of xenobiotics including the carbamate containing pesticides and therapeutic agents such as phenothiazines, ephedrine and N-methylamphetamine. Another important drug–oxidizing system is the prostaglandin synthetase–dependent co-oxidation.

$$\text{Prostaglandin } G_2 \text{ reduced} \rightleftharpoons \text{prostaglandin } H_2$$
$$\text{prostaglandin}$$
$$\text{synthetase}$$

Many xenobiotics including phenytoin can be co-oxidized along with the above reduction reaction. This pathway is of considerable toxicological importance as it often leads to generation of toxic reactive metabolites. Other enzymes that catalyze oxidation of xenobiotic include alcohol dehydrogenase, aldehyde dehydrogenase, xanthine oxidase and monoamine oxidase.

11.6.2. Reduction

Some drugs with azo-linkages (RN=NR, e.g. prontosil) and nitrogen groups (RNO_2, such as chloramphenicol) are transformed by reductive pathways. The Cyt P_{450} and NADPH–cyt P_{450}reductase enzymes that catalyze oxidation reactions are also involved in reduction reactions for drugs containing quinine moieties. These transformation results in the formation of semiquinone free radicals illustrated in Figure 8. The free radicals that are generated cause oxidative stress, lipid peroxidation, DNA damage, and hence cytotoxicity. These effects are particularly responsible for the antitumor property of a drug like doxorubicin.

11.6.3. Hydrolysis

Drugs containing ester functions (R_1COOR_2) such as procaine are hydrolyzed by a variety of non-specific esterases in liver, and plasma while drugs with amide bonds are hydrolyzed by amidases in the liver. The polypeptide drugs such as insulin and growth hormones are hydrolyzed by peptidases in the plasma and erythrocytes. The metabolites resulting from hydrolysis reactions are subjected to phase II biotransformation reactions before excretion in the bile or urine.

11.7. Mechanisms of phase II reactions

The phase II reactions generally involve coupling of drug/drug metabolite with an endogenous substance to enhance their removal from the body. They require participation of specific transferase enzymes and high energy activated endogenous substances.

Most of the conjugation reactions result in detoxification of the drug although in some cases conjugation reactions result in bioactivation of drugs. The following is a summary of the different types of phase II biotransformation reactions;

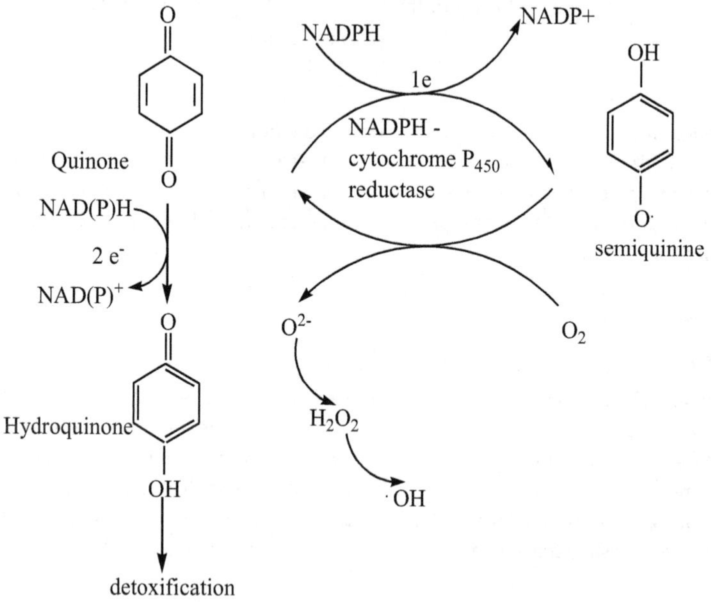

Figure 8. The transformation pathways for drugs with quinine moieties to generate free radicals.

11.7.1. Glutathione conjugation

Glutathione-S-transferases catalyze the enzymatic conjugation of xenobiotics with the endogenous tripeptide glutathione, glutamylcystenylglycine (GSH). The xenobiotics with suitable electrophilic centres such as the epoxides and nitro groups can be subjected to nucleophilic attack by glutathione (Figure 9). The final product, mercapturic acid is easily excreted from the body.

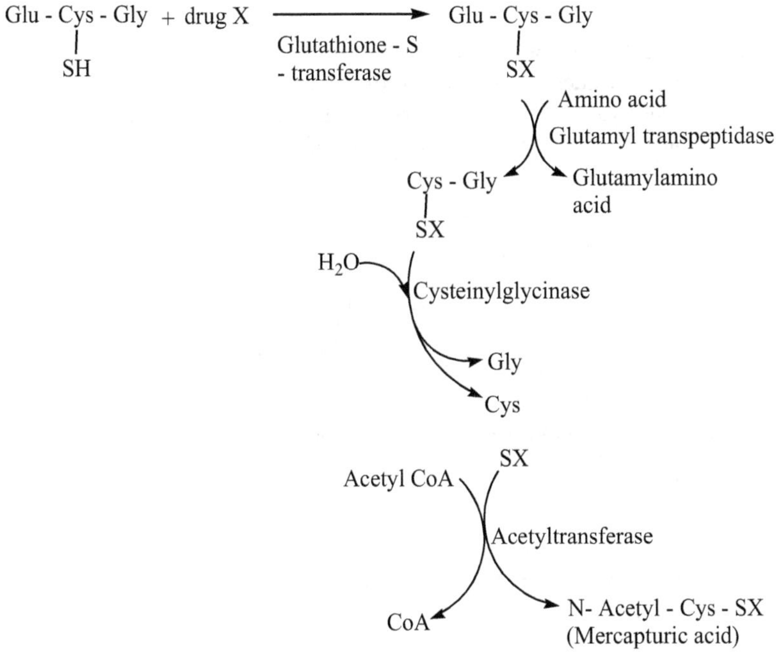

Glu - Cys - Gly + drug X ⟶ Glu - Cys - Gly
| Glutathione - S |
SH   - transferase   SX

Amino acid
Glutamyl transpeptidase

Cys - Gly ⟵ ⟶ Glutamylamino
| acid
SX

H₂O
Cysteinylglycinase

Gly
Cys

SX
Acetyl CoA
Acetyltransferase

CoA ⟵ ⟶ N- Acetyl - Cys - SX
(Mercapturic acid)

Figure 9. Glutathione conjugation reactions for a drug with a suitable nucleophilic centre leads to the formation of mercapturic acid which is easily excreted from the body

11.7.2. Glucuronidation

This is the conjugation of a drug or xenobiotic with glucuronic acid. Many functional groups are subject to glucuronidation. The benzoyl group in morphine, (an analgesic) and the amine group in meprobamate (a sedative) can undergo glucuronidation. A drug with a benzoyl group can undergo glucoronidation by a transferase as shown below:

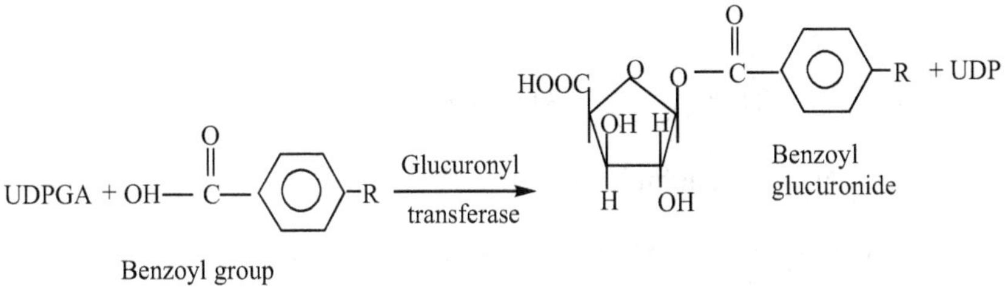

HOOC ... O-C-⟨ ⟩-R + UDP
Benzoyl
glucuronide

UDPGA + OH— C—⟨ ⟩-R   Glucuronyl
transferase

Benzoyl group

11.7.3. Epoxide hydration

A number of aromatic compounds are transformed by phase I reactions to form epoxide intermediates. The epoxides are reactive electrophilic species that can bind covalently to proteins and nucleic acids to bring about toxic effects. These epoxides are detoxified via the nucleophilic attack of water molecule on one of the electron deficient carbon atoms of the oxizane ring as shown below:

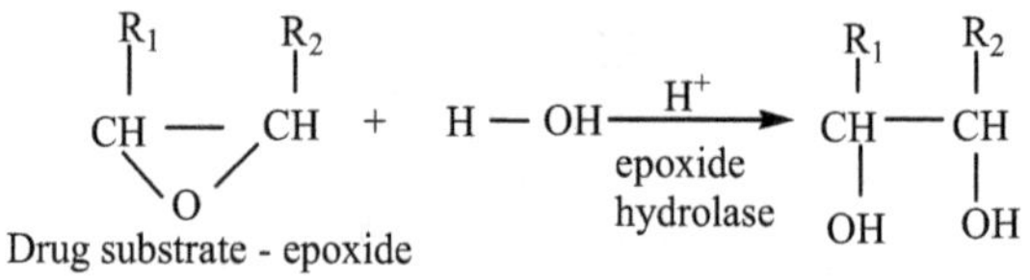

$$
\underset{\text{Drug substrate - epoxide}}{\overset{R_1 \quad\quad R_2}{CH - CH}} + H - OH \xrightarrow[\substack{\text{epoxide} \\ \text{hydrolase}}]{H^+} \underset{OH \quad OH}{\overset{R_1 \quad R_2}{CH - CH}}
$$

The glucuronide conjugates can be excreted via the bile or urine.

11.7.4. Acetylation

Acetylation is achieved by cytosolic enzymes known as N-acetyl transferases which catalyze transfer of acetate from acetyl co-enzyme A to primary aromatic amine or hydrazides (figure 10)

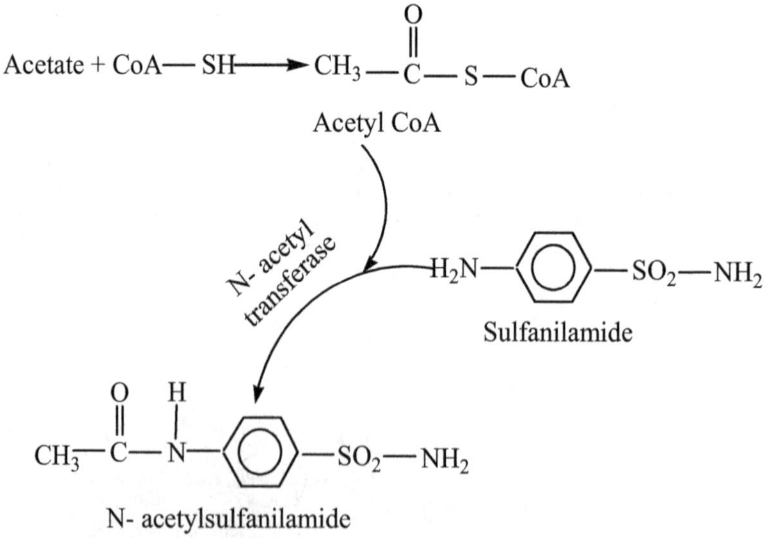

$$
\text{Acetate} + \text{CoA}-\text{SH} \longrightarrow \underset{\text{Acetyl CoA}}{CH_3 - \overset{\overset{O}{\|}}{C} - S - \text{CoA}}
$$

N-acetyl transferase

$$H_2N - \bigcirc - SO_2 - NH_2$$

Sulfanilamide

$$\underset{\text{N- acetylsulfanilamide}}{CH_3 - \overset{\overset{O}{\|}}{C} - \overset{\overset{H}{|}}{N} - \bigcirc - SO_2 - NH_2}$$

Figure 10. Acetylation reations leading to the formation of N– Acetylsulfanilamide, the final metabolite of the antimicrobial agent sulfanilamide which is secreted from the body

11.7.5. Methylation

Most of the methyl transferases are cytosolic enzymes. They utilize S-adenosyl methionine (SAM) as the methyl donor. The final metabolite, thiopurine, has antineoplastic properties and is used as an anticancer agent (Figure 11)

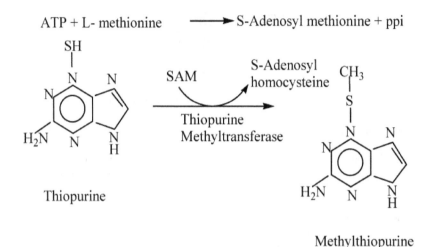

Figure 11. Methylation reactions leading to the formation of methylthiopurine

12. Adverse drug reactions associated with drug biotransformation reactions

Many adverse drug reactions can be traced to an improper balance between bioactivation and detoxification reactions. For example, when the analgesic acetaminophen is given at normal therapeutic doses, it undergoes glucuronidation and sulfation reactions that terminate the action of the drug and hasten its elimination. However, some of the drug is bioactivated via Cyt P_{450} to form N-acetylbenzoquinimine, a reactive intermediate that can be detoxified by conjugation with glutathione (GSH). When excessive doses of the drug are given, glucuronidation and sulfation reactions become saturated and more acetaminophen is bioactivated via Cyt P_{450}. This imbalance leads to high concentrations of N-acetylbenzoqunonine which cannot be sufficiently eliminated by the limited concentrations of gluthathione. This metabolite binds covalently to cellular protein thiols and initiates hepatotoxicity leading to hepatic necrosis.

12.1. Revision exercise 1

1. Discuss the absorption of á-D- Ribose-5-phosphate, given that the two ionizable hydroxyl groups of the monophosphate ester ribose have pKa values of 1.2. and 6.6. The fully protonated form of á-D-ribose 5-phosphate has the following structure;

2. Using specific examples of drugs, justify their various routes of administration.

12.2. Revision exercise 2

If the concentration of a drug in plasma decreases at a rate that is proportional to its initial concentration, give an expression that describes this relationship and hence show that $[C_t] = [C_0].e^{-kt}$

12.3. Worked examples

Problem 1: Describe how you can determine the partition coefficient of a labeled drug

Solution: The partition coefficient of a drug is its differential distribution between the hydrophobic and hydrophilic phases. The distribution of the drug between these two phases can be determined by allowing equilibration of a radioactively labeled drug between aqueous buffer containing the drug and a cell membrane preparation obtained by homogenization and fractionation of a tissue sample. The ratio of drug concentration in the membrane to the concentration in the aqueous phase gives the partition coefficient.

Problem 2: Describe how you can demonstrate transport across membranes

Solution: Erythrocyte 'ghosts' or self sealing micelles formed when the erythrocytes release cytoplasmic contents upon exposure into a hypotonic solution can be used to study the uptake or release of labeled molecules across erythrocytes. When the ghosts are prepared in ^{14}C glucose, it will be possible to monitor the rate of release or uptake of the labeled ^{14}C glucose from the membranes into the aqueous environment. These 'ghosts' can also be used to study the uptake of various molecules at various concentrations under different conditions of temperatures and the presence of inhibitors for specific molecular uptake.

Problem 3: A 120mg per kg dose of a drug was injected intravenously and its concentration (mg/L) monitored regularly over time. When $\log_{10} C$ was plotted vs time (h) a linear response was obtained with a slope of $- 0.08$ and an extrapolated y-intercept of 1.3. Calculate the following pharmacokinetic parameters;

i.   elimination rate constant (k)

ii.   initial concentration of the drug in blood plasma (C_o)

iii.   volume of distribution (V_d)

iv.   half-life of drug elimination ($t_{1/2}$).

Solution:

i.   Slope = - k/2.303, therefore, k = -2.303x -0.08 = 0.184

ii. C_o = Antilog of 1.3 = $10^{1.3}$ = 20 mg/L

iii.   Volume of distribution (V_d) = Do/Co = 120/20 = 6 L

iv.   The half-life of elimination $t_{1/2}$ = 0.693/k = 0.693/0.184 = 3.7 hours.

Once the apparent volume of distribution is known for a particular drug the amount of drug that must be given to achieve a desired concentration can be determined from

Do = Co.V_d

Problem 4: You have been given the following data based on a 65 kg patient; $t_{1/2}$ of drug X = 4.5hrs, V_d = 0.56L/kg, C_{min} the = 5mg/L, C_{tox} = 20mg/L and C_{ss} = 10mg/L; calculate:-

i.   Drug clearance from the body

ii.   Average rate of drug intake (Dosing rate)

iii.   Maintenance dose

iv.   Maintenance interval

v.   Initial loading dose

vi.   Loading dose at steady state concentration

Solution

Since $t_{1/2}$ = 0.693/ k; k= 0.693/ $t_{1/2 \, i.e.}$ 0.693/4.5=0.154, and V= 0.56 x 65 = 36.4.

i.   Total drug clearance = kV = 0.154 x 36.4 = 5.6L/h = 93.3ml/min.

ii.   Average rate of drug intake = rate elimination constant

= kxVxCss

= 0.154 x 36.4 x 10

= 56 mg/h

iii.   Maintenance dose

= (C_{tox} - C_{ther}). V

= (20 – 5) x 36.4 = 546 mg

iv.   Maintenance interval = maintenance dose/ rate of elimination

= 546/56

= 9.75 hrs

For a practical loading schedule, the maintenance interval should be lowered to say 8.0 hrs and the maintenance dose reduced proportionately: = 546 x 8/9.75 ~ 437 mg.

v.   The initial loading dose

$= C_{tox.} V$

= 36.4 x 20

= 728 mg

vi.   The loading dose at steady state

$= C_{ss} \times V$

= 36.4 x 10 = 364 mg

Practical problem 1

The analytical method of assaying paracetamol relies on the introduction of a nitro group into the molecule after the removal of plasma proteins through precipitation. The resultant nitrophenol compound which is formed has a deep yellow colour in an alkaline medium and absorbs at 430nm Figure 12.

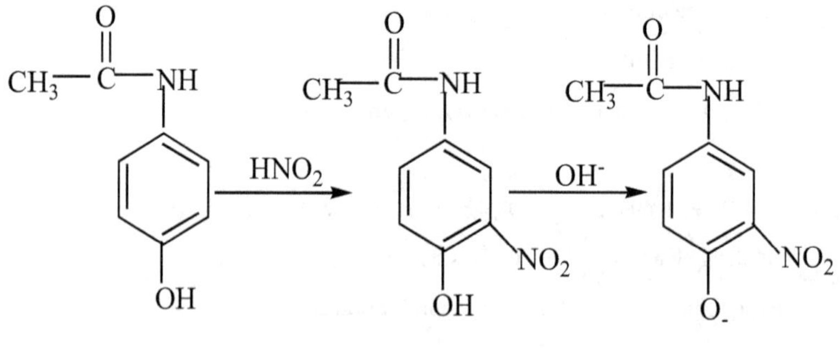

Figure 12. Formation of a chromogenic nitro compound from an analgesic Acetaminophen

i.   Describe how you would construct the standard curve for determination of parace-
         tamol concentration.

$K = \ln \frac{x_1}{\frac{x}{t1-t2}}$

2.   Design an experiment that would enable you to determine the $t_{1/2}$ of paracetamol

Practical problem 2

Liver damage can be induced by 20% w/v carbon tetrachloride. Given 10mg/ml pentobarbitone and 10mg/ml Phenolbarbitone, design an experiment that demonstrates that the duration of action of short acting barbiturates are dependent on the integrity of the liver.

13. Drug discovery and preclinical trials

The development of new drugs over the past 30 years has revolutionalized the practice of medicine and has for instance seen the increased use of new anti-hypertensives and drugs that reduce cholesterol synthesis or dissolve blood clots which led to a 50% reduction in the number of deaths from cardio-vascular diseases and stroke among other diseases.

13.1. Conventional approaches to drug discovery

These are the classical approaches to drug discovery that do not initially involve detailed scientific study they include the following;

Traditional knowledge approach

This is the discovery of drugs based on traditional medical knowledge. The best example is the documented analgesic effects of extracts from opium poppy that led to the isolation of morphine from the plant and the subsequent synthesis of related analgesics.

Discovery through serendipity

This is the accidental discovery of novel drugs based on the ingenuity of a scientist investigating a problem initially unrelated to the observed phenomenon; examples of such discoveries include the observation by Alexander Flemmings that penicilliummould could inhibit the growth of bacteria. This finding led to the discovery of antibiotics.

Discovery of therapeutic usefulness of a side effect e.g. clonidine originally used as a nasal decongestant was found to have antihypertensive properties while, the hypoglycemic effects of sulphonamides used in the treatment of typhoid fever led to the development of structurally related sulphonylureas as oral hypoglycemic drugs.

Discovery from effects of endogenous agents in test animals

An example of discovery arising from studies of endogenous agents in test animals is the anticoagulant action of the venom from the Malayan viper that led to the identification of the anticoagulant ancrod.

Modern approaches to drug discovery

These are those approaches that form a basis for the rational design of drugs and include the following;

Bioprospecting

This is the screening of a large number of natural products, chemical entities, large libraries of peptides, nucleic acids and other organic molecules for biological activity. This approach may lead to identification and development of new drug molecules.

Metabolomics

This is the profiling of natural products of related plant species screening using either liquid or gas chromatography mass spectrometry to determine active metabolites that may be present in novel crude herbal medical preparations.

In silico screening

This is the most advanced technique for drug discovery. It entails virtual screening or docking of compounds on the 3-D- structure of a known receptor based on homologies of the test drug molecules with a known test parent drug. *In silico* screening can form a basis for the modification of a known drug molecule to determine possible therapeutic applications and may lead to the development of putative drugs against new targets.

13.2. Screening of putative drug molecules

Selection of molecules for further study is usually conducted in animal models of human disease and the pharmacological tests include both the *in vitro* and *in vivo* studies after the initial screening for biological activity. For instance, antibacterial activity of drugs is assessed by their ability to inhibit growth of a variety of micro-organisms, while hypoglycemic drugs are tested for their ability to lower blood pressure.

The *in vitro* methods include incubation of a parent compound with various subcellular fractions such as microsomes, individual recombinant drug metabolizing enzymes from cells or tissue slices. The *in vivo* studies involve working on typical animal models such as dogs or rats. Some of the *invitro* and *invivo* studies that may be performed are shown in tables 1 and 2 below;

	Target	Specific or tissue in vitro studies	Biochemical measurement
a.	(i) Receptor binding	Cell membrane fraction / cloned receptors	Receptor affinity
	(ii) Receptor activity	Sympathetic nerves	Inhibition of nerve activity
	(iii) Enzyme activity e.g. tyrosine hydroxylase	Purified enzymes from adrenal glands	Inhibition of enzyme activity
b.	Cellular function	Cultured cells	Cell viability
c.	Isolated tissue	Blood vessels, heart lung or ileum from rat	Effects on vascular contraction and relaxation

Table 1. Screening of drugs for specific inhibitory effects on enzymes and isolated tissues.

	Disease model	Animal model	Route of administration	Physiological measurements
a.	Blood pressure	Hypertensive rat (conscious)	Parenteral	Systolic/diastolic
b.	Cardiac effects	Dog (conscious) Dog (anesthetized)	Oral / Parenteral	Electrocardiography (cardiac output)
c.	CNS	Mouse, rat	Parenteral	Degree of sedation
d.	Respiratory effects	Dog/guinea pig	Parenteral	Respiratory rate and amplitude
e.	GIT effects	Rat	Oral	GIT motility and secretions

Table 2. Putative animal models used in studying effects of drugs

If an agent possesses useful activity it would be further studied for possible adverse effects on other major organs. These studies might suggest the need for further chemical modification to achieve desirable pharmacokinetic/pharmacodynamic properties.

13.3. Preclinical trials

The data from animal studies form a basis for the calculation of the initial or starting doses to be used in the subsequent clinical studies. The human equivalent dose calculations for the maximum recommended dose are normally based on either the body surface area or body weight. The candidate drugs that survive initial screening and profiling must be carefully evaluated for potential risks before and during clinical testing. The main types of evaluation needed from safety and toxicity studies include:-

Acute toxicity

This involves looking at the effects of large single doses of therapeutic agent. Acute toxicity studies are usually performed in animal models such as mice and rats. These studies enable investigators to correlate any observed effects with the systemic level of the drug.

Sub-acute toxicity

This is similar to acute toxicity but measures the effects of multiple doses based on expected duration of clinical usage. It entails haematological, histology and electron microscope studies to identify organs which might be affected by toxicity. It usually lasts between one to three months. This enables the selection of putative compounds for subsequent studies.

Chronic toxicity testing

These studies are required when the drug is intended to be used in humans for prolonged periods. The goals of this investigation are mostly similar to those of sub-acute toxicity.

The reproductive performance

These are measurements intended to determine the effects of the drug agents on; mating behaviour, reproduction, parturition, progeny birth defects, and postnatal development.

Carcinogenicity studies

These studies are required to determine the effects of prolonged usage of the drug under investigation. They involve hematological and histological autopsy analysis.

Mutagenicity studies

These studies look at the genetic stability and mutations of bacterial or mammalian cells in culture. These studies are at the academic research level and are intended to provide data for future research.

Investigative toxicology

The main purpose of toxicology is to discover the pathways that are involved in toxic action. It includes studies on mechanisms of toxic action of drugs which may lead to the development of safer drugs.

14. Evaluation of new drugs and drug approval process

Toxicity testing is time consuming and expensive and may require two to five years to collect and analyze data before the drug can be considered ready for testing in humans.

Large numbers of animals are needed to obtain valid preclinical data.

Extrapolation of toxicity data from animals to humans may not be completely reliable.

The safety or efficacy of a drug must be thoroughly understood before the drug is administered to any group of individuals. Therefore regulations governing the development of new drugs have evolved to assure safety and efficacy of new medications. The clinical trials during drug development and post marketing experience form the scientific basis of patient response to a drug.

Once a drug is judged ready to be studied in humans, a notice of clinical investigational exemption for a new drug (IND) must be filled with the government body concerned with the regulation and registration of drugs. The IND includes manufacturing information, all data from animal studies, clinical plans and protocols and the names and credentials of physicians who will conduct the clinical trials.

14.1. Phase I clinical trials

The main goal in phase I is to determine whether test animals and humans show significant different responses to the drug and to establish limits of the safe clinical dosage range. The measurements carried out in phase I include, the rate of absorption, $t_{1/2}$ and metabolism of the candidate drug compound. The effects of the drug as a function of dosage are established in a small number 25 – 50 of healthy volunteers. When the drug is expected to have significant toxicity, as often the case with cancer and AIDS therapy, volunteer patients with the disease are used instead of the healthy volunteers. The requirements of clinical trials include the following:

i.   Homogenous populations of patients must be selected.

ii.   Appropriate controls for the investigation must be included.

iii.   Meaningful and sensitive indices for drug effects must be used i.e. well defined endpoints such as survival or pain relief should be used rather than surrogate or intermediate markers e.g. levels of enzymes involved in the process of survival/pain relief.

iv.   The experimental observations must be converted to data and then into valid conclusions.

v.   The accuracy of diagnosis and severity of the disease must be comparable between the groups being contrasted.

vi.   The dosages of the drugs must be chosen and individualized in a manner that allows relative efficacy to be compared at equivalent toxicities.

vii.   Compliance with experimental regimens should be assessed before subjects are assigned to experimental or control groups. Non-compliance may cause false estimates of the true potential benefits or toxicity of a particular treatment.

viii.   Ethical considerations. These may be the major determinants of the types of controls that can be used e.g. for therapeutic trials that involve life threatening diseases for which there is already in-effective therapy, the use of a placebo is considered unethical. In such cases, new treatments must be compared with standard therapies.

14.2. Study design of phase I trials

For clinical trials to have validity they must be based on a sound statistical basis. Some of the of the criteria that must be met include;

Randomization

Randomization is a design which ensures that there is no bias in allocation of treatments among the different groups. The purpose of randomization is to minimize the possibility that an observed treatment effect is due to inherent differences between groups. Randomization eliminates bias by avoiding recruiting patients who have a particular characteristic to one group and not the other e.g. only women/men and smokers/alcoholics. Randomization should not be carried out until immediately before treatment. The delay allows a patient to have second thoughts about taking part or the investigator to have to re-consider about admitting patients to the study. Simple methods of randomization can be designed using published tables of random numbers, where treatments are in a form of a square in which each treatment is contained only once in each row and column and the order of treatment is different in each group (Table 3).The presence of other diseases or risk factors should be taken into consideration i.e. need for careful selection and assignment of patients to each of the study groups.

	Group Treatment			
1	A	B	C	D
2	C	D	A	B
3	D	C	B	A
4	B	A	D	C

Table 3. A random number table array for assignment of various treatment regimes to various groups of patients in clinical trials

This approach eliminates systematic variation between groups since the patients are allocated at random order to group 1, 2, 3, or 4. A code list should be drawn up so that the main investigators may be kept blind to the treatment an individual is receiving but also so that it is possible to know the treatment by breaking the code. Coding should be such that when broken, it does not yield information about the treatments other patients are getting. The treatment information about all the patients should be left to one person preferably the pharmacist or trial co-ordinator.

Blindness

Blinding is a design which does not allow the investigator to know what treatment the patient is receiving. The purpose of blinding is to eliminate bias in reporting the outcome of the treatment since if an investigator knows what treatment the patient is taking, he/she may in some way influence a measurement or an outcome thus shifting the outcome in one direction or another consciously or unconsciously. The ideal trial should be double blind where neither the investigator nor the patient knows what treatment the patient is taking. Placebos or dummies are used in order to achieve blindness. The placebos should match the active treatment as closely as possible in terms of size, shape, color, texture, weight, taste and smell with the active formulation.

Number of testing centers

Clinical trial should be carried out in a defined centre so as to minimize variations in the popula-tion and in the investigators techniques. This also avoids problems of data collection, communi-cation and follows up. Multi-centre trials may become necessary when studying a rare disease hence scarcity of patients or when the effect being investigated is small one e.g. when one is looking out for an interaction effect between a major condition and a minor condition.

Clinical trials designed to evaluate efficacy of new drugs should always be prospective i.e. the characteristics of the population to be studied should be identified before the study begins. For example, if one randomized all patients with heart failure to treatment with either digoxin or a new drug X and then studied the outcome over six months that would be a prospective trial. In case of control study the outcome is first identified and then comparisons are made retrospectively between the characteristics of patients who did or did not have the outcome. Such a study for instance has shown that oral anticoagulants can reduce incidences of re-infarction in patients who have already had a myocardial infarction. The case control studies may be carried out some time, after the introduction of a drug therapy in order to get some idea of its place in the overall management of the disease since the results of a case control study may prompt formal prospective trials in order to confirm original findings.

14.3. Molecular markers in drug development

In vitro predictive efficacy and toxico-genomics should be carried out after phase 1 clinical trials in order to validate the results of the phase 1 clinical trials. This is achieved by using animal cell lines in which gene expression profiling and patterns of protein production are used to identity candidate biomarkers for the disease. The utilization of markers that are associated with the disease or those that indicate a known response to a therapeutic interven-tion or reflect a clinical outcome may yield information on efficacy or toxicity of a test drug. An example of a biological readout that has traditionally been used to determine efficacy during the treatment of diabetics is the determination of glucose in the urine of a diabetic patient. Reliable and specific biomarkers that act as predictors of efficacy or long-term toxicity are useful because they reduce the time, size and cost of clinical trials.

14.4. Phase II clinical trials

These are studies that recruit willing and informed patients and are designed to assess long term safety, refine pharmacokinetic data, determine optimal dose. The purpose of phase II studies is to determine efficacy. Typically, phase II trials require 100-150 subjects and take 9-12 months. An assessment of no effect or no worthwhile effect of a given drug demonstrates that it is futile to proceed with further clinical testing of the drug. It is therefore important to minimize type I errors or false negatives in the study design in order to minimize the risk of discontinuing a potentially effective drug. The data from well designed phase I and phase II trials are therefore critical in planning the subsequent trials. The phase III trials are large trials intended to determine whether a treatment is effective and to establish safety data.

Phase II clinical trials include inert placebos as negative controls and older active drugs as positive controls alongside the investigative compound. These studies are done in special clinical centers such as University Hospitals. A broader range of toxicities may be detected at this phase.

14.5. Phase III clinical trials

The drug is evaluated in a much larger number of patients (thousands) to further establish safety and efficacy. Phase III trials are performed in settings similar to those anticipated for the ultimate use of the drug. After successful phase III trials, the next step is the application for review of the new drug to seek approval to use the drug for clinical management of the disease condition.

14.6. Phase IV clinical trials

This phase is concerned with post-marketing surveillance and the main goal is to assess adverse reactions, patterns of drug utilization, discovery of additional indications. The interrelationships between the various studies in drug development are illustrated in Fig 13 below;

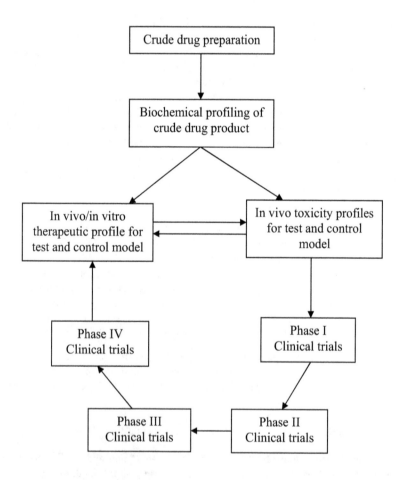

Figure 13. Illustration of the key steps in the development of a drug from a putative drug candidate extract

14.7. Pharmacogenomics and drug development

The personalized medication which takes into account the genetic make-up of individuals is known as pharmacogenomics. The pharmacogenomic differences that determine individualized therapy include genetic polymorphisms of drug transporters, drug receptors, and drug metabolizing enzymes. For example, genetic variation in Cyt P_{450} enzymes that are largely responsible for drug metabolism shows that different individuals respond differently to drug efficacy or toxicity. Genetic variants in the drug target, the disease pathway, genes or drug metabolizing enzymes could all be used as predictors of drug efficacy or toxicity. For example, drug monitoring using perpherazine, a Cyt P_{450} substrate, shows that there are three main categories of individuals; the efficient metabolizers obtained from the heterozygotes, the poor metabolizers from the homozygotes and the ultra-rapid metabolizers which carry two or more active genes in the same chromosome, a phenomenon known as gene duplication.

The information obtained from pharmacogenetic studies can be used to design new drugs that take the persons' genetic profile into consideration. The most common type of genetic variation are single nucleotide polymorphisms, therefore, a high resolution of single nucleotide map may expedite the identification of genes for various diseases. The molecular profiles of patients identified in phase I and II clinical trials as likely non-responders to the putative drug under investigation might present an opportunity to initiate new discovery programs for other pharmaceutical compounds.

14.8. Individualized drug therapy

Clinical usage of drugs requires a basic understanding of the pharmacokinetic and pharmacodynamic drug processes and an appreciation that a relationship does exist between the pharmacological effect or toxic response to a drug and the concentration of the drug. The interpatient and intrapatient variation in disposition of a drug must be taken into account in choosing a drug regimen.

A drug dosage regimen therefore is a recipe for the administration of a drug so as to produce a desired therapeutic effect with minimum toxic effects.

The regimen is described in terms of the following:

i.   Dose of the drug to be used and the formulation.

ii.   Frequency with which it is administered.

iii.   Route of drug administration.

The factors that determine the relationship between the prescribed drug dosage and drug effect operate at three levels; prescription level, drug administration level and at the physiological level of patient (Figure 14).

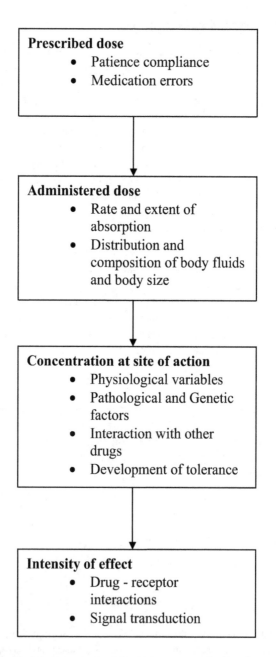

Figure 14. The operational levels that determine the relationship between prescribed drug dosage and the drug effect.

Drugs that are excreted primarily unchanged by the kidneys tend to have low variation among patients with similar renal function than do drugs which are inactivated by metabolism. For the extensively metabolized drugs, those with high metabolic clearance and large first pass elimination have marked difference in bioavailability, whereas those with low biotransformation tend to have largest variation in elimination rates among individuals.

14.9. Determination of drug dosage

The simplest way of determining a drug dosage regimen is to base it on the published recommended dosage. These are derived from the pharmacokinetics studies of the drug and the general procedure in using the published recommendations is to start at the lower end of the recommended dosage range and monitor the therapeutic effect. If the desired effect does not occur, the dosage can be increased gradually until one reaches the upper limit of the range. In certain conditions it may be necessary a sufficiently high dose for the drug to accumulate in the body to a satisfactory degree. This dose is known as the loading dose and is equal to the volume of distribution multiplied by the target concentration in the plasma. The reason for giving a loading dose is to circumvent the sometimes unacceptable time lag preceding the steady state levels. Once the correct loading dose is given, a steady-state concentration can be achieved rapidly and then maintained by giving a smaller maintenance dose.

Adjustment of dosage in individual patients is often as a result of the modification of pharmacokinetic parameters of which the three most important include; the bioavailability or the fraction of a drug that is absorbed into systemic circulation, its clearance and the volume of distribution.

For drugs with a high toxicity to therapeutic ratio, the loading dose can be given as a single dose and for drugs with a low toxicity: therapeutic ratio and a long half-life, the loading dose can be divided into several portions and given at intervals long enough to allow detection of adverse effects, but short enough to ensure that the loading dose is a true loading dose i.e. relatively little amounts of the drug is eliminated from the body during the period of loading.

14.10. Systemic drug availability

The extent of availability of a drug after oral administration is expressed as a percentage of the dose. The fractional availability (F) varies from 0 to 1. The extent of availability is more important parameter to measure rather than the rate of availability.

A true decrease in bioavailability could be due to several reasons including, a poorly administered dosage form that fails to disintegrate or dissolve in the GIT, interaction with other drugs in the GIT, metabolism of the drug in the GIT and/or first pass hepatic metabolism or biliary excretion.

Hepatic disease may in particular cause high availability because the metabolic capacity decreases or development of vascular shunts in the liver. Significantly high availability requires dosage adjustment by a factor of two, while significantly low in availability requires dosage adjustment by a factor of half.

14.11. Maintenance dose

In most clinical situations drugs are administered in such a way as to maintain a steady concentration i.e. just enough drug is given in each dose to replace the drug eliminated since the preceding dose. Therefore, clearance is the most important pharmacokinetic term to be considered in defining a rational steady-state drug dosage regimen.

The rate of elimination = Cl x Tc

Where, Cl is the rate of clearance and Tc is the target concentration of the drug.

The Dosing rate = Rate of elimination = Cl x Tc.

Therefore, if the target concentration is known, the prevailing clearance in that patient will determine the dosing rate and if the drug is given by a route that has a bio availability of less than 100%, then the dosing rate above can be modified using the formula:

$$\text{Dosing rate oral} = \frac{\text{Dosing rate}}{\text{Fractional availability}}$$

If intermitted doses are given, then maintenance dose = Dosing rate x Dosing interval.

14.12. Alteration of maintenance dose

The maintenance dose is usually altered when the clearance of the drug changes. For example, during renal impairment, the clearance of drugs which are predominantly cleared by the kidney is greatly reduced and therefore, the desired steady state concentration can only be achieved either through altering the dose or altering the dosing interval. Therefore, when a drug is cleared almost completely via kidneys, the dosage interval should be changed in proportion to renal clearance as follows:

The % eliminated in dosing interval should be proportional to creatinine clearance by a published constant to yield the percentage excreted in one dosage interval.

The quantities required for this adjustment are:

i.   Fraction of normal function remaining, and the

ii.   Fraction of drug usually excreted unchanged in urine.

The fraction of normal function remaining is equal to the ratio of patient's creatinine clearance to a normal value (120 ml/min/70kg).

The following equation is for adjustment of renal clearance

$rf_{pt} = 1 - fe_{nl}(1 - rfx_{pt})$

Where;

rf_{pt} = the adjusted total clearance of the patient,

fe_{nl} = fraction of drug excreted unchanged in normal individuals,

rfx_{pt} = fraction of renal clearance of the normal individual.

Clearance should also be adjusted for the size of the patient and for convenience, the published values are normalized to the metabolic rate = weight $^{0.75}$.

When clearance is low, $t_{1/2}$ is similarly high and when the volume of distribution is high, the $t_{1/2}$ is also high. Therefore, by using parameters for the individual patient, the dosing rate = Tc x Cl/F where, Tc = target concentration, Cl = clearance and F = fractional availability of the drug.

If a drug is relatively non toxic then the maximum loading strategy can be employed so that the dosing interval is much longer than $t_{1/2}$. For example t½, of penicillin is less than one hour but it is usually given in very large doses every six to twelve hours since it is non-toxic. The normal steady-state theophylline concentration can be determined using the equation:

$$Css, max = \frac{F.dose/V_{ss}}{1 - exp^{(-KT)}}$$

$$Css, min = \frac{F.dose/V_{ss}. \left(exp^{-KT}\right)}{1 - exp^{(-KT)}}$$

Where, Css, max and Css min are the maximum and minimum steady state concentrations,

$$T = dosage\ interval\ and\ K = \frac{0.693}{t½}$$

14.13. Drug dosage adjustment in old patients (geriatrics)

Drug absorption in the elderly is slightly different from the normal patients and therefore adjustment of the dosage should be taken into consideration during drug therapy. The rate of transdermal drug absorption may be diminished in elderly because of reduced tissue blood perfusion. Compounds that permeate the intestinal epithelium by carrier mediated transport mechanisms may be absorbed at lower rates in the elderly.

14.14. Drug distribution

In geriatrics the 'body mass' declines with age and the total body water content falls by between 10 – 15%. The volume of distribution of hydrophilic drugs will therefore decrease while plasma concentration will increase and the likelihood of toxic drug effects will also increase. When geriatric patients use diuretics, the extracellular space reduces even further leading to a higher likelihood of drug toxicity. The total body fat in the elderly increases by 12 – 18%, therefore, for hydrophobic drugs, the higher volume of distribution implies an increase in half life of distribution and the time needed to reach steady-state serum concentration. Therefore, for geriatrics a once or twice daily drug administration is optimal. This can be achieved though delayed release or fixed drug combinations.

14.15. Patient compliance and rational use of drugs

Drug treatment of any kind is often compromised by lack of full compliance by the patient. The common errors of compliance to a regimen by a patient include; omission in taking the drug, wrong timing of dosages, premature termination of therapy or using additional medications. In order to improve patient compliance, the patient should be made to understand the nature and prognosis of the illness and what to expect from the medication by detailing both the acceptable and undesirable unwanted effects as well as signs of efficacy that may help enforce compliances.

Patients frequently discontinue taking a medication such as septrin because they have not been told the necessity of continuing with the drug after the acute symptoms have subsided.

The effectiveness of physician-patient communication is inversely related to the error rate in the taking of drugs. A physician might prescribe a drug to be taken three times a day with meals for a patient who either eats only twice a day or sleeps all day and works at night. Therefore, an exploration of the patients eating, sleeping and working habits is necessary before a prescription is given.

The educational level of a patient may also require that the prescription is carefully worded and oral instructions given in the primary language of the patient since when such patients take three or more medications they are less likely to use them properly. It is therefore important to provide identifying symbols for each medication e.g. "Heart pill" or "sugar pill"and to reduce the doses into once or twice daily regimens.

14.16. Adverse drug reactions

Pharmacological formulations are potentially harmful to the individuals taking the drugs. There is need to ascertain the safety of new drugs before allowing them to be marketed. The following figures highlight the magnitude of the problem: ~ 10 – 20% of hospitalized patients suffer adverse drug reactions, while 0.3 – 5.0% inpatients admissions and ~ 0.3% deaths in hospital are due to adverse drug reactions. Adverse drug reactions can be classified into two main categories: They may be dose related or non dose related with each being short-term or long-term.

14.17. Dose related adverse reactions

Adverse drug reactions can occur because of the changes in the systemic availability of a formulation. For instance, the change of excipients in phenytoin capsules from $CaSO_4$ to lactose leads to high availability and hence adverse drug reactions. Sometimes, adverse drug reactions can occur due to the presence of contaminants like bacteria if quality control breaks down. Out-of-date formulations may also cause adverse drug reactions because of degradation products arising from the drug e.g. outdated tetracycline may cause Faconis Syndrome (a type of rickets) because of the transformation product,epiandrotetracycline. Dose related adverse reactions may also arise from pharmacokinetic variations in the individuals taking the drug. Pharmacokinetic variations may also arise due to hepatic disease like advanced cirrhosis which lowers the clearance of drugs such as phenytoin and morphine. The pharmacological variations could be environmental such as diet or smoking, while others are genetic.

14.18. Non-dose related adverse drug reactions

These include immunologic reactions and are related to the surface proteins present on β-humans lymphocytes (HLA antigens) which are important in the function of T-lymphocytes. The association of HLA antigens with foreign antigens stimulates T-lymphocytes. Some of these antigens expressed by major histocompatibility complex (MHC) genes have been associated with an increased risk of adverse drugs e.g. nephrotoxicity from penicillamine is increased in patients with HLA types B8 and DR 3 while patients with HLA- DR, 7 are protected against adverse drug effects.

14.19. Types of drug allergies

Drug allergies can be classified into five categories:

Type I

This anaphylaxis or immediate hypersensitivity reactions; the body reacts within five to thirty minutes. The IgE molecules fixed to mast cells and basophil leucocytes release histamine and other pharmacological mediators such as kinins. Drugs likely to cause are anaphylactic shock include;-penicillins, streptomycin, local anaesthetics etc.

Type II

In these reactions, the circulating antibody of 1gG, 1gM or 1gA interacts with the drug combined with a cell membrane protein to form a hapten-protein/antigen-Ab complex. This leads to the activation of the complement leading to cell lysis of phagocytic attack of the cell with the complex. Drugs such as the cephalosporins, penicillins, quinine and transfusion of improperly matched blood can yield this type of reactions.

Type III

In this type of allergy, the immune complex reactions initiate an inflammatory response due to the combination of the excess drug- protein complex with the IgG in circulation. The complex thus formed is deposited in the tissues and causes activation of the complement and damage of capillary endothelium. This type of reaction is manifested mostly as fever, arthritis, and/or enlarged lymph nodes. Penicillins, sulphonamides and streptomycin may elicit type III allergic reactions.

Type IV

This is the cell-mediated or delayed hypersensitivity reactions in which the T - lymphocytes are sensitized by a hapten to form protein-antigenic complex such that when the lymphocytes come into contact with the antigen, an inflammatory response ensues. Type IV reactions are exemplified by contact dermatitis caused by local anaesthetic areas, antihistamine areas, topical antibiotics and antifungal drugs.

Type V

These are pseudo allergic reactions, that resemble allergic reactions clinically, but for which no immunological basis can be found, e.g. asthma and skin rashes caused by aspirin. Administration of ampicillin or amoxicillin causes a skin rash which resembles the one caused by penicillin hypersensitivity. The ampicillin-caused rash can be distinguished from penicillin hypersensitivity on the basis of two features; it has a later onset, typically ten to fourteen days, compared to penicillin sensitivity which comes between seven to ten days. Furthermore, the sensitivity does not recur following re-exposure to ampicillin and is not as serious as the one caused by penicillin.

14.20. Clinical evaluation of adverse drug reactions

The two basic approaches for clinical evaluation of adverse drug reactions include the cohort studies (or follow-up studies) of patients taking the drug and the case control studies which record the incidences of adverse drug effects retrospectively.

Cohort or prospective studies

In cohort studies, drugs are identified and incidences of adverse effects recorded. The weaknesses of these studies include; the relatively small number of patients likely to be recruited, and lack of suitable control groups to assess the background incidence of any apparent adverse reaction noted.

Case control or retrospective studies

The approach here is to start with the incidence of adverse reaction(s) and then look for the drug and the individuals with symptoms which could be due to an adverse drug reaction. These individuals are screened to see if they had taken the drug. The prevalence of drug taking in the group is then compared with the prevalence in a reference population which did not take the drug. This approach is excellent for validation and assessment of adverse drug effects, but it may not detect new adverse effects. Furthermore, it requires a very large number of patients and is very expensive to undertake hence difficult to justify and organize for every new product.

14.21. Worked examples

Problem 5

Drug clearance must always be adjusted for alterations of renal function using the formula: $rf_{pt} = 1 - fe_{nl}(1 - rfx_{pt})$, where $fe_{nl} =$ fraction of the drug excreted unchanged in normal individuals, $rf_{pt} =$ adjustment factor for total clearance in patient, $rfx_{pt} =$ patients' clearance as a fraction of normal clearance and $Cl_{nl} =$ normal clearance.

Given that an asthmatic patient has a creatinine clearance of $40 \text{mlmin}^{-1} 70 \text{kg}^{-1}$ and that the fraction of terbutaline excreted unchanged, $fe_{nl} = 0.56$, the normal clearance, $Cl_{nl} = 3.4$ ml/min/kg, calculate the clearance of the drug in the patient.

Solution

The patient has depressed renal function: $rfx_{pt} = (40 \text{ ml/min})/ (120 \text{ ml/min}) = 0.33$

$rf_{pt} = 1 - fe_{nl}(1 - rfx_{pt})$

inline formula $rf_{pt} = 1 - 0.56 (1 - 0.33) = 0.62$

$$Cl_{pt} = Cl_{nl}.rf_{pt}$$

inline formula $= 3.4 ml.min^{-1}kg^{-1} \times 0.62$

$= 2.1 ml.min^{-1}kg^{-1}$

Problem 6

Given the following characteristics of drug A; $t_{\frac{1}{2}}$ = 8h, given at a dosage of 450mg every 12h, has V_{ss} = 0.5 L/kg, effective concentration is 12mg/L and that

$$C_{ss} min = \frac{F \ x \ dose \,/\, V_{ss}(exp^{-kt})}{1 - exp^{(-KT)}}$$

$$C_{ss}, max = \frac{F \ x \ dose / V_{ss}}{1 - exp^{(-kT)}}$$

Determine the C_{ss}min and C_{ss}max for a 60 kg patientif F = 1 and exp^{KT} = 0.35. Explain how changing of the dosage interval to 6 hours would affect C_{ss}min.

Solution

The term $exp^{(-KT)}$ is the fraction of the last dose that remains in the body at the end of a dosing interval and is equal to 0.35 and C_{ss} min = C_{ss} max.exp($^{-kt}$). Therefore,

$$C_{ss} min = \frac{450/30 \ x \ 0.35}{1 - 0.35} = 15/0.65 \ x \ 0.35 \sim 8.0 \ mg/L \ while \ C_{ss}max = 15/0.65 = 23 \ mg/L$$

The predicted minimum of 8.0mg/L is below the effective concentration to achieve efficacy. Therefore the dosing interval should be reduced. A reduction of the interval to, say, six hours, increases denominator and therefore causes an increase of C_{ss}min. Since $t_{1/2}$ = 0.693/K, K = 0.086 i.e. $1 - e^{-KT} = 1 - 2.71^{-0.086 \ x \ 6} = 1 - 0.596 = 0.4$.

The new C_{ss} minimum becomes; = 450/30 x 0.4 = 15 mg/L which is within the required therapeutic concentration.

Review exercise

1. Write an essay on statistical considerations that guide clinical evaluation of new drug agents

2. Write an essay on bioprospecting for new antimicrobial agents.

3. Drug clearance must always be adjusted for alterations of renal function using the formula: rf_{pt} = 1- fe_{nl} (1- rfx_{pt}), explain what each term in the above equation represents. Consequently, calculate the clearance of acetaminophen (panadol) in a 70 kg patient with depressed renal function given the following; normal clearance = 350 ml min $^{-1}$70 kg; f_{enl} = 0.56. The patient creatinine clearance = 80 mlmin^{-1} 70 kg. Normal creatinine clearance = 120 ml min^{-1} 70 kg. What effect would the impaired renal function have on dosing interval?

4.　Given that fe_{nl} for drug X = 0.42, and the normal creatinine clearance is 120 ml/min/70 kg, calculate the clearance rate of the drug by a patient with creatinine clearance of 75 ml/min/ 70 kg.

5.　Write an essay on adverse drug reactions associated with the use of macrolide antimicrobial agents.

Author details

Gabriel Magoma

Department of Biochemistry, Jomo Kenyatta University of Agriculture and Technology. Nairobi, Kenya

References

[1]　Christoph & F., Heike Brotz-Oesterhelt (2005). Functional genomics in antibacterial drug discovery. *Today Targets* DD. 10

[2]　David, A. L. and Michael P. W. (2004). Molecular biomarkers in drug development. *Research Focus* DDT. 9, 22

[3]　Di Bernardo, A.B. and Cudkowicz, M.E. (2006). Translating preclinical insights into effective human trials in ALS. *Biochemicaet Biophysica Acta*1762, 1139 -1149.

[4]　Harvey A, L. (2007). Natural products as screening source. *Current Opinions in Chemical Biology*.11, 480 - 484.

[5]　Jaennefer M. F., Paul, A. L. (2000) Emerging novel antifungal agents. *Therapeutic focus.* DD. 5, 1 January 2000

[6]　Iris, R. (2008). PK/PD Modelling and simulations: utility in drug development. *Drug Discovery Today*.348, 1 - 6.

[7]　Klaus, T. (2003).When drug therapy gets old: pharmacokinetics and pharmacodynamics in the elderly. *Experimental Gerontology*38 843-853.

[8]　Kieran, F. R., Eric S. and Philip H. W. (2001).Modelling and simulation in clinical drug development. *Research Focus* DD Vol. 6, 15

[9]　Lindpaintner, K. (2002). The Impact of pharmacogenetics and pharmagenomics on drug discovery. *Naure Review on Drug Discovery*.1, 463 - 469.

[10]　Sundbergh, M. I. (2001). Genetic susceptibility to adverse effects of drugs and environmental toxicants. The role of the CYP family of enzymes *Mutants Researh* 482. 11-19

[11] Timothy, D. R., Steven R.G., Herve, T., Brian A.D. (2001). Finding drug targets in microbial genomes. *Drug Discovery Today*6, (17): 887-892.

[12] Tim, R. C. and Marc L. (2007). Pharmacogenitics of antiretroviral drugs for the treatment of HIV-infected patients: An update. Infection, Genetics and Evolution 7, 333-342

[13] Turnheim, K. (2003). Why drug therapy gets old Pharmacokinetics and pharmacodynamics in the eldery. *Experimental Gerontology* 38 843-853.

[14] Paul, B. (2003). Toxicokinetics in preclinical evaluation. *Research Focus* DD Vol. 8

[15] Ulrich, R., Friend, S. H. (2000). Toxicogenomics and drug discovery: Will new technologies help us produce better drugs? *Nat. Rev. Drug Discov.* 1, 84 – 88.

[16] Werbovetz, K. A. (2000). Target based drug discovery for Malaria, Leishmania and Trypanosomiasis. *Current medicinal Chemistry* 7 (8) 835 – 860.

[17] Aungst B. (2000). Intestinal permeation enhancers. *Journal of Pharmacological Sciences*,89 (4), 429-442.

[18] Salama, N.N. Eddington N.D. Fasano, A. (2006).Tight junction modulation and its relationship with drug delivery. *Advanced Drug Delivery Reviews*.58: 15-28.

[19] Guengerich F. P. (2001). Common and uncommon cytochrome P_{450} reactions related to metabolism and chemical toxicity. *Chemical Research and Toxicology*.14: 611 - 650.

[20] Blanka R., (1998). Receptor-mediated targeted drug or toxin delivery. *Advanced Drug Delivery Reviews* 29: 273-289.

[21] John R. C. (2005). Some distinctions between flavin-containing and cytochrome P_{450}monooxygenases.*Biochemical and Biophysical Research Communications* 338: 599-604.

[22] Xiaoling L. William K. C. (1999). Transport, metabolism and elimination mechanisms of anti-HIV agents. *Advanced Drug Delivery Reviews*29: 273-289 39, 81-103.

[23] Brown, M.J., Bennet, P.N., Lawrence, D.R. (1997). Clinical pharmacology (8th Edition) Wesley, Longman China Ltd.

[24] Hardman J.G., Gilman A.G., Limbird L. E.(1996). *The pharmacological basis of therapeutics* (9[th]Edition) McGraw-Hill.

[25] Katzung B. G.,(2004). *Basic and clinical pharmacology* (9th Edition) Mcgraw Hill Inc.

Chapter 2

Anticancer Drug Discovery — From Serendipity to Rational Design

Jolanta Natalia Latosińska and
Magdalena Latosińska

Additional information is available at the end of the chapter

1. Introduction

Cancer is nowadays used as a generic term describing a group of about 120 different diseases, which can affect any part of the body and defined as the state characterized by the uncontrolled growth and invasion of normal tissues and spread of cells [1]. According to WHO reports cancer is a leading cause of premature death worldwide, accounting for 7.6 million deaths (around 13% of all deaths) only in 2008 [2]. The deaths from cancer worldwide are projected to continue rising, reaching an estimated 13.1 million in 2030 (WHO 2012). The number of all cancer cases around the world reached 12.7 million in 2008 and is expected to increase to 21 million by 2030. Approximately one in five people before age 75 will suffer from cancer during their lifetime, while one in ten in this age range is predicted to die due to cancer [2]. About 70% of all cancer deaths occurred in low- and middle-income countries. Cancer statistics indicate that most common new cancer cases (excluding common non-melanoma skin cancer) include lung, breast, colorectum, stomach, prostate and liver. These statistics are affected by a few factors including the increase in the number of carcinogens in daily life conditions (food, alcohol, tobacco etc.; high levels of chemicals and pollutants in environment, exposure to UV and ionizing radiation and viruses), genetic disposition [1] but also higher effectiveness of the treatment regimes. The number of recognized carcinogens (agents, mixtures, oncoviruses, environmental factors) increased from 50 in 1987 to 108 in 2012. Although it seems small, this number increases continually with the evidence of new (probably and possibly) carcinogens (64 and 271 in 2012) to humans [3]. What is significant only one compound is listed as probably not carcinogenic - caprolactam. Moreover, since not all chemicals have been tested yet, the number of human carcinogens is undervalued and will increase in the near future. Although mortality rates for some cancers (e.g. leukaemia, testicular or ovarian cancer) are reduced and the overall survival time increased significantly, especially in high-developed countries, but in fact the metastases, not the cancer itself, are the major cause of death. In 1971, only 50% of people diagnosed with the cancer went on to live at least five years, while nowadays, the five-year survival rate is 63% [2]. However if a cancer has spread the chances of survival are only scarcely better than in the 1970s. These numbers indicate that although the knowledge about cancer in the last two decades raised, even to a larger degree than in all preceding centuries, but the problem of cancer diseases persists and our knowledge is still insufficient to solve it. Despite the remarkable progress in cancer prevention, early detection, and treatment, made during the last few decades, the methods of cancer diagnosis and treatment are still not sufficiently specific and effective thus cancer still takes a heavy toll.

Not so long ago in the beginning of 20th century, neither carcinogens nor cellular targets were identified while the treatment was carried out exclusively by surgeries or natural products selected by trial and error. Modern cancer therapy based on the so-called holistic approach - the combined use of surgical methods, radiotherapy, chemotherapy, hormonal therapy and immunotherapy - is applied in the treatment of cancer at most stages. In fact this approach originated from the ancient Sumerian, Akkadian, Babylonian, Assyrian and Egyptian medicine, and was largely influenced by the Roman and Greek ideas concerning anatomy, physiology as well as the achievements of practical medicine and natural science. The chemotherapy, hormonal therapy, immunotherapy and radiotherapy as the methods of cancer treatment joined to the oldest surgical one only in the 20th c. An important component of the combined therapy, but sometimes when cancer had already metastasised, the only available therapeutic method, is chemotherapy using natural or synthetic anticancer drugs and treated as curative, palliative, adjuvant or neoadjuvant. Over the centuries anticancer drugs evolved from natural products, discovered mainly from green plants and minerals to fully chemically synthesized chemotherapeutic agents. However, even today drugs of natural origin play an important role in the treatment of cancer as 14 of them were on the list of the top 35 drugs worldwide sales [4]. The process of anticancer drug discovery leading from natural products to chemotherapeutic agents, often illicitly limited only to cytostatic and antiproliferative, has evolved from serendipity to rational design based on advances in chemistry, physics and biology in a long and complicated process. Nowadays both cancer itself and anticancer drugs are investigated at the molecular level thus methods of drug discovery have changed diametrically. The dominant direction of contemporary aniticancer drug discovery is the search for the possibilities to influence the pathogenetic mechanisms specific of the tumour structures at the cellular and molecular levels, which require the knowledge of cancer origins.

This chapter will focus on the factors which influenced the direction of anticancer drug discovery methods from guessing to the targeted search i.e. from serendipity to rational design.

2. Cancer origins

Cancer (proper medical name - malignant neoplasm) commonly considered to be a civilization disease, has in fact been traced to occur even before the ancestral species of man [5]. The oldest evidence of cancer dates back to several million years ago and has been found in fossilized remains (bones) of a dinosaur in Wyoming. The oldest specimens of cancer, a hominid malignant tumour (probably Burkitt's lymphoma) and bone cancer - were found in the remains of a body of either Homo erectus or an Australopithecus and in the remains of a female skull dating to the Bronze Age (1900-1600 B.C.), respectively. Bone cancers have been also discovered in mummies in the Great Pyramid of Giza and in mummified skeletal remains of Peruvian Incas. The earliest written records differentiating between benign and malignant cancers date back to ancient times (3000-1500 B.C., Mesopotamia and Egypt). Seven Egyptian Papyruses including the Edwin Smyth (2500 B.C.), Leyde (1500 B.C.), and George Ebers (1500 B.C.) described not only the symptoms but also the first primitive forms of treatment, i.e. the removal of a malignant tissue. The Hindu epic, the Ramayana (500 B.C.), mentioned not only cancer cases but also the first medicines in the form of arsenic pastes, for treatment of cancerous growth. Ancient Greek physician Hippocrates of Kos (ca. 460-370 B.C.) described many different types of cancer (breast, uterus, stomach, skin, and rectum) recognised the difference between benign and malignant tumours and formulated the humoral theory of cancer genesis. As the veins surrounding the tumour resembled the crab claws, he named the disease after the Greek word *carcinos*. Cornelus Celsus (ca. 25 B.C.-50 A.D.), who described the first surgeries on cancers, translated Greek carcinos into now commonly used Latin term cancer. Claudius Galen (129-216 A.D.), the most famous Roman Empire physician, who wrote about 500 medical treatises, left a comprehensive descriptions of many neoplasms. He introduced the Greek word *oncos* (swelling) to describe tumours. Nowadays the use of Hippocrates and Celsus term is limited to describe malignant tumours, while Galen's term is used as a part of the name of the branch of medicine that deals with cancer - that is oncology. Followers of his works in Constantinople, Alexandria, Athens explained the appearance of cancer as a result of an excess of black bile. This idea prevailed through up to the 16th century.

The intensive studies in the field of anatomy and physiology during the Renaissance, resulted in advancement of surgery and development of rational therapies based on clinical observations. Based on autopsies William Harvey (1578-1657) described the systemic circulation of blood through the heart and body. Although cancers were still incurable, their temporary inhibition was often observed thanks to complementary remedies including the most common arsenic-based creams and pastes. In the beginning of the 16th c. Zacutus Lusitani (1575-1642) and Nicholas Tulp (1593–1674) formulated the contagion theory and proposed isolation of patients in order to prevent the spread of cancer. Throughout the 17th and 18th centuries, this theory was so popular that the first cancer hospital founded in Reims, France, was forced to move outside the city. Nowadays, we know that their certain viruses, bacteria, and parasites can increase a risk of developing cancer. Gaspare Aselli (1581-1625), who discovered the lymphatic system, suggested a connection between the lymphatic system and cancer. Georg Ernst Stahl (1660-1734) and Friedrich Hoffman (1660-1742) proposed a concept that tumours grow from degenerating lymph constantly excreted by the blood. This idea was accepted by John Hunter (1728-1793), who described methods to identify surgically removable tumours. At that time the so-called humoral theory of cancer was replaced by the lymph theory. Claude-Deshasis Gendron (1663-1750) was convinced that cancer arises as a solid and growing mass untreatable with drugs, and must be completely removed. The discovery of a microscope by

Antonie van Leeuwenhoek (1632-1723) in the late 17th century extended the knowledge about the cancer formation process and accelerated the search for the origin of cancer. It was realised that the progress in cancer treatment critically depends on the ability to distinguish between normal and malignant cells. Giovanni Battista Morgagni (1682-1771), father of pathomorphology, related the illness to pathological changes that laid the foundation for scientific oncology. This observation in connection with discovery of anaesthesia in 1844 by Horace Wells (1815-1848) enabled development of precise diagnosis of cancer and modern radical cancer surgery. In 1838, Johannes Peter Muller (1801-1858) indicated cells as basic units of tumours and proposed the blastema theory that cancer cells developed from budding elements (blastema) between normal tissues. In 1860, Karl Thiersch (1822-1895), showed that cancers metastasize through the spread of malignant cells and described establishment of secondary cancer as a result of their spread by lymph. Rudolf Virchow (1821-1902), the founder of cellular pathology, recognized leukaemia cells. He showed that cancer cells can be differentiated from surrounding normal cells from which they originated and the stage of cancer can be determined using microscopic images. Virchow also properly recognized chronic irritation as one of the factors favouring cancer development. Nowadays, we are aware that cancers arise from sites of infection, chronic irritation and inflammation. The next key step in understanding the mechanism of cancer development was the discovery of chromosome and mitosis credited to German botanist Wilhelm Hofmeister (1824-1877). In 1902 Theodor Boveri (1862-1915) reasoned that a cancerous tumour begins with a single cell, which divided uncontrollably, while David Paul von Hansemann (1858–1920), included multipolar mitoses among the factors responsible for the arise of abnormal chromosome numbers in cells leading to tumour formation. In fact Hansemann formulated chromosomal theory of cancer, while Boveri proposed the existence of cell-cycle checkpoints, tumour suppressor genes, and oncogenes and speculated that uncontrolled growth might be caused by physical (radiation), chemical (some chemicals) or biological (microscopic pathogens) factors. Thomas Hunt Morgan (1866-1945) made a key observations of chromosomal changes and demonstrated in 1915 the correctness of this theory. But still the carcinogens like chemical agents or irradiation could not explain the fact that sometimes cancer seemed to run in families. Already in the 17th c. Lusitani and Tulp observed the appearance of breast cancer in whole families.

A rapid progress in understanding the cancer origins was possible thanks to the scientific progress and appearance of instruments required to solve complex interdisciplinary problems of chemistry and biology. The turning points in the research on cancer were the mapping of locations of the fruit fly (Drosophila melanogaster) genes by Alfred Sturtevant (1891-1970), the discovery that DNA is the genetic material by Oswald Avery (1877-1955), Colin Munro MacLeod (1909-1972) and Maclyn McCarty (1911-2005) and the resolution of the exact chemical structure of DNA, the basic material in genes, by James Watson and Francis Crick (1916-2004). Their results indicated that DNA was the cellular target for carcinogens and that mutations were the key to understanding the mechanisms of cancer. In 1970 the first oncogene (SRC, from sarcoma) a defective proto-oncogene i.e. gene which after mutation, predispose the cell to become a cancerous (stimulate cell proliferation) was discovered by G. Steve Martin in a chicken retrovirus. One year later, but long before the human genome was sequenced, Alfred George Knudson identified first tumour suppressor gene, the Rb gene, located on a region of long arm of chromosome 13 at position 14.2 in humans. Its mutation results in retinoblastoma juvenile eye tumour. On the basis of the earlier (dated to 1953) findings of Carl Nordling, he has formulated the accepted till now "two-hit hypothesis" which assumes that both alleles coding a particular protein must be affected before an effect is manifested. Knudson provided an explanation of the relationship between the hereditary and non-hereditary origins of cancer and predicted the existence of tumor suppressor genes that can suppress cancer cell growth. It was later discovered that both classes of genes proto-oncogenes and tumor-suppressor genes encode many kinds of proteins controlling cell growth and proliferation and the mutations in these genes can contribute to carcinogenesis.

In 1976 John Michael Bishop and Harold Elliot Varmus discovered the presence of oncogenes in many organisms including humans. Nowadays, after human genome sequencing in 2004, we know that human DNA contains approximately 20,500 genes [6]. About 50 of them are known to be proto-oncogenes, while 30 tumour suppressor genes. The proto-oncogenes (c-onc) initiate the process of cell division and code enzymes which control grows and division of cells. Proto-oncogenes can be activated to oncogenes by many factors including chromosome rearrangements, gene duplication, mutation or overexpression. For example, a chromosome rearrangement results in formation of BCR-ABL gene which leads to chronic myeloid leukaemia [7], acquired mutation activate the KIT gene which results in gastrointestinal stromal tumour [8], while inheritance of BRCA1 or BRCA2 increase the risk of breast, ovarian, fallopian tube, and prostate cancers [9]. To cause cancer most oncogenes require an additional step, for example mutations in another gene or introduction of foreign DNA (e.g. by viral infection). Infection and inflammation significantly contribute to about 25% of cancer cases. During the inflammatory response to viral infection the free radicals - reactive oxygen and nitrogen species - are generated as a physiological protective response. During chronic inflammation the mechanism is different - free radicals induce genetic and epigenetic changes including somatic mutations in cancer-related genes and posttranslational modifications in proteins involved in DNA repair or apoptosis. However, irrespective of the origins, the tumour microenvironment created by inflammatory cells, is an essential factor in the whole neoplastic process. It facilitates proliferation and survival of malignant cells, promotes angiogenesis and metastasis, subverts adaptive immune responses, and alters responses to chemotherapeutic agents. If a cell accumulates critical mutations in a few of these proto-oncogenes (five or six), it will survive instead of undergoing apoptosis, will proliferate and become capable of forming a tumour. The protecting mechanism involves the tumour suppressor genes, "anti-oncogenes", which protect from developing or growing cancer by repairing DNA damages (mutations), inhibiting cell division and cell proliferation or prevent reproduction by stimulating apoptosis. Mutation of these genes may lead to cessation of the inhibition of cell division. As a result the cell will divide uncontrollably, and produce daughter cells with the same defect. For example, mutation in the TP53 gene (initially after discovery in 1979 by Arnold Levine, David Lane and William Old incorrectly believed to be an oncogene), one of the most commonly mutated tumour suppressor genes which encoding tumour protein - so called p53 protein, a key element in stress-induced apoptosis, is involved in the pathophysiology of leukaemias, lymphomas, sarcomas, and neurogenic tumours [10,11]. Homozygous loss of p53 is found in 70% of colon cancers, 50% of lung cancers and 30–50% of breast cancers. Other important tumour suppressor genes include p16, BRCA-1, BRCA-2, APC or PTEN [12]. Mutation of these genes may lead to melanoma (p16), breast and ovarian cancer in genetically related families (BRCA), colorectal cancer (APC) or glioblastoma, endometrial cancer, and prostate cancer (PTEN).

In general cancerogenesis is a multistep process thus it is usually a combination of proto-oncogene activation and tumour suppressor gene loss or inactivation is required. However, in a few cases (only 5-10% of cancer cases) this abnormal change in gene can be inherited, passed from generation to generation, in most cases it is a result of sporadic or somatic mutation acquired during a person's lifetime. Although cancer is generally believed to arise as a result of slow accumulation of multiple mutations, but in some cases (2-3%) massive multiple mutation can also arise in a single event. Thus cancer is described as a disease of abnormal gene function, genetically caused by the interaction of two factors: genetic suscept-ibility and environmental mutagens and carcinogens. Of key importance for the recognition of the molecular mechanism underlying cancer treatment - cell apoptosis - was the discovery of telomeres and telomerase. In the early 1970s, Alexei Olovnikov, on the basis of the Leonard Hayflick's concept of limited somatic cell divisions (Hayflick limit), suggested that chromo-somes cannot completely replicate their ends. In 1978 Elizabeth Blackburn discovered the unusual nature of stretches of DNA in the ends of the chromosomes of protozon *Tetrahyme-na* - the so-called telomeres. The sequence of human telomere was established 10 years later, in 1988, by Robin Allshire. Blackburn described telomere-shortening mechanism which limits cells to a fixed number of divisions and protect chromosomes from fusing each other or rearranging that can lead to cancer. Shortened telomeres have been found in many cancers, including pancreatic, bone, prostate, bladder, lung, kidney, and head and neck. In 1985, Carol Greider isolated the enzyme telomerase, controlling the elongation of telomeres. Four years later, in 1989, Gregg B. Morin reported the presence of telomerase in human tumour cells and linked its activity with the immortality of these cells (inability to apoptosis), while Greider discovered the lack of active telomerase in normal somatic cells apart from stem cells, kerati-nocytes, intestines, and hair follicle. It was discovered that deactivation of telomerase prompts the apoptosis of human breast and prostate cancer cells. These results indicated the important role of telomerase in the process of oncogenesis.

Carcinogenesis have been found a complex and multi-step (preinitiation, initiation, promotion and metastasis) biological process characterised by independence from growth factors, insensitivity to inhibitors of growth, unlimited potential for replication (reactivation of telomerase), invasiveness, the ability to metastasis and to sustain angiogenesis, and resistance of apoptosis [13]. DNA mutation inherited and caused by exposure to carcinogens (chemical: compounds including drugs, physical: radiation, or biological: the introduction of new DNA sequences by viruses) have been found to be the true origin of uncontrolled growth of cells coupled with malignant behaviour: invasion and metastasis (Fig. 1).

The knowledge of the molecular mechanisms involving the above mentioned factors, espe-cially apoptosis and cancer resistance to it, can improve cancer therapy through resensitization of tumour cells. Fundamental method of cancer treatment - classical chemotherapy (and radiotherapy) which is harmful also to normal cells, act primarily by inducing cell apoptosis either locally, in tumour, or globally, when cancer metastasize. Any disturbance in apoptosis results in a decrease in the effectiveness of the therapy. The recent targeted therapies instead of interfering with rapidly dividing cells, interfere with selected targets in the cell and use small molecules to interfere with abnormal proteins (required for carcinogenesis and tumour growth) or cell receptors, or use monoclonal antibodies, which destroy malignant tumour cells and prevent tumour growth by blocking specific receptors. Targeted cancer therapy, which may be more effective and less harmful than classical chemotherapy but still are based on the use of chemical compounds is perceived as modern chemotherapy or chemotherapy of the future.

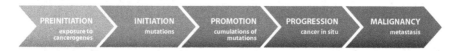

Figure 1. Multi-step process of carcinogenesis.

3. Cancer risk — Carcinogens and co-carcinogens

Currently we are aware that apart of inherited mutations, an important role in carcinogenesis play the factors connected with the expression to carcinogens [14]. This includes environmental factors (pollutions), lifestyle factors (tobacco smoking, diet, alcohol consumption, obesity, sedentary life), occupational factors (e.g. synthesis, dyes, fumes) and other factors (excessive exposure to sunlight, radiation, viruses, etc). Carcinogens (of chemical, physical or biological origin) include chemicals or non-chemical agents, which under certain conditions are able to induce cancer. Co-carcinogens, are not carcinogenic themselves but with other chemicals or non-chemical carcinogens, such as for example UV or ionizing radiation, promote the effects of a carcinogen in carcinogenesis. Carcinogens as well as co-carcinogens can be of natural or synthetic origins. In general, their carcinogenic action relay on direct or indirect action in the cellular DNA. Carcinogens acting directly can initiate the carcinogenesis by yielding highly reactive species that bind covalently to cellular DNA, while those acting indirectly can induce mutations to cellular DNA. Thus carcinogens are able to distort the conformation or function (replication/transcription) of DNA, which results not only in oncogene activation but also DNA amplification, gene transposition or chromosome translocation. Carcinogens may induce carcinogenesis directly by mutational activation of protooncogenes and/or inactivation of tumour suppression genes. Indirect action is realised through the mechanisms that generate chemical species (free radicals, reactive oxygen species, carcinogenic metabolites) which are capable of entering the nucleus of the cell.

Over 80% of carcinogenic substances are of environmental origins [15]. Restriction of the exposition to carcinogens can substantially reduce the risk of cancers also those of occupational type, which make approximately 4-5% of all human cancers. Thus evaluation and classification of the carcinogens is required from the cancer prevention point of view. Although there are many international and national organizations that classify carcinogens, but only a few are highly influential, the oldest and setting the standards, World Health Organization of the United Nations (WHO) International Agency for Research on Cancer (IARC) headquartered in Lyon, France, established in 1965; United Nations initiative from 1992 called Globally Harmonized System of Classification and Labelling of Chemicals (GHS), National Toxicology Program of the U.S. Department of Health and Human Services established in 1978, professional organization American Conference of Governmental Industrial Hygienists, founded in 1938 in Washington and reorganized in 1946, European Union directives Dangerous Substances Directive (67/548/EEC) and the Dangerous Preparations Directive (1999/45/EC) and Safe Work Australia (Independent Statutory Agency) which evolved from National Occupational Health and Safety Council (NOHSC) established in 1985. One of the prime roles of these organizations is to evaluate and classify the chemical, physical and biological carcinogens targeted to develop strategies for cancer prevention and control used by international and national health and regulatory agencies to protect public health. Since 1971 IARC evaluated the carcinogenicity of approximately 400 and collected data about 900 agents and published them in a series (101 till 2012) of Monographs on the Evaluation of Carcinogenic Risks to Humans [3]. Up to now IARC has identified 108 definitely, 66 probably, 284 possibly carcinogens, 515 not classifiable as carcinogens and 1 probably not carcinogenic, Table 1. Alternative to IARC, a complex GSH classification system, collects data from tests, literature, and practical experience [16]. Since 2003 four editions of GHS have been published, but only most recent one, dated to 2011, has the form convenient for worldwide implementation. GSH delivers a global system of classification of chemicals (substances, alloys, mixtures) divided into three groups of hazards: physical (16 classes), health and environmental (12 and 2 classes, respectively) and a unique system of labelling and collecting the information in the form of safety data sheets (SDS). GSH requires the use of the harmonized classification scheme and the harmonized label elements for any carcinogenic chemical. Within the GSH system, the class of carcinogens was clearly separated as health hazard risk factor and divided to two categories: known and presumed carcinogens (subcategories 1A and 1B, respectively) and suspected carcinogens (category 2), Table 2. Irrespective of the classification system, the epidemiological evidence indicates that many drugs, including antineoplastic, sex hormones, antithyroid, antibacterial, antiparasitic, immunosuppressive ones used as single agents or in combinations as well as radiation (γ, X or UV) are known carcinogens.

3.1. Carcinogens of chemical/environmental origins

As early as in 16th c. Phillippus Aureolus Theophratus Bombastus von Hohenheim (1493-1541) known as Paracelsus suggested that the "wasting disease of miners" might be linked to exposure to realgar (tetra-arsenic tetra-sulphide). Since the 17th c. cancer was associated with the presence of some chemicals. For example John Hill (1716-1775) linked tobacco use with nasal cancer, while Percivall Pot (1814-1788) described occupational risk of epithelial cancer of the scrotum connected with soot, in chimney sweepers. In 1795 Samuel Thomas von Soemmerring (1755-1830) cautioned that pipe smokers were excessively prone to cancer of the lip. Since then epidemiological evidence has been important in detecting carcinogens. In 1858, a Montpellier surgeon Etienne-Frédéric Bouisson (1813-1884) found that 63 of his 68 patients suffering from oral cancer were pipe smokers. Shortly after replacement of natural dyes b synthetic aromatic amine dye in German industry, Ludwig Rehn (1849-1930) reported an increased incidence of bladder cancer in workers exposed to it. Many years later exact carcinogen, 2-naphthylamine, was recognized. In the 1930s the first company in American dye industry, DuPont, reported first cases of occupational cancer connected with the use of dyes, bladder cancer, at the Chambers Works plant. In 1935, Takaoki Sasaki and Tomizo Yoshida (1903-1973) induced malignant tumours (hepatoma) in a digestive organ by feeding rats by one of the azo dyes - o-aminoazotoluene.

IARC classification	Effect	Criteria	No	Agents and groups of agents/mixtures/ the exposure circumstance
Group 1	definitely carcinogenic	sufficient evidence of carcinogenicity to humans, epidemiologic evidence, occupational exposure, and animal studies; strong evidence that the agent acts through relevant mechanisms of carcinogenicity to humans	108	chlorambucil, cyclophosphamide, chlornaphazine, melphalan, tamoxifen5, thiotepa, sulfur mustard
				ultraviolet radiation (UV-A, UV-B, UV-C), X-radiation, γ-radiation, radiation, radionuclides, neutron radiation, solar radiation
Group 2A	probably carcinogenic	limited evidence of carcinogenicity to humans, but sufficient evidence of carcinogenicity in experimental animals; strong evidence that the carcinogenesis is mediated by mechanisms that are also operate in humans	66	azacitidine, cisplatin, nitrogen mustard, doxorubicin
Group 2B	possibly carcinogenic	limited evidence in humans; less than sufficient evidence in experimental animals; inadequate evidence in humans but sufficient or limited in experimental animals	284	aziridine, dacarbazine, daunomycin, thiouracil, bleomycin
Group 3	not classifiable as carcinogenic	inadequate evidence in humans; inadequate or limited to experimental animals; mechanisms of carcinogenesis in animals does not operate in humans.	515	ifosfamide, isophosphamide, actinomycin D
Group 4	probably not carcinogenic	negative evidence of carcinogenicity, not used	1	caprolactam

Table 1. Classification of carcinogens according to IARC, 2012

But the first chemical carcinogen - coal tar - was identified as early as in 1915 by Katsusaburo Yamagiwa (1863-1930) and Koichi Ichikawa (1888-1948) who induced cancer in laboratory animals by prolonged application of coal tar to rabbit skin. Inflammation accompanying the coal tar application and cancer formation was in a good agreement with Virchow findings. The search for specific chemical carcinogens led to the discovery of pure carcinogenic chemicals including polycyclic aromatic hydrocarbons PAHs (e.g. benzo[a]pyrene, 1,2,5,6-dibenzanthracene) by Ernest Lawrence Kennaway (1881-1958) and Izrael Hieger (1901-1986), which were shown to be carcinogenic in mouse skin by Hieger et al. in 1933 [17]. Nowadays, we know that PAHs, mainly benzo[a]pyrene and heterocyclic amines (HCAs) belong to definite carcinogens which appear in smoke as a result of incomplete combustion [18] and thus are present not only in tobacco smoke but also in a fried/smoked meat as well as barbeque. PAHs often induce stomach cancer.

Category	Effect	Criteria	Signal word	Hazard statement	Symbol/Pictogram
1A	known human carcinogen	known to have carcinogenic potential for humans – largely based on human evidence	Danger	may cause cancer	
1B	presumed human carcinogen	presumed to have carcinogenic potential for humans – largely based on animal evidence	Danger	may cause cancer	
2	suspected human carcinogen	evidence from animal and/or human studies is limited	Warning	suspected of causing cancer	

Table 2. Classification of carcinogens according to GSH, 2011

Although cancer-causing substances are often considered to be exclusively synthetic, there are numerous natural carcinogens, chemical compounds that occur in environment, and in food plants [19]. Isaac Berenblum (1903-2000) discovered the potent inflammatory agent, croton oil extracted from *Croton Tiglium* L. native or cultivated in Asia (India, Ceylon, China), Malay Argipelago and Africa (Zanzibar, Tanzania), and its most active ingredient, 12-O-tetradecanoylphorbol-13-acetate (TPA) in 1941 [20]. Both agents now belong to classic tumour promoters. In 1956, John Barnes (1913-1975) and Peter Magee, reported an example of synergistic interaction of chemical carcinogens with proinflammatory agents. i.e. liver tumors in rats induced by N-nitrosdimethylamine (NDMA) [21]. In 1972, another case, the influence of chronic respiratory infection with influenza virus on the development of lung cancer in rats induced by carcinogenic N-nitrosamine was reported [22], which occurs in some foodstuffs, latex, cosmetics. Since then about 90% of nitrosamine derivatives including hydrazines from raw mushrooms *Agaricus bisporus* (Lange) Imbach and *Gyromitra* (Pers.) Fr. have been deemed to be carcinogenic and promoters of benign hepatomas, liver cell carcinomas, angiomas and angiosarcomas of blood vessels, adenomas and adenocarcinomas of lungs.

One of the most potent naturally occurring microbial carcinogen is Aflatoxin B_1, which is produced as secondary metabolite by the fungi *Aspergillus flavus* and *Aspergillus parasiticm* [23] growing on stored grains, nuts and peanut butter and found worldwide as a contaminant in food. The discovery of Alfatoxin B$_1$ followed upon "Turkey X Disease" (a liver disease) which killed over 100,000 turkeys in the UK in the early 1960s. The major metabolite of Aflatoxin B1, Aflatoxin B1-8,9-epoxide, exerts hepatotoxic effect, but synergistic interaction between Aflatoxin B1 and hepatitis B virus results in hepatocellular carcinoma. Another fungal contaminant is mycotic toxin Ochratoxin-A (OTA) produced by *Penicillium viridicatum* discovered during laboratory studies in the mid-1960s and encountered as a natural contaminant in maize in 1969 in the USA [24]. Large group of carcinogens are tannins and tannic acid, which occur widely in plants (tea, coffee, and cocoa) but in concentrated doses reveal hepatocarcinogenic properties in both animals and humans. They have been found capable of causing liver tumours in experimental animals and oesophageal, throat & mouth cancers in humans. Cycads, important food sources in tropical regions, contain unique toxines cycasin and macrozamin that cause liver and kidney tumours in rats [25]. Safrole, 5-Allyl-1,3-benzo-dioxole found in sassafras tea, cinnamin, cocoa, nutmeg, black pepper, and other herbs and spices as well as isosafrole, 1,2-(Methylenedioxy)-4-propenylbenzene belong to liver carcinogens in rats, they produce liver tumours following their oral administration [26]. Dihydrosafrole is also carcinogenic in rats and mice, in which it produces tumours of the oesophagus, and liver tumours in males and lung tumours in both males and females, respectively. There is an evidence of the carcinogenic properties of estragole from anise, star anise, basil, bay, tarragon, fennel, marjoram or American wood turpentine oil, which proceeds through a genotoxic mechanism identical to that of safrole and also induce liver cancer in mice [27]. Black pepper (*Piper nigrum* L.), apart of tannic acid and safrole contains secondary amines pyperadine and alpha-methylpyrroline, which can be nitrosated to N-nitroso-piperidine, a strong carcinogen, carcinogenic to experimental mice. It has been known since the 1960s that Comfrey (*Symphytum officinale* L.) contains carcinogenic hepatoxines belonging to pyrrolizidine alkaloids (PAs) e.g. lasiocarpine and symphatine, which can interfere with RNA and DNA synthesis within the liver cells and cause liver damage, cancer, and death [28].

Some chemical carcinogens have been discovered as a result of industrial or environmental accidents. For example in 1976, notoriety was gained by Seveso disaster - an explosion occurred in a TCP (2,4,5-trichlorophenol) reactor at the ICMESA chemical plant located about 20 km north of Milan, Italy. A mixture of different chemicals including dioxin was released into the atmosphere. This industrial accident caused the highest known exposure to 2,3,7,8-tetrachlorodibenzo-p-dioxin (TCDD) in residential populations and linked dioxin exposure to chloracne, genetic impairments and excessive risk of lymphatic and hematopoietic tissue [29-32]. Another environmental disaster related to dioxines was contamination of a landfill of Love Canal in the Niagara Falls, New York, USA. This region was turned in 1920 to municipal and industrial chemical dumpsite by Hooker Chemica and in 1942-1953 it was contaminated by eleven highly toxic carcinogens including TCDD. In 1978 a record amount of rainfall in Love Canal resulted in leaching the chemicals from corroding waste-disposal drums in this area which caused environmental disaster, a drastic increase in birth defects, nervous disorders, high white-blood-cell counts in residents, a possible precursor of leukaemia and cancers [33-35]. Many years later probable carcinogenic action of triclosan, an antibacterial agent added to soaps, toothpastes etc., has been linked to its degradation to TCDD in chlorinated water [36]. In the early 1980s the high risk of lung, skin, kidney and bladder cancer due to chronic low level arsenic poisoning of water in different countries (Bangladesh, Vietnam, Cambodia, Tibet, Argentina, Chile, China, India, Mexico, Thailand, and US) caused by contamination of water by pesticides and various alloys containing arsenic, which resemble and thus substitute phosphorus in chemical reactions, was discovered [37]. In 1980 it was realized that exposure to formaldehyde (a hazard in embalming and production of plastics and vinyl chloride, from which PVC is manufactured) could cause nasal cancer in rats [38]. In the early 1970s, the carcinogenicity of vinyl chloride was linked to occupational angiosarcoma cancers in workers in industry. A few years later PVC was classified as a carcinogen [39-41]. Since then specific substances: aniline and benzidine, asbestos, wool/wood/leather dust have been linked to different types of cancer in humans bladder cancer, sinuses and lung cancer, mesothelioma, nasal sinuses, respectively [3]. Many drugs, including chemotherapeutic anticancer agents, diuretics, hormones have been recognized as a source of secondary cancers and thus classified as definite carcinogens. Most of anticancer drugs is classified as group 1 agents in IARC classification [3].

3.2. Carcinogens of biological origins (Oncogenic viruses/bacteria/parasites)

The hypothesis that cancer can originate from a virus comes from Danish scientists Oluf Bang (1881-1937) and Vilhelm Ellerman (1871-1924), who was the first to show, in 1908, that avian erythroblastosis (chicken leukaemia) can be transmitted by cell-free extracts. In 1911, Francis Peyton Rous (1879-1970), American pathologist, described a solid cancer, sarcoma, in domestic chickens caused by exposing the healthy bird to a cell-free filtrate containing retrovirus later became known as the *Rous sarcoma virus* [42]. Abbie Lathrop (1868-1918) and Leo Loeb (1869-1959) described breast cancer in mice caused by a transmissible agent as early as in 1915 [43]. Since then several oncoviruses have been linked to different types of cancer [44]. In 1933 Richard Edwin Shope (1901-1966) discovered the first mammalian tumour caused in cottontail rabbit by fibroma virus and papilloma virus (*Shope papilloma virus*). Shortly later, in 1936, a geneticist and cancer biologists John Joseph Bittner (1904-1961) discovered a mouse mammary tumour virus (MMTV), the so-called Bittner virus, causing a breast cancer, which is a promoter in models of human breast cancer [45]. In 1957, Sarah Elizabeth Stewart (1905-1976) and Berenice E. Eddy (1903-1989), pioneers in the field of viral oncology research, discovered the Stewart-Eddy polyoma virus, which produced several types of cancer in a variety of small mammals [46]. John J. Trentin (1908-2005) and others were the first to report of cancer (sarcoma) produced in animals (hamsters) by inoculation of virus of human origin (*Adenovirus*) [47]. Michael Anthony Epstein, Bert Achong (1928-1996) and Yvonne Barr identified the first human cancer virus (Epstein-Barr Virus or EBV) from Burkitt lymphoma cells in 1964 [48]. Baruch Blumberg (1925-2011) isolated Hepatitis B virus (HBV), a cause of hepatitis, and suggested that it contributed to liver cancer hepatocellular carcinoma. It was confirmed to be an oncovirus in the 1980s. Hepatitis C virus (HCV) was shown to be a major contributor to liver cancer (hepatocellular carcinoma) by Michael Houghton and Daniel W. Bradley in 1987. The first human retroviruses, Human T-lymphotropic virus 1 (HTLV I) and 2 (HTLV 2), linked to T-cell lymphoma/T-cell leukaemia and Hairy-cell leukaemia, respectively, were discovered by Bernard J. Poiesz, Robert Charles Gallo and Mistuaki Yoshida. In 1984 Harald zur Hausen and Lutz Gissman discovered that the human papillomaviruses HPV16 and HPV18 were responsible for approximately 70% of cervical cancers, while Alan Storey, Kit Osborn and Lionel Crawford in 1990 indicated that HPV types 6 and 11 were responsible for 90% of genital warts. Valerie Beral, Thomas A. Peterman, Harold W. Jaffe related Kaposi's sarcoma-associated herpesvirus (KSHV) with AIDS [49], which prompted Patrick S. Moore, Yuan Chang, Frank Lee and Ethel Cesarman to isolate Kaposi sarcoma-associated herpesvirus (KSHV or HHV8) in 1994 [50]. Very recently in 2008, Chang and Moore developed a new method to identify oncoviruses called digital transcriptome subtraction (DTS) and isolated DNA fragments of Merkel cell polyomavirus from a Merkel cell carcinoma, considered to be responsible for 70–80% of these cancers [51].

There is also evidence of a link between the bacteria Helicobacter pylori (HP) responsible for development of gastric and duodenal ulcers and cancer risk [52,53]. The human oncogenic viruses, which include HBV, HCV, HIV, HPVs, EBV, KSHV, HTLV-I and HTLV-II and HP are associated with nearly 20% of the human cancer cases. The elimination of these pathogens would decrease by 23.6% the cases of cancer in developing countries and by 7.7% in developed countries [54]. The commonly omitted advantage of the discovery of oncoviruses was the possibility of transplantation of carcinogen-induced tumour systems in mice, which delivered models for the studies on anticancer drugs.

Rare source of cancer are also parasitic diseases caused by *Clonorchis sinensis* (Japan, Korea, Vietnam) and *Opisthorchis viverrini* (Thailand, Laos, and Malaysia) or *Schistosomas species* (Africa, Asia). All of them are known to be carcinogenic and linked with biliary tract cancer (cholangiocarcinoma) and bladder cancer, respectively [55]. Most of the biological carcinogens are classified as group 1 agents in IARC classification [3].

3.3. Carcinogens of physical origins (Radiation)

Shortly after the discovery of chemical carcinogens, i.e. factors that suppress and activate the cell growth and division, the first physical carcinogens were identified. After discovery of X-rays by Wilhelm Roentgen (1845-1923) in 1895 and radioactive radiation by Henri Becquerel (1852-1908) in 1896, the exposure to radiation has been identified as one of the causes of cancer. Working with early X-ray generators resulted in the acute skin reactions and the first radiation-induced cancer arising in an ulcerated area of the skin was reported in 1902. In 1910 to 1912, Pierre Marie, Jean Clunet and Gaston Raulot-Lapointe reported the induction of sarcoma in rats by the application of X-irradiation. As early as in 1911 the first report of leukaemia in radiation workers appeared [56]. The 20th century pioneers in X-Ray/radium studies fell victims to their work; surgeon Robert Abbe (1851-1928), physicist Marie Skłodowska-Curie (1867-1934) and physician Jean Bergonie (1857-1925) died due to leukaemia. The use of uranium/plutonium based bombs against Hiroshima/Nagasaki during World War II revealed that ionising radiation irrespective of its origin is a cause of cancer [57]. Increased incidence of cancer of bone marrow and essentially all organs was noted in Japan years to decades later. Some physical carcinogens have been discovered as a result of nuclear disasters. In 1957, the cooling system failed and the radioactive wastes chemical explosion of at Mayak nuclear fuel reprocessing plant, Ozyorsk/Mayak, Russia caused radiation contamination which spread over hundred kilometres and pollution of the Techa River. This accident called Kyshtym disaster belongs to three most serious nuclear accidents ever recorded, although it was revealed only in 1976 [58]. The scarce epidemiological studies suggest very different numbers of cancer deaths among residents associated to radiation exposure. In 1979 the cooling system of Three Mile Island nuclear power plant near Harrisburg, Pennsylvania failed and the reactor core was partially melted. Radiation from the reactor contributed to the premature deaths and cancers in local residents, but the disaster was relatively small [59]. There is still vivid discussion about the carcinogenic effects of nuclear power plant explosion in 1986 in Chernobyl located 80 miles from Kiev, Ukraine, which was the greatest source of long-lived radioactive plutonium and short-lived radioactive caesium (^{137}Cs), iodines (particularly ^{131}I) and strontium (^{90}Sr). The major health effect of Chernobyl was an elevated thyroid-cancer incidence due to iodine absorption by the thyroid gland in adolescents and children some of whom were not yet born at the time of the accident, and drastic increase in leukaemia cases caused by distribution the strontium incorrectly recognized by the body as calcium throughout the bone structure [60]. Radioactive isotopes of barium, caesium, iodine and tellurium were detected in a radiation plume released by damaged nuclear reactors at the nuclear plant in Fukushima, Japan in 2011. Fukushima Daiichi disaster was the most serious accident in global scale. As the prolonged exposure to radiation in the air, ground and food can result in leukaemia and other cancers thus about 160,000 people were evacuated from the region surrounding the plant. According to theoretical 3-D global atmospheric models this nuclear disaster may cause as many as 2,500 cases of cancer, mostly in Japan. Only recently, in the 1990s, much-less energetic UV radiation has been also recognized as carcinogen causing not only genetic mutations but also melanoma or non-melanoma cancers. In 2011 WHO/IARC classified radiofrequency electromagnetic fields as possibly carcinogenic to humans (Group 2B), on the basis of an increased risk of glioma, a malignant type of brain cancer, associated with wireless phone use [3]. Nowadays we are aware that exposure to radiation can be incidental like in Hiroshima, Nagasaki, Chernobyl, Fukushima [1,61] or systematic due to repeated doses of radiation like UV during sun-bathing or MW during phone-cell use. Anyway the most common radiation induced cancers are basal cell carcinoma and squamous carcinoma of the skin, leukaemia and thyroid cancer. The first two can arise from excessive exposure to UV radiation, while the other are mainly result of ionising radiation e.g. γ, X-Ray [1]. The controlled use of ionising radiation in medicine and industry and annual limits of doses for each individual [62] has reduced the risk connected with ionising radiation but the awareness of UV or MW related risk is still low. Common feature of cancers induced by physical factor is late onset and long period of risk persisting. Most of the physical carcinogens are classified as group 1 or 2 agents in IARC classification [3].

4. Chemotherapeutical agents

4.1. Drugs of natural origin

In the second half of the 20th century, one more type of cancer therapy was added to surgery, irradiation and hormonotherapy, which was chemotherapy. Nowadays this term primarily refers to the treatment of cancer with an antineoplastic drug or a combination of drugs, but when it was introduced in 1909 by Paul Ehrlich (1854-1915) it had a broader meaning as it referred as well to antibacterial chemotherapy and treatment of autoimmune diseases, in general use of chemicals to treat disease. Chemotherapy, generally assumed as the youngest method of cancer treatment, is in fact rooted in ancient times. Although cutting out the cancer changed tissue was early found as the main treatment, it was not always effective. Thus various substances of natural origin were applied as complementary medications. Many even ancient cultures had proposed theories explaining the cause of cancer. These theories influenced the search for medicaments. For example Egyptians believed that natural substances similar in look or function to human organs can be used to treat ailments in those organs, thus the use of mixtures of pigs eyes or ears was popular.

Although the products of animal and mineral origin had made an important contribution to drug development, the main source of drugs for millennia have been green plants. The most frequently used included castor oil plant (*Ricinus communis* L.), exploding cucumber (*Ecballium elateritum* L.), belladonna (*Atropa belladonna* L.), myrrh (dried sap from trees *Commiphora Myrcha* L.), incense (dried sap from trees *Boswellia thurifera* L., *Boswellia frereana* Birdw., *Boswellia bhawdajiana* Birdw.), stinging nettle (*Urtica dioica* L.), gingers (*Zingiber Boehm.* L.), red clover (*Trifolium pratense* L.) and autumn crocus (*Colchicum autumnale* L.). Although, in nature most of them cause sickness, but in small doses or after chemical modifications, they revealed therapeutic effects. Some of them were rediscovered by modern medicine. For example from *Colchicum autumnale* L. described by Pedanius Dioscorides (40-90 A.D.) in De Materia Medica a toxic alkaloid colchicine was extracted in 1820 by Pierre Joseph Pelletier (1788-1842) and Joseph Bienaimé Caventou (1795–1877). Albert Pierre Dustin (1914-1993), described its antimitotic properties in 1934 [63]. In 2009 it was accepted by Food and Drug Administration (FDA) as a drug for gout and Familial Mediterranean Fever. Another interesting case described by Dioscorides is red viscous sap called the dragon's blood mostly collected from *Dracaena cinnabari* Balf. f or *Croton lechleri* L. and used as a dye and anti-inflammatory, antimicrobial and anticancer folk remedy not only by ancient Greek but also Romans and Arabs. Recently methanolic extract of *Croton lechleri* was shown to exert cytotoxic effects on HeLa (Human epithelial carcinoma cell line) cells and its antitumor effect in HeLa tumour in mice was documented [64]. Two other commonly used antileukemic drugs, vinblastine and vincristine, were extracted in 1950 from the species of Madagascar periwinkle (*Catharanthus roseus* L.), for centuries known as folk remedy, and shortly after approved by FDA. Nowadays vinblastine, which binds tubulin, thereby inhibiting the assembly of microtubules, is an important component of a number of chemotherapy regimens, including ABVD for Hodgkin lymphoma, advanced testicular cancer, breast and lung cancers, and Kaposi's sarcoma [65]. Realgar widely used in Chinese traditional medicine because of its anti-inflammation, antiulcer, anticonvulsion, and anti-schistosomiasis activity was recently found capable to induce cell apoptosis and thus effective in the treatment of hematological malignant diseases [66]. As early as in 1021, Avicenna described the medicinal use of *Taxus baccata* L. (Zarnab) as cardiac remedy in The Canon of Medicine. Various parts of *Taxus brevifolia* Peattie, *Taxus Canadensis* Marshall, *Taxus baccata* L. have been used by several Native American Tribes mainly for the treatment of non-cancerous diseases [65] but the use for the treatment of cancer was noted only in the Hindu Ayurvedic medicine. Paclitaxel (Taxol®), used in treatment for breast, ovarian, small and non-small cell lung cancer and Kaposi sarcoma, was isolated in 1967 by Monroe E. Wall and

Mansukh C. Wani from the bark of the 200-years old Pacific yew (*Taxus brevifolia* Nutt.) tree [67]. Its structure was elucidated in 1971 [67,68]. Its cytostatic mechanism of action (mitosis inhibition) was discovered by Susan B. Horowitz in the late 1970s, but only the discovery of total chemical synthesis of Paclitaxel in 1994 by Robert A. Holton widespread its use [69]. Camptothecin isolated from the Chinese and Tibetan ornamental joy tree Decne (*Camptotheca acuminata* var. rotundifolia B. M. Yang & L. D. Duan), *Nyssaceae* Arnott family, was discovered in 1966 by Wall and Wani in systematic screening of natural products [70]. Although it is a potent topoisomerase inhibitor, it was dropped in the 1970s from clinical trials because of severe bladder toxicity [71]. But two of its semi-synthetic derivatives - topotecan and irinotecan are used for the treatment of ovarian and small cell lung and colon-rectal cancers, respectively [72,73]. Epipodophyllotoxines also belong to active anti-tumour agents derived from plants. Podophyllotoxin and deoxypodophyllotoxin were obtained from the roots of American mandrake or May apple (*Podophyllum peltatum* L.), Himalayan mayapple (*Podophyllum emodi* Wallich ex Hook. f. & Thomson) and Chinese or Asian Mayapple (*Podophyllum pleianthum* L.), respectively [74], all belongs to *Berberidaceae* Juss. family. *Podophyllum peltatum* and *Podophyllum emodii* were used by the Native American Tribes for the treatment of cancer including skin-cancers. Podophyllotoxin was isolated from the rhizome in 1880 by V. Podwyssotski [75]. More cytotoxic 4-deoxypodophyllotoxin was isolated from Cow Parsley (*Anthriscus sylvestris* L.) and Korean pasque flower (*Pulsatilla koreana* Y.Yabe ex Nakai). Although native epipodophyllo-toxines are not used but its synthetic analogues - etoposide and teniposide, which belongs to topoisomerase II inhibitors, are effective in the treatment of lymphomas and bronchial and testicular cancers [65,76]. Another example is bruceantin isolated from a tree, *Brucea antidy-senterica* Mill from *Simaroubaceae* DC family, used traditionally for the tumour treatment in Ethiopia [77]. Recently it was discovered that bruceantin can be an effective agent for the treatment of hematological malignancies (leukaemia, lymphoma and myeloma). Its activity has been linked with the down-regulation of a key oncoprotein. Omacetaxine mepesuccinat (Homoharringtonine), alkaloid isolated from the Cowtail Pine called Japanese Plum Yew (*Cephalotaxus harringtonia* Koch), is one more example of plant-derived anticancer agent [78,79]. Its racemate (harringtonine mixed with homoharringtonine) which induces apoptosis by inhibition of protein synthesis, particularly Mcl-1 (induced myeloid leukemia cell differentia-tion protein), is used for the treatment of chronic leukaemia - acute lymphoblastic leukaemia and chronic myelogenous leukaemia [65]. Elliptinium acetate, a derivative of ellipticine, which was isolated from a Fijian plant *Bleekeria vitensis* A.C. Sm., is used for the treatment of breast cancer [65]. Recently numerous potential anticancer compounds have been isolated from different plants. A few of them are currently in clinical or preclinical trials but most require further investigation. A case of considerable interest is indirubine extracted from Mu Lan (*Indigofera tinctoria* L.) from *Leguminosae* Lindl. family called Indigo plant a main component of traditional Chinese herbal remedy called Dang Gui Long Hui Wan used to treat chronic myelogenous leukaemia. Synthetic agents flavopiridol derived from the indirubins - plant alkaloid rohitukine, which was isolated from *Dysoxylum binectariferum* Hook. f. (*Meliaceae* Juss.) [80] and roscovitine derived from olomucine, which was isolated from *Raphanus sativus* L. (*Brassicaceae* Burnett), are respectively in Phase I and II of clinical trials [65,81] against a broad range of cancers including leukaemia, lymphomas and solid tumours [82]. Both are belongs to inhibitors of cyclin-dependent kinases (Cdks), key regulatory proteins in the cell cycle. Most recent studies indicate that drugs of the indirubin family may block brain tumour and thus improve survival in glioblastoma. Other synthetic derivatives of indirubins (3'-monooxime and 5-bromo) reveal comparable activity to other Cdk inhibitors and thus are promising for drug development [83]. Unique source of indirubines are gastropod molluscs: *Bolinus brandaris* L. and *Hexaplex trunculus* L. (*Muricidae* L.) used for over 2,500 years to obtain purplish red dye known as "Tyrian Purple". The 6-bromoindirubine treated as impurity to indigo dye and its synthetic derivative show selective inhibition of glycogen synthase kinase-3 (GSK-3) [81]. The discovery of GSK-3 functions resulted in the search for its inhibitors as potential drugs against neurodegenerative diseases, inflammation and cancer. Combretastatin isolated from the bark of the South African "bush willow", tree *Combretum caffrum* (Eckl. & Zeyh.) Kuntze (*Combretaceae* Loefl. familly) [84] belongs to the most cytotoxic phytomolecules isolated so far [85,86] and is promising in the treatment of colon, lung cancers, lymphomas and leukaemias. Combretastatins belongs to stilbenes, which are anti-angiogenic agents, causing vascular shutdown resulting in tumour necrosis. *Combretum* was widely used in African and Hindu medicine for the treatment of a variety of diseases, but *Terminalia* L. flowering plant from the same family *Combretaceae* Loefl., have been used traditionally for cancer treatment. Another promising stilbene is trans-Resveratrol natural phenol produced by several plants (eg. *Vitis vinifera* L., *Vitis labrusca* L., *Vitis rotundifolia* Michx.), when under attack by pathogens (bacteria or fungi like Botrytis cinerea (De Bary) Whetzel). It was extracted from False Helleborine (*Veratrum Album* L.) by Michio Takaoka in 1939. More than 60 years later in 1997, Ming-Hua Jang reported that trans-Resveratrol prevented skin cancer development in mice treated with a carcinogen, which gain attention to its potential anticancer applications. It was shown that trans-Resveratrol acts on all steps of the process of carcinogenesis [87]. It triggered apoptosis in uterine, colon cancer cell line, colon, human breast, prostate, lung cancer and pancreatic cancer cell lines in vitro, but is also able to arrest the cell cycle or to inhibit kinase pathways. The inhibition in the development of oesophageal, intestinal, and breast cancer after oral administration of resveratrol was revealed in studies on animal models. The human clinical trials for cancer have not been reported. A few promising substances betulinic acid, lupeol have been obtained from white part of *Betula species* (*Betulaceae* Gray) bark. The alcohol precursor of betulinic acid - betulin - was isolated as long ago as in 1788 by Tobias Lowitz (1757-1804). Betulinic acid, a pentacyclic triterpene, is a common secondary metabolite of plants, it was isolated also from *Ziziphus zizyphus* L. H. Karst. species, e.g. *Ziziphus Mauritiana* Lam., *Ziziphus Rugosa* Lam. and *Ziziphus Oenoplia* (L.) Mill. [88,89], while lupeol was found in a variety of plants, including mango (*Mangifera L.*) and acacia visco (*Acacia visite* Griseb.). All of them are potent anti-inflammatory agents and displayed selective cytotoxicity against human melanoma cell lines [90]. A case of considerable interest is birch polypore fungus Chaga (*Inonotus obliquus* Pers. Pill.), which belongs to *Basidiomycetes* R.T. Moore. It forms black perennial woody growth called a conk on birch trees. It is traditionally used in Russia for the treatment of a number of conditions including cancer, gastritis and ulcers. Two phenolic compounds, hispidin and hispolon extracted from Chaga but also from Japan, Chinese and Korean medicinal fungus *Phellinus linteus* (Japanese *meshimakobu*, Chinese *song gen*, Korean *sanghwang*) were reported to be cytotoxic against human cell line HeLa [91], while the polysaccharides ß (1→3)-D glucopyrans and ß (1→6)-D-glucosyl, found also in ornamental plant *Pteris ensiformis* Burm., originating from tropical Africa, Asia and Pacific region, have prom-ising anticancer activity against a number of different cell lines.

Claims for another efficient plant derivative - *Tabebuia* Gomes (*Bignoniaceae* Juss.) used traditionally by the indigenous people in the Amazonian region for the treatment of variable diseases, appeared in the 1960s. Numerous bioactive compounds including naphthaquinones, particularly lapachol and ß-lapachone have been isolated from the stem bark and wood of *Tabebuia impetiginosa* (Mart. Ex DC.) Standl., *Tabebuia rosea* Bertol., and *Tabebuia serratifolia* (Vahl) Nicholson. Lapachol revealed potent in vivo anti-tumour activity, but was dropped out because of unacceptable level of toxicity [92]. ß-lapachone was recently found active against breast cancer, leukaemia, prostate tumour and several multidrug resistant (MDR) cell lines and more promising than lapachol [93]. It is a potent inhibitor of Cdc25 phosphatases enzyme that play a key role in cell cycle progression [83]. Another potent and promising in the field of MDR is pervilleine A, aromatic ester tropane, selectively cytotoxic against oral epidermoid cancer cell line which was isolated from the roots of the Madagascar tree *Erythroxylum pervillei* Baill. from *Erythroxylaceae* Kunth family [94,95]. In the early 1970s another plant originated substance, maytansine was isolated from the Ethiopian plant, *Maytenus serrata* (Hochst. Ex A. Rich.) Wilczek from *Celastraceae* R. Br. family. Although the results of preclinical animal tests were very promising but the lack of efficacy in clinical trials in the early 1980s resulted in dropping it out from further study. However, related compounds, the ansamito-cins, isolated from actinomycete *Actinosynnema pretiosum* shed some light on its possible microbial origin [96]. Its synthetic derivative - cytotoxic Mertansine is a component of human-ized monoclonal antibodies: Cantuzumab mertansine, Bivatuzumab mertansine, Lorvotuzu-mab mertansine and Trastuzumab emtansine effective in colorectal, squamous cell carcinoma, small-cell lung or ovarian cancer and breast cancer, respectively. Another case of considerable interest is thapsigargin isolated from the umbelliferous plant, *Thapsia garganica* L. (*Apiaceae* Lindl.) from Mediterranean island of Ibiza [97]. Thapsigargin, induces apoptosis in prostate cancer cells and synthetic prodrug derived from it called "G-202" is in Phase II clinical trials. Silvestrol isolated from the fruits of *Aglaila sylvestre* Roemer from *Meliaceae* Juss. family [98], exhibit cytotoxicity against lung and breast cancer cell lines [65]. Its synthetic analogue 4'-desmethoxyepisilvestrol is cytotoxic against lung and colon cancer cell lines. Two alkaloids, schischkinnin and montamine isolated recently from the seeds of *Centaurea schischkinii* Tzvelev and *Centaurea montana* L. [99,100] exhibit significant cytotoxicity against HCCLs (human colon cancer cell lines). The essential oil of *Salvia officinalis* L., most popular folk remedy in Middle East known for its antitumor effects, which contains monoterpenes thujone, β-pinene, and 1,8-cineol was shown to be cytotoxic against squamous human cell carcinoma cell line of the oral cavity [101]. There are many other natural substances like extracts of unknown composition from *Colubrina macrocarpa* (Cav.) G. Don., *Hemiangium excelsum* (Kunth) A.C. Sm, *Acacia pennatula* (Schltdl. & Cham.) Benth., *Commiphora opobalsamum* Jacq., *Astragalus* L., *Paris polyphylla* Sm., *Teucrium polium* L., *Pistacia lentiscus* L. used as anticancer remedies on folk medicine in China, Israel, Plestina, Saudi Arabia etc.

In general, over 120 currently prescribed drugs including anticancer ones being the basis of modern chemotherapy were first extracted from plants. About 60% of the anticancer drugs available prior to 1983 were of natural origin [65]. As much as 40% of anticancer drugs developed from 1940 to 2002 had natural or natural-product origins, while another 8% were natural-product mimics. Although nowadays about 300,000 different plant species are known but less than 5,000 have been studied for their potential drug usefulness. Since 1989, the National Cancer Institute (NCI) has screened up to 10,000 potential anticancer agents per year including minerals, exotic plants from tropical rain forests and animal venoms and toxins.

Animal venoms and toxins which has been used as therapeutics in ancient Ayurvedic, Unani, Chinese folk medicine as well as in Homeopathy are also screened. Venoms of snakes, scorpions, toads, frogs and their derivatives protein or non-protein toxins, peptides, enzymes are promising and show some potential in cancer treatment. Léon Charles Albert Calmette (1863-1933) a French physician, bacteriologist and immunologist, was the first to describe an antitumor effect of the venom of Indian cobra Naja naja sp. on adenocarcinoma cells. Thereafter many reports have established the anticancer potential of venoms of different species of Elapidae, Viperidae, Crotalidae snakes [102-107] and Hydrophis spimlis sea snake [108,109] and assigned it to phospholipase activity. Scorpions venom has been used by traditional and folk medicine in India, China, Africa and Cuba. Chinese red scorpion (Buthus martensi Karsch) venom and skin extracts, known as Chan Su in China and Senso in Japan, have been used by traditional Chinese medicine for as long as 2000 years also as anti-leukaemia agents. 4',6-diamidino-2-phenylindole extracted from Buthus martensi Karsch induced cell apoptosis in malignant glioma cells in vitro [110], while serine proteinase and hylauronidase have promising anticancer activity against a number of different cell lines including breast ones [111]. Bengalin protein isolated from Hindu black scorpion is suspected to have anti-leukemic properties [112]. Chlorotoxin and Charybdotoxin, 36- and 37-amino acid peptides, respectively isolated from the venom of death stalker scorpion (Leiurus quinqestriatus Hebraeus) are promising for the treatment of several types of cancers including glioma and human breast cancer [113,114]. The anticancer effect of the venom of Cuba red scorpions (Rhopalurus junceus) was discovered 20 years ago in Guantanamo, but after 15 years of studies Vidatox drug was announced in 2011. The skin extract from Hindu toads (Bufo melanostictus, Bufo gargarizans Cantor), Chan Su used by Chinese traditional medicine, was discovered to contain a few bufadineolides showing specific activity against human leukemic, liver carcinoma and melanoma cell lines. Species belonging to the families Bufonidae (toads), Lampyridae (fireflies) and Colubridae (snakes) as well as mammalian tissues contain bufadienolides, but the richest source of them are toad species. Although all the bufadienolides showed potent cytotoxicity in vitro, but the evidence of their activity in vivo is limited to human hepatocellular carcinoma and HeLa human cancer cells in mice and require further investigation.

Some hope rises with the use of minerals as a source of anticancers drugs. Most important example is sodium bicarbonate, $NaHCO_3$, which was originally derived from Nahcolite (thermokalite) carbonate mineral. The ancient Egyptians used natural natron, a mixture of sodium carbonate decahydrate, and sodium bicarbonate as a soap and embalming tool. Recently it has been shown that sodium bicarbonate administered orally causes a selective increase in the pH of tumour and reduces the formation of spontaneous metastases in mouse models of metastatic breast cancer [115,116]. Another interesting case is selenite known since ancient times but recently revealed as a promising anticancer agent capable of inducing apoptosis in malignant mesothelioma and sarcoma cells [117].

As yet none of the new natural venom, toxin or minerals derived anticancer agents have reached the status of the clinical drug, but a number of agents are still in study or in preclinical development.

4.2. Synthetic drugs

The first steps toward chemical synthesis of drugs were undertaken by iatrochemistry, a branch of chemistry and medicine concerned with seeking chemical solutions to diseases and ailments. Paracelsus pioneered the use of chemicals and minerals in medicine. He introduced alcohol, arsenic, copper, lead and silver salts into medicine, and developed rules for drug administration and dosages of drugs. Paracelsus also devised methods of extracting the arcanum (active ingredient) from plant materials. For this reason he is considered to be the father of phytochemistry and pharmacognosy. Ehrlich, the father of chemotherapy, developed the animal model to screen a series of chemicals for their potential activity against diseases, which had a major influence on the direction of cancer drug development. He also studied the usability of aniline dyes and the first primitive alkylating agents in cancer treatment. The first overall cancer treatment programme was the work of another pioneer of modern chemotherapy - George Clowes (1915-1988). He developed the first transplantable carcinogen-induced tumour systems in mice, which allowed the standardization of models for cancer drug testing. These early model systems including Sarcoma 37 (S37), Sarcoma 180 (S180), Walker 256, and Ehrlich's ascites tumour have been used for several decades [118]. In 1935 Murray Shear developed the most organized program for cancer drug screening. About 3,000 compounds including natural ones, were screened with S37 as a model system. The reason for the failure of this first systematic attempt to search for anticancer drugs - only two drugs have been subjected to clinical trials, but finally dropped because of unacceptable toxicity - was the lack of knowledge on how to test cytotoxic effects in humans. An extension of the number of tumour systems available for studies by the Yoshida's ascites sarcoma model and a murine leukaemia induced by a carcinogen, Leukaemia 1210, described by Lloyd Law allowed fast progress.

4.3. Cell Cycle Non Specific Agents (CCNSA)

4.3.1. Alkylating agents

The first real breakthrough in the search for chemotherapeutics was the chemical synthesis of nitrogen mustards [4,119]. Sulphur mustard was synthesised much earlier, in 1822, but its harmful effects were not known until 1860. It was first used as chemical warfare weapon agent during the latter part of the First World War but its therapeutic activity against squamous cell carcinoma was discovered by accident. In fact most of the first so-called true synthetic chemotherapeutics, were discovered by serendipity, the special term *Serendipity* for accidental discoveries was introduced by Horace Walpole (1717-1797) in the 18th c. Nitrogen mustard, an analogue of the highly toxic sulphur mustard gas, was introduced in 1942 as the first alkylating agent and a true chemotherapeutic. Alfred G. Gilman, Louis S. Goodman and Thomas Dougherty, examined the potential therapeutic effects of nitrogen mustard in rabbits and mice bearing a transplanted lymphoid tumour, while Gustaf E. Lindskog (1903-2002), a thoracic surgeon, administered it to patients with non-Hodgkin's lymphoma. Many cases of cancer regression succeed intensive screening of related alkylating compounds and discovery of busulphan by L.A. Elson, G.M. Timmis, and David A. G. Galton (1922-2006) in 1951, Chlorambucil by James Everatt in 1953, melphalan by Frank Bergel and John Stock in 1954, Cyclophosphamide by Herbert Arnold, Friedrich Bourseaux and Norbert Brock in 1956, Lomustine and Carmustine by John A. Montgomery, George S. McCaleb, Thomas P. Johnston in 1966. While many different classes of alkylating agents (nitrogen mustards, nitrosoureas, alkyl sulphonates, triazines, and ethylenimines) are known, the chemical mechanism of their action is common and based on three different mechanisms all of which achieve the same end result - disruption of DNA function and apoptosis. The first mechanism of DNA alkylation results in its fragmentation by repair enzymes to prevent DNA synthesis and RNA transcription from the affected DNA. The second mechanism is the formation of intrastrand or interstrand cross-links by an alkylating agent, which prevents DNA from being separated for synthesis or transcription. The third mechanism of action is the induction of mispairing of the nucleotides, which leads to mutations, even permanent ones.

Alkylating agent acts on a cancer cell in every phase of its life cycle, Fig. 2, thus can be used in the treatment of a wide range of cancers from various solid tumours to leukaemia. However strong adverse effect is their ability to induce secondary cancers, which is reflected by their classification as definite carcinogens by IARC [3].

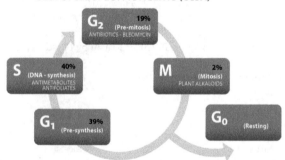

Figure 2. Cell replication occurs in the cell cycle (G_0, G_1, S, G_2 and M). The cell cycle nonspecific agents (alkylating agents, platinum compounds, cytotoxic antibiotics) are able to kill a cell during any phase of the cycle, while cell cycle specific (antimetabolites, antifoliates, planta alkaloids, some cytotoxic antiniotics line bleomycin) are only able to kill only during a specific phase.

4.3.2. Cytotoxic antibiotics

A number of cytotoxic antibiotics that have been derived from natural sources such as gram-positive bacteria in soil and water, belonging to genus *Streptomyces* (phylum *Actinobacteria*) [4,119]. They produce secondary metabolites, many of which have been successfully isolated and used as antifungals, antibiotics and anticancer drugs. The large-scale screening of fermentation products by the pharmaceutical industry which resulted in the discovery of antibiotics to treat wound infections is one more example of finding anticancer drugs by serendipity. Although penicillin, which was the basic compound for the above mentioned studies has no antitumor properties itself, but the chromo oligopeptide actinomycin D, isolated from *Streptomyces antibioticus* by Selman Abraham Waksman (1888-1973) and Boyd Woodruff in the 1940s as a result of search for drugs to treat tuberculosis, has significant antitumor properties and was applied in the 1950/1960s in paediatric oncology. This antibiotic was approved by the U.S. Food and Drug Administration (FDA) in 1964. In 1950, the search for anticancer compounds from soil-based microbes in the area of Castel del Monte, Italy, resulted in the discovery of an antibiotic - Daunorubicin (red pigment) - independently by Aurelio di Marco, Arpad Grein and Celestino Spalla from bacterium *Streptomyces peucetius* and by M. Dubost from *Streptomyces caeruleorubidus*. It was found to be active against murine tumours (Yoshida sarcoma). Although clinical trials which began in the 1960s suggested its significant activity against acute leukaemia and lymphoma, but shortly after, in 1967, it was recognized that daunorubicin had significant cardiac toxicity. In general, many antibiotics produced by *Streptomyces* are too toxic for use as antibiotics in humans, but their activity towards specific cells lines makes them useful in chemotherapy. The search for more effective antitumor antibiotics over 2,000 analogues of slightly modified structures yielded in a series of compounds, some of which are in common use till today. In 1969, Federico Arcamone developed a derivative of Doxorubicin which in the same year was tested against animal tumours by di Marco. Daunroubicin and Doxorubicin belongs to inhibitors of the topoisomerase II, one of two enzymes that regulate overwinding/underwinding of DNA. Inhibition of the topoisomerase II block cleavage of both strands of the DNA which ultimately leads to cell death. An important antibiotic of a wide spectrum of anticancer activity is Mitomycin C isolated from *Streptomyces caespitosu* in 1955 and *Streptomyces lavendulae* in 1958 and clinically used since the first successful trials against childhood leukaemia reported by Charlotte Tan in 1965. Mitomycin C belongs to bifunctional alkylating agents, whose biological activity mode is DNA alkylation and cross-linking. It has a broad activity against a range of tumours. In 1966 Hamao Umezawa discovered an important unique antibiotic in this group - bleomycin - a glycopeptide showing anticancer activity, while screening a culture filtrates of *Streptomyces verticullus*. Bleomycin is used to treat many types of cancer, including testicular cancer, non Hodgkin's lymphoma, Hodgkin's lymphoma and cancers of the head and neck. Anticancer antibiotics, apart from Bleomycin, act on a cancer cell in every phase of its life cycle and prevent cell divisions, but Bleomycin is considered as cell cycle agent specifically working in G2 and M phase, Fig. 2. However, the risk connected with the use of cytotoxic antibiotics classified as group 2 or 3 agent in IARC classification is smaller than that related to alkylating agents [3].

4.3.3. Platinum compounds

Cisplatin was synthesized in 1845 but its potential as an antitumour agent was not recognized until 1965 when its capabilities were discovered by Barney Rosenberg, Loretta van Camp and Thomas Krigas. The inhibition of growth caused by platinum complex of ammonia and chloride (Peyrone's salt i.e. Cis-platinum) was discovered by serendipity during the studies of the influence of electric current on bacterial growth. The positive result during the studies of murine tumours in vivo confirmed its antitumor activity and prompted the studies of other compounds from this class [4,56,119]. It was introduced into clinical practice one decade later in the 1970s [120]. By 1978 about 1,000 platinum complexes had been screened, but only seven were selected for detailed pharmacological evaluation on rats and only two - Carboplatin and Oxaliplatin - were non-toxic at effective antitumour dose. Although Cisplatin belongs to three most commonly used chemotherapeutics, progress made to improve its use since its discovery is in fact limited. The mechanism of action of Cisplatin and other platinum compounds resemble that of the alkylating agents. They interact covalently with DNA and form intrastrand (within the same DNA molecule; >90%) or interstrand (between two different DNA molecules; <5%), cross links between adjacent guanine molecules [121]. The formation of DNA adducts results in an inhibition of DNA synthesis and transcription. Platinum compounds act on a cancer cell in every phase of its life cycle, Fig.2. Their use is widespread and includes the treatment of bladder and colorectal cancer, upper gastrointestinal disease, germ cell tumours, head and neck malignancies, lung and ovarian cancer. Their ability to induce secondary cancers reflected by their classification as definite carcinogens by IARC is high [3].

4.4. Cell Cycle Specific Agents (CCSA)

4.4.1. Antifolates

Antimetabolites (folic acid, pyrimidine or purine analogues), which structurally resemble naturally occurring molecules necessary for DNA and RNA synthesis and either inhibit enzymes needed for nucleic acid production or induce apoptosis during the S phase of cell growth, Fig. 2, were among the first effective chemotherapeutics discovered. In the early 1940s, Sidney Faber (1903–1973) studied the effect of folic acid (pteroylglutamic acid; Vitamin B9) first isolated from spinach leaves. In 1945, Rudolf Leuchtenberger reported that folic acid inhibited tumour growth in mice, while Richard Lewisohn reported complete regression of spontaneous breast in mice observed with folic acid. Farber, Robert D. Heinle, and Arnold D. Welch tested folic acid in leukaemia and concluded spuriously that deficiency of Vitamin B9 accelerates leukaemia cell growth. Efforts to treat leukaemia resulted in pharmacological folic acid analogues with effects antagonistic to those of Vitamin B9. Shortly after Sidney Farber and Harriet Kilte developed a series of foliate antagonists including highly active aminopterin (4-amino-pteroylglutamic acid). Its analogue 4-amino-4-deoxy-10-N-methyl-pteroylglutamic acid, known nowadays as Methotrexate, was discovered by Yellapragada Subbarao (1895-1948) and successfully applied by Sidney Farber in 1947 to induce remissions in children with leukaemia. In 1958 Min Chiu Li, reported fully effective treatment of a very rare tumour of the placenta, choriocarcinoma with Methotrexate, which was the first-ever intentionally discovered synthetic anticancer drug i.e. first true chemotherapeutic. Starting from the 1950s, Methotrexate has replaced the more toxic aminopterin and is still in widespread clinical use. In general folate antagonists mechanism of action is linked with competing with folates for uptake into cells and inhibition of the formation of folate co-enzymes or reactions that are mediated by them. Only one of those mechanisms is clinically important, it is the prevention of formation of tetrahydrofolate by inhibition of the enzymes: dihydrofolate reductase (DHFR) or thymidylate synthase (TS). Methotrexate inhibits only DHFR, while a new-generation antifolate Pemetrexed developed by Edward C. Taylor in 1992 inhibits DHFR, TS and also transformylases (GAR and AICAR), but primarily acts as a TS inhibitor. Thus both act similarly by hindering enzymes needed for de novo synthesis of the thymidine and purine nucleotides but show different spectrum of activity. Methotrexate is effective mainly in the treatment of leukaemia, lymphoma and choriocarcinoma but also cancers of breast, head and neck, colorectal, osteosarcoma and bladder, while Pemetrexed is approved for the treatment of mesothelioma and non–small cell lung cancer, active in solid tumours treatment, especially those drug resistant. The risk connected with the use of Methotrexate classified as group 3 agent in IARC classification is smaller than that of alkylating agents [3].

4.4.2. Antimetabolites

The discovery of nitrogen mustard and Methotrexate and their success in medical applications was a breakthrough and stimulated the search for the other antimetabolites as well as new classes of cell cycle specific synthetic anticancer drugs [4,56,119]. In 1944, Richard O. Roblin and James W. Clapp synthesised 8-azaguanine (8-AZA), while 5 years later George W. Kidder and Virginia C., reported that 8-AZA was a guanine antagonist in the metabolism of *Tetrahymena geleii* (S) (*Colpidium campylum* L.) and inhibited the growth of transplanted mammary adenosarcoma in mice. Since 1944, George Herbert Hitchings (1905-1998) and Gertrude Belle Elion (1918-1999) have investigated the role of purines in nucleic acid metabolism and methods to prevent them from being incorporated to DNA synthesis along the metabolic pathway that would lead to interruption of cell reproduction. By the early 1950s, Hitchings & Elion synthesized more than 100 purine analogues including 2,6-diaminopurine, 6-thioguanine (6-TG), 6-mercaptopurine (6-MP) and Azathioprine (AZA) as a result of their rational approach to drug development. 6-TG, 6-MP and AZA although categorized as growth inhibitory antimetabolites, exert their functions more like a genotoxic methylating agents, such as alkylating drug Temozolomide, which methylates DNA. 6-MP, one of the early analogues, is widely used not only for acute leukaemias but also in gout and herpes viral infections, and as immunosuppressive agents in the organ transplantations, 6-TG is predominantly used as antileukaemic agent, while AZA as an immunosuppressive. The discovery of a few purine analogues Fludarabine (FLU), Cladribine (2CDA), and Pentostatin (DCF) was a result of further targeted studies performed within a NIH programme. Fludarabine discovered by John Montgomery and Kathleen Hewson in 1968 was the first halogenated ribonucleotide reductase inhibitor, a new-generation pro-drug of the purine class successfully used in treating refractory chronic lymphocytic and chronic B cell leukaemias, non-Hodgkin's lymphoma and T-cell lymphoma. Cladribine, resembling deoxyadenosine and remarkably active in hairy cell leukaemia was synthesised in 1972 by L.F. Christensen, A. Broom, M.J. Robins, and A.J. Bloch and in 1978 selected by Dennis A. Carson as the most potent enzyme adenosine deaminase (ADA) inhibitor from many candidate congeners. Pentostatin, which also inhibits ADA and similarly to 2CDA is active in hairy cell leukaemia and chronic lymphocytic leukaemia was synthesised by Hollis D.H. Showalter and David C. Baker in 1983. Recently, three new purine antimetabolites nerlabine, clofarabine, and forodesine have been found highly promising. Although these compounds belong to purine antimetabolites and reveal activity against specific types of leukaemia, they differ in metabolic properties and mechanism of action. As long ago as in 1964 Elmer Reist and Leon Goodman synthesized 9-β-Darabinofuranosyl guanine (ara-G), which despite of its antitumor properties in in-vitro canine leukaemia models evaluated by Elion & Kurtzberg was rejected because of inadequate solubility. In 1988, nelarabine, the 6-methoxy derivative of Ara-G, which is 10-fold more soluble than Ara-G, was synthesized by Thomas A. Krenitsky. In 2012, 48 years after synthesis of Ara-G, Nelarabine entered phase II of clinical studies with indication to T-cell acute lymphoblastic leukaemia or T-cell lymphoblastic lymphoma treatment. Clofarabine, a hybrid of Fludarabine and Cladribine, was synthesised by Mongomery in 1992. It also recently entered phase II of clinical studies with indication as antileukemic agent active in acute lymphoblastic leukaemia as well as in myeloid disorders in paediatrics. The third intensively studied purine antimetabolite is forodesine, synthesised by Peter C. Tyler and Vern L. Schramm in 1998. Forodesine, which is not incorporated into DNA and has unexplored mechanism of action is effective for the treatment of relapsed B-cell chronic lymphocytic leukaemia.

In the 1950s Robert Duschinsky synthesised the first pyrimidine analogue, 5-fluorouracil (5-FU). His discovery was based on the observation of the role of greater uptake of uracil in rat hepatoma metabolism, thus it was the first known case of "targeted" studies. 5-FU introduced into the clinic in 1957 by Charles Heidelberger has broad-spectrum activity against non-hematologic cancers, thus is now widely applied for treatment of many kinds of solid tumours of breast, head and neck, adrenal, pancreatic, gastric, colon, rectal, oesophageal, liver and G-U (bladder, penile, vulva, prostate). Even nowadays, 5-FU apart of its analogue Floxuridine, remains a fundamental drug in the treatment of colorectal cancer. Discovery of 5-FU was not only the first example of targeted studies but also the first targeted therapy, which later attracted much attention in current cancer drug development. However, the target in this case was understood not as a molecular target but as a biochemical pathway. In 1950 two spongo-nucleosides (spongouridine and spongothymidine) were isolated by Werner Bergman and Robert Feeney from a Caribbean sponge *Cryptotethya crypta*. It inspired Richard Walwick, Walden Roberts, and Charles Dekker to synthesise Cytarabine and Vidarabine in 1959. In 1964, John Evans tested activity of Cytarabine using in-vitro murine S180 model while four years later Rose Ruth Ellison introduced it into clinic for the B-cell leukaemia treatment. Cytarabine is effective in acute non-lymphocytic, lymphocytic, myelogenous, chronic myelocytic leukae-mias, as well as leptominingeal carcinomatosis and non-Hodgkin's lymphoma, Other pyri-midine antagonists include Capecitabine, which is an oral 5-FU pro-drug adjuvant in colon and breast metastasis therapy, Gemcitabine which is a prodrug of Cytarabine, effective in pancreatic, metastatic breast, bladder, ovarian and non-small cell lung cancers and Decitabine, used in myeloplastic syndrome. The antimetabolites of purines and pyrimidine compounds acts on a cancer cell in S phase of its life cycle, Fig.2 and are classified as a group 3 agents in IARC classification.

4.4.3. Plant alkaloids

A true breakthrough in chemotherapeutics came by in the 1950s as the discovery of the activity of plant alkaloids from Madagascar periwinkle plant *Vinca rosea* (*Catharanthus roseus* (L.) G. Don) by Canadian scientists Robert Laing Noble, Charles T. Beer and Gordon Sloboda [56]. The vinca alkaloids extracted from *Vinca rosea* consist of a subset of structurally similar compounds comprising two multiringed units, vindoline and catharanthine. Initially, they were investigated because of putative hypoglycaemic properties, but strong marrow suppression observed in rats and significant antileukaemic effects *in vitro* decided about their clinical use shortly after the discovery of their properties, in 1959. Nowadays, vinca alkaloids are produced synthetically and only four major ones - Vinblastine, Vincristine, Vinorelbine and Vindesine - are in the oncological clinical use. Vinblastine is most often applied in Hodgkin's disease, non-Hodgkin's lymphoma, breast cancer, and germ cell tumours, Vincristine is effective against leukaemia and Hodgkin's, Vinorelbine has significant antitumor activity in patients with breast cancer and antiproliferation effects on osteosarcoma, while Vindesine is used in the treatment of leukaemia, lymphoma, melanoma, breast cancer, and lung cancer. All vinca alkaloids have a unique mechanism of action; they bind to the microtubular proteins of the mitotic spindle, which leads to crystallization of the microtubule and mitotic arrest or apoptosis.

Another group of novel cytotoxic agents from plant alkaloids, taxane diterpenes, was discovered during long-term screening in the 1970s. The main compound in this class, Paclitaxel, was the first taxane introduced into clinical practice for the treatment of recurrent ovarian cancer metastatic, breast cancer, often in combination with Cisplatin. Nowadays, Paclitaxel is totally synthesized, but less popular than vinca because of its poor solubility. Both plant alkaloids vinca and taxanes are mitotic inhibitors M phase specific, Fig. 2, but they act in different ways. Their principal mechanism of action is the disruption of microtubule function, but in contrast to the vinca alkaloids, taxanes do not destroy mitotic spindles. The plant alkaloids are classified as a group 3 agents in IARC classification [3].

4.4.4. Combination regimens

In 2005, conventional chemotherapeutics still made the majority of the Top 20 Cancer Therapeutics. Their popularity was dictated not only by wide spectrum of activity and also long history of use in oncology but also their key role in the multidrug treatment programs. In the early 1960s, single alkylating agents were basic for all cancer treatment programmes. Although the remissions were observed for example up to 25% in advanced Hodgkin's disease but they were still incomplete and temporary. Increasing resistance of the cancer cells to classical drugs and numerous side effects forced new strategies. After Jacob Furth and Morton Kahn discovery that a single leukemic cell was sufficient to cause the death of an animal, Howard E. Skipper formulated "Cell Kill" hypothesis, according to which a given dose of drug is able to kill only a constant fraction of tumour cells. This hypothesis favoured search for more aggressive chemotherapeutics but also resulted in the use of drug combinations. In 1965 Emil Frei and Emil J. Freireich developed the new treatment program for children leukaemia known as "VAMP" (Nethotrexate, 6-MP, Vincristine and Prednisone). The use of multiple drugs: Methotrexate, which disrupt folic-acid uptake, 6-MP which inhibits synthesis of purine, both critical in cell division, Vincristine which interfered with cell division by binding to spindle protein and Prednisone, anti-inflammatory steroid resulted in the remission rate level as high as 60%. Further modifications like "MOMP" (nitrogen mustard, Vincristine, Methotrexate, and Prednisone), "MOPP" (Procarbazine, nitrogen mustard, Vincristine, and Prednisone) and C-MOPP (Procarbazine, Cyclophosphamide, Vincristine, and Prednisone) resulted in the 80% complete remission rate in advanced Hodgkin's disease in the 1970s. On the basis of the above mentioned first programs dedicated exclusively to leukaemias many modifications - e.g. four drug EBVP (Epirubicin, Bleomycin, Vinblastine, Prednisone) and ABVD (Adriamycin, Bleomycin, Vinblastine and Dacarbazine) and six-drug STANFORD-V (Cyclophosphamide/ Mechlorethamine/Ifosfamide, Doxorubicin, Vinblastine, Vincristine, Bleomycin, Etoposide) - have been developed. Nowadays, some cancer diseases like Hodgkin's or acute lymphocytic leukaemia are curable in 90% within the modern protocols using aggressive chemotherapy programs. Despite the reasonable position of classical chemotherapeutics in multidrug combined regimens, their capabilities inevitably decrease because of multidrug resistance (a major factor in the failure of many forms of treatment) and secondary effects (adverse or paradoxically carcinogenic). Significant limitation is also the need for multiple chemotherapy in long-term, sequential multidrug regimens and in-hospital administration.

4.4.5. Modern chemotherapeutics

At the beginning of the 20th c., Paul Ehrlich postulated the idea of a "Magic Bullet" (Zauber-kugel) i.e. drugs that reach directly intended cell-structural targets. To some extent this idea is the driving force behind the development of modern targeted chemotherapeutics. Conventional chemotherapeutics are cytotoxic, but affect all cells and work in the so-called statistical manner. Because cancer cells multiply faster than normal, the cancerous cells are killed by the drug with a higher ratio than the normal ones, which are not spared. Therefore the principal criterion applied in the modern anticancer drug design is the principle of selective toxicity, which require activity restricted exclusively to the cancer cells. From the point of view of selective activity directed on tumour cells and mechanisms of carcinogenesis, a few different classes of modern drugs can be distinguished: inhibitors of cytokine stimulating cell prolifer-ation, dissociation, motility; cytokine receptor blockers; intracellular kinases inhibitors; transcription factors inhibitors; cell cycle inhibitors; cell adhesion inhibitors and proteasome inhibitors.

Short-lived hopes were raised in the 1990s at the discovery of the inhibitors of angiogenesis, which hold back the growth of capillary vessels in cancer. Avastin, humanized monoclonal antibody, discovered by Napoleone Ferrara in 1997 was the first drug from this class approved by FDA in 2004 to use for several types of metastatic cancer, but the approval of the breast cancer indication was revoked in 2011. Two other inhibitors of angiogenesis include Cetuxi-mab invented by Joseph Schlessinger, Michael Sela in 1988, approved for by FDA in 2009 to use in colorectal cancer therapy and Sunitinib discovered by Joseph Schlessinger and Axel Ullrich approved by FDA in 2006 to use for renal cell carcinoma and gastrointestinal stromal tumour. Recent progress in genetic sequencing has led to the discovery of Vemurafenib by Fritz Hoffmann, approved by FDA in 2011. It targets the B-Raf gene that signals the growth of new blood cells in melanoma tumours, which are extremely difficult to treat.

Recently widespread attention has been given to inhibitors of protein kinases, enzymes that catalyze phosphorylation reactions, a principal mechanism of signal transduction governing various cellular processes including growth, division, migration and apoptosis. Imatinib, developed in the late 1990s by Nicholas Lydon, introduced to clinic by Brian Druker and approved to treat chronic myelogenous leukaemia by FDA in 2001 was the first drug of this new class of small active molecules. It inhibits the oncogene BCR-ABL1 and blocks the signals for cell proliferation, controlling tumour growth. Many imatinib analogues: including Nilotnib, Dasatinib, Bosutinib, Ponatinib, Bafetinib were obtained further by rational drug design. Gefitinib invented by ASTRA/ZENECA (approved by FDA in 2003 but withdrawn in 2005) and Erlotinib invented by OSI (approved by FDA in 2004), were the first selective inhibitors of epidermal growth factor receptor among the kinase inhibitors used for treatment of lung cancer.

Monoclonal antibodies that allow the cytotoxin to reach a target required to kill the malignant cells (induce apoptosis), without harming normal cells belong to the unique class of chemo-immunotherapeutics. In contrast to small molecule drugs which have a direct impact on their targets, the monoclonal antibodies stimulate the immune system i.e. re-direct targets to the immune system. Most popular includes: Gemtuzumab ozogamicin invented by Wyeth Ayerst and used for the treatment of acute myelogenous leukaemia, but withdrawn from the market in 2010 due to its toxicity, Ibritumomab tiuxetan developed by IDEC Pharmaceuticals used for the treatment of non-Hodgkin's lymphoma, but known to cause serious side effects, Panitu-mumab used for the treatment of colon cancer but ineffective, Rituximab developed by IDEC Pharmaceuticals and still used for the treatment of B-cell non-Hodgkin's lymphoma and tositumomab developed by Mark Kaminski and Richard Wahl used for the treatment of non-Hodgkin's lymphoma (mainly follicular lymphoma), currently in the clinical trials.

Although modern targeted therapies provide a new approach to cancer therapy and similarly to conventional ones are able to suppress tumour growth, but they also have drawbacks and limitations, while true cancer treatment is still a challenge for oncology.

5. Summary

Throughout history of medicine the process of new drug discovery has been based on natural sources and drugs have been discovered by serendipity (sheer luck) or in a trial-and-error process. While until the mid-1980s new drugs were discovered mainly by serendipity, over the next decade, till mid-1990s, the knowledge of structure was the basis for research, then the starting point was to identify a target and a relationship between structure and function [122]. Nowadays a few major classes of drugs useful in cancer treatment have been defined: (1)

General Chemotherapy Drugs (the alkylating agents, anti-neoplastics, anti-metabolites), (2) Steroids, (3) Bisphosphonates, (4) Hormone therapies and (5) Biological therapies/Immunotherapy. This modern classification reflects the fact that anticancer drugs evolved from classical chemotherapeutics discovered mostly by serendipity to drugs acting directly against abnormal proteins in cancer cells designed by rational drug design. All of them have remarkable influence on the growth of cancer cells and on the mechanisms whereby cells replicate, transmit, and translate genetic information.

Current research are so multidirectional that it is impossible to discuss all of them in a short chapter. New directions in this field include the search for the improved pharmaceutical forms, new analogues of currently used drugs, new chemical compounds (natural or synthetic) of anticancer activity, selective anticancer agents (acting on the basis of pathophysiological mechanisms), the search for drugs among old-known drugs currently used for other indications than cancer, search for the methods of precise delivering the anticancer drugs to cancer tissue and stroma or to stimulate the immune system to generate anti-tumor immune responses and protect against cancer.

Even nowadays precursors or generic drugs are frequently discovered by serendipity, while their analogues are developed by purely rational design. Often the newly synthesised drug proved effective in quite different than expected applications. For example Aminoglutethimide was found to be effective in breast cancer treatment instead of being an antiepileptic, Cisplatin, an electrolysis product, was discovered to be cytotoxic or Tamoxifen antiestrogenic activity of *cis*-isomer was discovered as unexpected bonus in the search for drugs to treat mania in bipolar disorder. Sometimes surprisingly a new field of activity is revealed for a long known drug. For example potassium-sparing diuretic Amiloride is effective in glioma; sedative Thalidomide, linked to birth defects, slows the propagation prostate cancer; Tebrophen, antiviral drug, slows the propagation of breast cancer; S-dimethylarsin-gluthathione, an organic form of arsenic, slow solid tumours expansion; anti-epileptic Valproic and Rapamycin, immunosuppressor in organ transplantation are valuable in antitumor therapy; Gossypol, potential male contraceptive overcome resistance to Cisplatin; antimalarial chloroquine may address a critical cell nutrition issue with proliferating cancer cells while insecticide benzoyl-phenylurea helps understand the microtubule assembly process important for growth of the pancreatic cancer cell. Anticancer properties have been ascertained to be shown by aspirin used commonly as analgesic, antipyretic and an anti-inflammatory medication, 9-aminoacridine used as an antiprotozoa and antibacterial agent and Quinacrine commonly used antimalarial drug. The use of long know drugs fasten modern process of drug discovery, which involves the identification of candidates, synthesis, characterization, screening, and assays for therapeutic efficacy and proceeds through many stages including discovery, product characterisation, formulation, pharmacokinetics, preclinical toxicology testing and IND (Investigational New Drug) application, bioanalytical testing and clinical trials. The new drugs (new completely or a long known one) often have many adverse effects. Sometimes in the final step the new drug proves toxic, ineffective or even carcinogenic. Many widely applied chemotherapeutic anticancer agents (nitrogen mustards, HN2 and HN3, treatamine, Chlorambucil,

Sacrolysin, Melphalan, and Busulphan), have been recognized as a source of secondary cancers and thus classified as definite carcinogens.

Sometimes known carcinogens have became invaluable drugs widely applied in clinical oncology. The most impressive example is arsenic - a component of the well known Poison of Kings (As_2O_3). It was used in traditional Chinese medicine in the treatment of promyelocytic leukaemia and acute myelogenous leukaemia. Reaglar containing arsenic was used by Hipocrates as a component of antitumor liniment. Avicenna in the 11th c. recommended it for cancer, both internally and topically. In the 16th century Paracelsus used it as a drug but linked with a cancer disease. In 1786 Thomas Fowler discovered Fowler's Solution (a 1% aqueous solution of potassium arsenite, $KAsO2$),which was applied as first chemotherapeutic in chronic myeloid leukaemia treatment in 1865 by Lissauer and persisted till the introduction of the first modern cytotoxic drugs in the 1940s. In 1931, its use in chronic myeloid leukaemia was described. In the late 1960s in China, an arsenic containing liniment was rediscovered for use as an effective anticancer treatment in melanoma. First reports of the intravenous administration of Fowler's Solution in acute promyelocytic leukaemia appeared in the 1990s, also in China. But in the 1990s IARC classified arsenic compounds as definite carcinogens. Despite this, in 2001 Fowler's Solution was accepted by FDA for the treatment of relapsed or refractory acute promyelocytic leukaemia in children. After being abandoned for decades, arsenic trioxide in the 21st c started to be prescribed as a drug for acute promyelocytic leukaemia, and still it is classified as definite anticancer. Recently some hope rises with realgar as well as new arsenic-based compounds (e.g. C-glycosides), which have been intensively studied. On the other hand, a very recent studies performed by Peter S. Nelson et al. indicated that chemotherapy can damage healthy cells which secrete a protein WNT16B that sustains tumour growth and results in a resistance to further treatment [123]. This proves that chemotherapy itself can boost cancer growth. The paradox drug/carciogen concerns not only chemotherapeutics but also the methods, which revolutionized the treatment of cancer, being on the other hand carcinogenic, like X-Ray widely used in the diagnosis of cancer cells, cancer treatment and anticancer drug design, UV radiation being a basis of the photodynamic therapy. Paracelsus, father of toxicology already wrote *"All substances are poisons: there is none which is not a poison. The right dose differentiates a poison and a remedy."* Paraphrasing him - the method and conditions of the use differentiates a carcinogen and anticancer drug. Thus the search for new drugs among carcinogens seems quite reasonable, while the protection against contact with or exposure to a carcinogen is a necessity.

The recent advances in genomics and proteomics deliver a promise of understanding the true internal mechanisms of cancerogenesis - a basis for cancer diseases. They cover the knowledge of genes alteration caused by cancer, its influence on the proteins encoded by them, the interaction of these proteins with each other in living cells, the resulting changes in the specific tissues and finally the effect on the entire body. The achievements in this field delimit new fully rational directions in anticancer drug discovery and development of drugs addressing the specific needs (targeted drugs).

Author details

Jolanta Natalia Latosińska* and Magdalena Latosińska

*Address all correspondence to: jolanta.latosinska@amu.edu.pl

Faculty of Physics, Adam Mickiewicz University, Poznań, Poland

References

[1] Yarbro C.H.; Goodman M.; Frogge M.H. (Eds.) (2005). Cancer Nursing Principles and Practice (6th edition); Boston, Jones & Bartlett Publishers. pp. 1879. ISBN 0815169906.

[2] Ferlay J.; Shin H.R.; Bray F.; Forman D.; Mathers C.; Parkin (2010). D.M. GLOBOCAN 2008 v1.2. Cancer Incidence and Mortality Worldwide: IARC CancerBase No. 10. Lyon, France: International Agency for Research on Cancer, Available from: http://globo-can.iarc.fr, accessed on day/month/year.

[3] IARC monographs on the evaluation of carcinogenic risks to humans, vol. 100 (A,B,C,D,E,F) 2012, Available from: http://monographs.iarc.fr/ENG/Classification. ISBN 9283213297.

[4] Olson J.S. (1989). The History of Cancer: An Annotated Bibliography (Bibliographies and Indexes in Medical Studies), Greenwood Press, Inc. pp. 434. ISBN 0313258899.

[5] Butler M.S. (2004). The role of natural product chemistry in drug discovery. *Journal of Natural Products*. 67:2141-2153. *ISSN 0163-3864*.

[6] Ensemble Human Genome. Available from: http://www.ornl.gov/sci/techresources/ Human_Genome/project/hgp.shtml

[7] Morris C.; Kennedy M.; Heisterkamp N.; Columbano-Green L.; Romeril K.; Groffen J.; Fitzgerald P. (1991). A complex chromosome rearrangement forms the BCR-ABL fusion gene in leukemic cells with a normal karyotype. Genes Chromosomes Cancer. 3:263-71. ISSN 1098-2264

[8] Hirota S.; Isozaki K.; Moriyama Y.; Hashimoto K.; Nishida T.; Ishiguro S.; Kawano K.; Hanada M.; Kurata A.; Takeda M.; Muhammad Tunio G.; Matsuzawa Y.; Kanakura Y.; Shinomura Y.; Kitamura Y. (1998). Gain-of-function mutations of c-kit in human gastrointestinal stromal tumors. Science. 279:577-580. ISSN 1095-9203.

[9] Burke W.; Daly M.; Garber J. (1997). Recommendations for follow-up care of individuals with an inherited predisposition to cancer. II. BRCA1 and BRCA2. The Journal of the American Medical Association. 277:997-1003. ISSN 0002-9955.

[10] Haupt S.; Haupt Y. (2006). Importance of p53 for cancer onset and therapy. Anticancer Drugs. 17:725–32. ISSN 1473-5741.

[11] Vazquez A.; Bond E.E.; Levine A.J.; Bond G.L. (2008). The genetics of the p53 pathway, apoptosis and cancer therapy. *Nature Reviews Drug Discovery*.7:979–87. *ISSN 1474-1776*.

[12] Jorde L.B.; Carey J.C.; Bamshad M.J.; White R.L. (2000). Cancer genetics. In: Schmitt W. (ed.), Medical Genetics, 2nd ed. St Louis: Mosby, pp. 221–238. ISBN 9780323040358.

[13] Hanahan D.; Weinberg R.A. (2000). The hallmarks of cancer. *Cell* 100: 57–70. ISSN 0969-2126

[14] Pohanish R.P. (2011). Sittig's Handbook of Toxic and Hazardous Chemicals and Carcinogens, William Andrew, 6 edition. pp. 3096. *ISBN 1437778690*.

[15] Baba A.I.; Câtoi C. (2007). Comparative Oncology. Bucharest: The Publishing House of the Romanian Academy. ISBN 9732714573.

[16] United Nations (UN) (2003) Globally harmonized system of classification and labelling of chemicals (GHS). New York and Geneva. Available from: http://www.unece.org/trans/danger/publi/ghs/ghs_rev00/00files_e.html

[17] Cook J.W.; Hewett C.L.; Hieger, I. (1933). Isolation of A Cancer-producing Hydrocarbon from Coal Tar II. Isolation of 1,2- and 4,5-Benzopyrenes, Perylene, and 1,5-Benzoanthracene, Journal of the Chemical Society. 396-8. ISSN 0368-1769.

[18] Pott F.; Stöber W. (1983). Carcinogenicity of airborne combustion products observed in subcutaneous tissue and lungs of laboratory rodents. Environmental Health Perspectives. 47: 293–303. ISSN 0091-6765.

[19] Concon, J.M. (1988). Food Toxicology, Parts A and B. Marcel Dekker, New York. ISBN: 0824777360.

[20] Berenblum I. (1941). The mechanism of carcinogenesis. A study of significance of cocarcinogenic action and related phenomena. *Cancer Research*. 1:807-814. *ISSN 0008-5472*.

[21] Magee P.N.; Barnes J.M., (1956). The production of malignant primary hepatic tumours in the rat by feeding dimethylnitrosamine, British Journal of Cancer. 10:114-22. ISSN 0007-0920.

[22] Schreiber, H.; Nettesheim, P.; Lijinsky W.; Richter, C. B.; Walburg, H. E., Jr. (1972). Induction of lung cancer in germ-free specific-pathogen-free, and infected rats by N-nitrosoheptamethyleneimine: Enhancement by respiratory infection. Journal of the National Cancer Institute. 49: 1107-1114. ISSN 0027-8874.

[23] Dvorackova, I. (1990). Aflatoxins and Human Health. Boca Raton, FL: CRC Press. *ISBN 0849346282*.

[24] van Walbeek W.; Scott P.M.; Harwig J.; Lawrence J.W. (1969). Penicillium viridicatum Westling: a new source of ochratoxin A. Canadian Journal of Microbiology. 11:1281–1285. ISSN 1480-3275.

[25] Laqueur G. L.; Mickelsen O.; Whiting M. G.; Kurland L. T. (1963). Carcinogenic Properties of Nuts from Cycas Circinalis L. Indige nous to Guam. Journal of the National Cancer Institute. 31: 919-951. ISSN 0027-8874.

[26] Homburger F.; Boger E. (1968). The Carcinogenicity of Essential Oils, Flavors, and Spices: A Review. *Cancer Research*. 28: 2372-2374. ISSN 0008-5472.

[27] McDonald T.A. (1999). Evidence on the carcinogenicity of estragole, Environmental Protection Agency. Available from: http://oehha.ca.gov/prop65/pdf/estragf.pdf

[28] Mei N.; Guo L.; Fu P.P.; Fuscoe J.C.; Luan Y.; Chen T. (2010). Metabolism, genotoxicity, and carcinogenicity of comfrey. *Journal of Toxicology and Environmental Health*. 13:509-26. ISSN 1528-7394.

[29] Caramaschi F.; del Corno G.; Favaretti C.; Giambelluca S.E.; Montesarchio E.; Fara G.M. (1981). Chloracne following environmental contamination by TCDD in Seveso, Italy. *International Journal of Epidemiology*. 10:135–43. ISSN 1464-3685.

[30] Bertazzi P.A.; Bernucci I.; Brambilla G.; Consonni D.; Pesatori A.C. (1998). The Seveso studies on early and long-term effects of dioxin exposure: a review. Environmental Health Perspectives. 106: 625–633. ISSN 0091-6765.

[31] Pesatori A.C.; Consonni D.; Rubagotti M.; Grillo P.; Bertazzi P.A. (2009). Cancer incidence in the population exposed to dioxin after the "Seveso accident": twenty years of follow-up. *Environmental Health*. 47, 8:39. ISSN 1476-069X.

[32] Viluksela M.; Bager Y.; Tuomisto J.T. (2000). Liver tumor-promoting activity of 2,3,7,8-tetrachlorodibenzo-p-dioxin (TCDD) in TCDD-sensitive and TCDD resistant rat strains. *Cancer Research*. 60:6911–20. *ISSN 0008-5472.*

[33] Gibbs L. M. The Citizen's Clearinghouse for Hazardous Wastes (Arlington Va.) (1995). Dying from dioxin : a citizen's guide to reclaiming our health and rebuilding democracy. Boston, MA, South End Press. ISBN 049608-187-7.

[34] Paigen B.; Goldman L.R.; Magnant M.M.; Highland J.H.; Steegmann A.T. (1987). Growth of children living near the hazardous waste site, Love Canal. Human Biology. 59: 489-508. ISSN 1520-6300.

[35] Rahill A. A. (1989). The effects of prenatal environmental toxin exposure (dioxin): A case study. Psychosocial effects of hazardous toxic waste disposal on communities. D. L. Peck. Springfield, Illinois, Charles C. Thomas, Publisher.

[36] Canosa P.; Morales S.; Rodríguez I.; Rubí E.; Cela R.; Gómez M.(2005). Aquatic degradation of triclosan and formation of toxic chlorophenols in presence of low concentrations of free chlorine. Analytical and Bioanalytical Chemistry 383:1119-26. ISSN 1618-2650.

[37] Ravenscroft P.; Brammer H.; Richards K. (2009). Arsenic Pollution: A Global Synthesis Wiley. *ISBN 9781405186025.*

[38] Infante, P.F. (1976). Oncogenic and Mutagenic Risks in Communities with Polyvinyl Chloride Production Facilities. Annals of the New York Academy of Sciences. 271:49 - 57. ISSN 1749-6632.

[39] Hathway, D.E. (1977). Comparative Mammalian Metabolism of Vinyl Chloride and Vinylidene Chloride in Relation to Oncogenic Potential. Environmental Health Perspectives. 21:55 - 59. ISSN 0091-6765.

[40] Emmerich K.H.; Norpoth K. (1981). Malignant Tumors after Chronic Exposure to Vinyl Chloride. Journal of Cancer Research and Clinical Oncology. 102:1 - 11. ISSN 1432-1335.

[41] Allsopp M.W.; Vianello G. (2012). Poly(Vinyl Chloride): Ullmann's Encyclopedia of Industrial Chemistry, 2012, Wiley-VCH, Weinheim. ISBN 9780494193815.

[42] Rous F.P. (1911). Transmission of a malignant new growth by means of a cell-free filtrate. Journal of the American Medical Association. 56:198. ISSN 1538-3598.

[43] Lathrop A.E.; Loeb L. (1915). Further Investigations On The Origin Of Tumors In Mice : I. Tumor Incidence And Tumor Age in Various Strains of Mice. The Journal of Experimental Medicine. 22:646–673. ISSN 1540-9538.

[44] Brower V. (2004). Connecting Viruses to Cancer: How Research Moves from Association to Causation. Journal of the National Cancer Institute. 96:4. ISSN 1540-9538.

[45] Bittner J.J. (1942). The Milk-Influence of Breast Tumors in Mice. Science. 95:462–463. ISSN 0036-8075.

[46] Eddy B.E.; Stewart S.E. (1959). Characteristics of the SE Polyoma Virus. American Journal Public Health Nations Health. 49:1486–1492. ISSN 0090-0036.

[47] Trentin J.J., Yabe Y., Taylor G. (1962). The quest for human cancer viruses. Science .137: 835-841. ISSN 0036-8075.

[48] Epstein M.A., Achong B.G., Barr Y.M. (1964). Virus Particles in Cultured Lymphoblasts from Burkitt's Lymphoma. Lancet. 7335:702–3. ISSN 0140-6736.

[49] Beral, V., Peterman T., Berlelman R., Jaffe H. (1990). Kaposi's sarcoma among persons with AIDS: a sexually transmitted infection? Lancet. 335:123–127. ISSN 0140-6736.

[50] Chang Y.; Cesarman E.; Pessin M.S.; Lee F.; Culpepper J.; Knowles D.M.; Moore P.S. (1994). Identification of herpesvirus-like DNA sequences in AIDS-associated Kaposi's sarcoma. Science. 266:1865-9. ISSN 0036-8075.

[51] Feng H.; Shuda M.; Chang Y.; Moore P.S. (2008). Clonal integration of a polyomavirus in human Merkel cell carcinoma. Science. 319:1096–100. ISSN 0036-8075.

[52] Caruso M.L.; Fucci L. (1990). Histological identification of Helicobacter pylori in early and advanced gastric cancer. Journal of Clinical Gastroenterology. 12:601-2. ISSN 0192-0790.

[53] Ruggiero P. (2012). Helicobacter pylori infection: what's new. Current Opinion in Infectious Diseases. 25:337-44. ISSN 1473-6527.

[54] Parkin, D.M. (2006). The Global Health Burden of Infection-Associated Cancers in the Year 2002. International Journal of Cancer. 118:3030-3044. ISSN 1097-0215.

[55] Samaras V.; Rafailidis P.I.; Mourtzoukou E.G.; Peppas G.; Falagas M.E. (2010). Chronic bacterial and parasitic infections and cancer: a review. Journal of Infection in Developing Countries. 4:267-281. ISSN 19722680.

[56] Upton, A.C. (1986). Historical perspectives on radiation carcinogenesis. In Upton A.C.; Albert R.E.; Burns F.J. and Shore R.E. (Eds) Radiation Carcinogenesis. Elsevier, New York, 1–10. ISBN 0444008594.

[57] Goodman M.T.; Mabuchi K.; Morita M.; Soda M.; Ochikubo S.; Fukuhara T.; Ikeda T.; Terasaki M. (1994). Cancer incidence in Hiroshima and Nagasaki, Japan, 1958-1987. The European Journal of Cancer. 30A:801-7. ISSN 09615423.

[58] Gyorgy, A. (1980). No Nukes: Everyone's Guide to Nuclear Power. South End Press. *ISBN 0896080064.*

[59] Parenti Ch. (2011). After Three Mile Island: The Rise and Fall of Nuclear Safety Culture, The Nation, March 22, 2011, http://www.thenation.com/article/159386/after-three-mile-island-rise-and-fall-nuclear-safetyculture.

[60] Brenner A.V.; Tronko M.D.; Hatch M.; Bogdanova T.I.; Oliynik V.A.; Lubin J.H.; Zablotska L.B.; Tereschenko V.P.; McConnell R.J.; Zamotaeva G.A.; O'Kane P.; Bouville A.C.; Chaykovskaya L.V.; Greenebaum E.; Paster I.P.; Shpak V.M.; Ron E. (2011). I-131 Dose-Response for Incident Thyroid Cancers in Ukraine Related to the Chornobyl Accident. Environmental Health Perspectives. 119:933-9. ISSN 0091-6765.

[61] Walter J. (1977) Radiation hazards and protection: Cytotoxic chemotherapy. In: Walter J. (Ed.), Cancer and Radiotherapy: A short guide for nurses and medical students. London: Churchill Livingstone. ISBN 0443015333.

[62] Palmer A. (2001). Understanding radiotherapy and its applications. In: Gabriel J. (Ed.), Oncology Nursing in Practice. London: Whurr, pp. 30-51. ISBN 9780470057599.

[63] Dustin, A. P. (1934). Action de la colchicine sur le sarcome greffe de la souris. Bulletin et Académie Royale de Médecine de Belgique, 14:487-502. ISSN 0377-8231.

[64] Alonso-Castro A.J.; Ortiz-Sánchez E.; Domínguez F.; López-Toledo G.; Chávez M.; De Jesús Ortiz-Tello A.; García-Carrancá A. (2012). Antitumor effect of Croton lechleri Mull. Arg. (Euphorbiaceae). Journal of Ethnopharmacology .140:438-442. ISSN 0378-8741.

[65] Cragg G.M.; Newman D.J. (2005). Plants as source of anticancer agents. Journal of Ethnopharmacology. 100:72-79. ISSN 0378-8741.

[66] Chen S.; Zheng L.; Liu J.; Li J.; Zhang L.; Gu J.; Li X.; Shen W.; Ma F.; Yao Y.; Wu G.; Chen Q. (2011). Effects of realgar (tetra-arsenic tetra-sulfide) on malignant tumor cells. Journal of Clinical Oncology 29: e13525. ISSN 0732-183X.

[67] Wani M.C.; Taylor H.L.; Wall M.E.; Coggon P.; McPhail A.T. (1971). Plant anti-tumor agents. VI. The isolation and structure of taxol, a novel anti-leukemic and anti-tumor agent from Taxus brevifolia. Journal of the American Chemical Society. 93:2325-27. ISSN 0002-7863.

[68] Rowinsky E.K.; Onetto N.; Canetta R.M.; Arbuck S.G. (1992). Taxol-the 1st of the texanes, an important new class of anti-tumor agents. Seminars in Oncology.19: 646-62. ISSN 0093-7754.

[69] Holton R.A.; Somoza C.; Hyeong Baik Kim; Feng Liang; Biediger R.J.; Douglas Boatman P.; Mitsuru Shindo; Smith C. C.; Soekchan Kim (1994). First total synthesis of taxol. 1. Functionalization of the B ring. Journal of the American Chemical Society.116:1597–1598. ISSN 0002-7863.

[70] Wall, M.E.; Wani M.C.; Cook C.E.; Palmer K.H.; McPhail A.T.; Sim G.A. (1966). Plant antitumor agents. 1. The isolation and structure of camptothecin, a novel alkaloidal leukemia and tumor inhibitor from Camptotheca acuminata. Journal of the American Chemical Society. 88:3888-3890. ISSN 0002-7863.

[71] Potmesil M.; Pinedo H. (1995). Camptothecins: new anticancer agents. Boca Raton, Florida, CRC Press. 149-150. ISBN 0849347645.

[72] Creemers G.J.; Bolis G.; Gore M.; Scarfone G.; Lacave A.J.; Guastalla J.P.; Despax R.; Favalli G.; Kreinberg R.; VanBelle S.; Cuendet M.; Pezzuto J.M. (2004). Antitumor activity of Bruceantin. An old drug with new promise. Journal of Natural Products. 67:269–272. ISSN 0163-3864.

[73] Bertino J.R. (1997). Irinotecan for colorectal cancer. Seminars in Oncology. 24:S18-S23. ISSN 0093-7754.

[74] Stahelin H. (1973). Activity of a new glycosidic lignan derivative (VP 16-213) related to podophyllotoxin in experimental tumors. *The European Journal of Cancer*. 9:215-21. *ISSN 0959-8049*.

[75] Podwyssotski V. (1880). Pharmakologische Studien uber Podophyllum peltatum. Archiv für Experimentelle Pathologie und Pharmakologie. 13:29–52. ISSN 0028-1298.

[76] Harvey A.L. (1999). Medicines from nature: are natural products still relevant to drug discovery. Trends in Pharmacological Sciences. 20:196-98. ISSN 01656147.

[77] Creemers G.J.; Bolis G.; Gore M.; Scarfone G.; Lacave A.J.; Guastalla J.P.; Despax R.; Favalli G.; Kreinberg R.; VanBelle S.; Cuendet; M.; Pezzuto J.M. (2004). Antitumor activity of Bruceantin. An old drug with new promise. Journal of Natural Products. 67:269–272. ISSN 0163-3864.

[78] Itokawa H.; Wang X.; Lee, K.H. (2005). Homoharringtonine and related compounds. In: Cragg, G.M., Kingston, D.G.I., Newman, D.J. (Eds.), Anticancer Agents from Natural Products. Brunner-Routledge Psychology Press, Taylor & Francis Group, Boca Raton, FL, pp. 47–70. ISBN 1439813825.

[79] Powell R.G.; Weisleder D.; Smith C.R. Jr; Rohwedder W.K. (1970). Structures of harringtonine, isoharringtonine, and homoharringtonine. *Tetrahydron Letters*. 11:815-818. *ISSN 0040-4039*.

[80] Kelland L. R. (2000). Flavopiridol, the first cyclic-dependent kinase inhibitor to enter the clinic: current status. *Expert Opinion on Investigational Drugs*. 9: 2903-11. ISSN 1354-3784

[81] Meijer L.; Skaltsounis A.L.; Magiatis P.; Polychronopoulos P.; Knockaert M.; Leost M.; Ryan X.P.; Vonica C.A.; Brivanlou A.; Dajani R.; Crovace C.; Tarricone C.; Musacchio A.; Roe S.M.; Pearl L.; Greengard P. (2003). GSK-3-selective inhibitors derived from Tyrian purple indirubins. Chemistry & Biology. 10:1255-66. ISSN 1074-5521.

[82] Christian M.C.; Pluda J.M.; Ho P.T.; Arbuck S.G.; Murgo A.J.; Sausville E.A. (1997). Seminars in Oncology 24:219-40. ISSN 0093-7754.

[83] Newman D.J.; Cragg G.M.; Holbeck S.; Sausville E.A. (2002). Natural products as leads to cell cycle pathway targets in cancer chemotherapy. Current Cancer Drug Targets. 2:279–308. ISSN 1873-5576.

[84] Pettit G.R.; Singh S.B.; Boyd M.R.; Hamel E.; Pettit R.; Schmit J.M.; Hogan F. (1995). Antineoplastic agents. 291. Isolation and synthesis of combretastatins A-4, A-5 and A-6. The Journal of Medicinal Chemistry. 38: 1666-72. ISSN 0022-2623.

[85] Ohsumi K.; Nakagawa R.; Fukuda Y.; Hatanaka T.; Morinaga Y.; Nihei Y.; Ohishi K.; Suga Y.; Akiyama Y.; Tsuji T. (1998). New combretastatin analogues effective against murine solid tumors: design and structure-activity relationship. The Journal of Medicinal Chemistry .41: 705-06. ISSN 0022-2623.

[86] Pettit G. R.; Herald C. L.; Hogan F. (2002). In *Anticancer Drug Development*. B. C. Baguley and D. J. Kerr (Eds.), pp. 203–235, Academic Press, San Diego

[87] Delmas D.; Lançon A.; Colin D.; Jannin B.; Latruffe N. (2006). Resveratrol as a Chemo-preventive Agent: A Promising Molecule for Fighting Cancer.*Current Drug Targets*. 7 ISSN 1389-4501

[88] Pisha E.; Chai H.; Lee I.S.; Chagwedera T.E.; Farnsworth N.R.; Cordell G.A.; Beecher C.W.; Fong H.H.; Kinghorn A.D.; Brown D.M.; Wani M.C.; Wall M.E.; Hieken T.J.; Das Gupta T.K.; Pezzuto J.M. (1995). Discovery of betulinic acid as a selective inhibitor of human melanoma that functions by induction of apoptosis. *Nature Medicine*.1: 1046-51. ISSN 1078-8956.

[89] Nahar N.; Das R.N.; Shoeb M.; Marma M.S.; Aziz M.A.; Mosihuzzaman M. (1997). Four triterpenoids from the bark of Zizyphus rugosa and Z. oenoplia. Journal of Bangladesh Academy of Sciences. 21: 151-56. ISSN 0378-8121.

[90] Balunas M.J.; Kinghorn A.D. (2005). Drug discovery from medicinal plants. *Life Sciences*. 78: pp. 431-41. *ISSN 0024-3205*.

[91] Rzymoska J. (1998). The effect of aqueous extracts from Inonotus obliquus on the mitotic index and enzyme activities. *Bollettino Chimico Farmaceutico.* 137:13-5. ISSN. 0006-6648

[92] Suffness M.; Douros J. (1980). Miscellaneous natural products with antitumor activity. In: Cassady, J.M., Douros, J.D. (Eds.), Anticancer Agents Based on Natural Product Models. Academic Press, New York, p. 474 (Chapter 14). *ISBN* 0121631508.

[93] Ravelo A.G.; Estevez-Braun A.; Chavez-Orellana H.; Perez-Sacau E.; Mesa-Siverio D. (2004). Recent studies on natural products as anticancer agents. Current Topics in Medicinal Chemistry. 4:241–265. ISSN 0929-8673.

[94] Silva G.L.; Cui B.; Chavez D.; You M.; Chai H.B.; Rasoanaivo P.; Lynn S.M.; O'Neill M.J.; Lewis J.A.; Besterman J.M.; Monks A.; Farnsworth N.R.; Cordell G.A.; Pezzuto J.M.; Kinghorn A.D. (2001). Modulation of the multidrug-resistance phenotype by new tropane alkaloid aromaticesters from Erythroxylum pervillei. Journal of Natural Products. 64,1514–1520. ISSN 0163-3864.

[95] Mi Q.; Cui B.; Silva G.L.; Lantvit D.; Reyes-Lim E.; Chai H.; Pezzuto J.M.; Kinghorn A.D.; Swanson S.M. (2003). A new tropane alkaloid aromatic ester that reverses multidrug resistance. Anticancer Research. 23:3607–3616. ISSN 0250-7005.

[96] Yu T.W.; Floss, H.m(2005). The ansamitocins. In: Cragg, G.M., Kingston, D.G.I., Newman, D.J. (Eds.), Anticancer Agents from Natural Products. Brunner-Routledge Psychology Press, Taylor & Francis Group, Boca Raton, FL, pp. 321–338. ISBN 1439813825.

[97] Denmeade S.R.; Jakobsen C.M.; Janssen S.; Khan S.R.; Garrett E.S.; Lilja H.; Christensen S.B.; Isaacs J.T. (2003). Prostate-specific antigen-activated thapsigargin prodrug as targeted therapy for prostate cancer. *Journal of the National Cancer Institute.* 95: 990–1000. ISSN 0027-8874.

[98] Hwang B.Y.; Lee J.H.; Koo T.H.; Kim H.S.; Hong Y.S.; Ro J.S.; Lee K.S.; Lee J.J. (2001). Kaurane diterpenes from Isodon japonicus inhibit nitricoxide and prostaglandin E2 production and NF-nB activation in LPS-stimulated macrophage RAW264.7 cells. Planta Medica. 67:406–410. ISSN 0032-0943.

[99] Shoeb M.; Celik S.; Jaspars M.; Kumarasamy Y., MacManus S., Nahar L., Kong T.L.P., Sarker S.D. (2005). Isolation, structure elucidation and bioactivity of schischkiniin, a unique indole alkaloid from the seeds of Centaurea schischkinii. Tetrahedron. 61: 9001-06. *ISSN 0040-4020.*

[100] Shoeb M.; MacManus S.M.; Jaspars M.; Trevidadu J.; Nahar L.; Thoo-Lin P.K.; Sarker S.D. (2006). Montamine, a unique dimeric indole alkaloid, from the seeds of Centaurea montana (Asteraceae), and its in vitro cytotoxic activity against the CaCo2 colon cancer cells. Tetrahedron. 62:11172-77. *ISSN 0040-4020.*

[101]   Sertel S.; Eichhorn T.; Plinkert P.K.; Efferth T. (2011). Cytotoxicity of Thymus vulgaris essential oil towards human oral cavity squamous cell carcinoma. Anticancer Research. 31:81-7. ISSN 1791-7530.

[102]   Tu A.T.; Giltner J.B. (1974). Cytotoxic effects of snake venoms on KB and Yoshida sarcoma cell. Research Communications in Chemical Pathology and Pharmacology. 9:783–786. ISSN 0034-5164.

[103]   Iwaguchi T.; Takechi M.; Hayashi K. (1985). Cytolytic activity of cytotoxin isolated from Indian cobra venom against experimental tumor cells. Biochemistry International. 10:343–349. ISSN 0158-5231.

[104]   Chaim-Matyas A.; Ovadia, M. (1987). Cytotoxic activity of various snake venoms on melanoma, B16F10 and chondrosarcoma. *Life Sciences*. 40:1601–1607. *ISSN 0024-3205.*

[105]   Zhong X.Y.; Liu G.F.; Wang Q.C. (1993). Purification and anticancer activity of cytotoxin-14 from venom of Naja naja atra. Zhongguo Yao Li Xue Bao. 14:279–282. ISSN 0253-9756.

[106]   Lipps B.V. (1999). Novel snake venom proteins cytolytic to cancer cells in vitro and in vivo systems. Journal of Venomous Animals and Toxins including Tropical Diseases. 5:173–183. ISSN 16789199.

[107]   Jokhio R.; Ansari A.F. (2005). Cobra snake venom reduces significantly tissue nucleic acid levels in human breast cancer. The Journal of the Pakistan Medical Association. 55:71–73. ISSN 0030-9982.

[108]   Araya C.; Lomonte B. (2007). Antitumor effects of cationic synthetic peptides derived from Lys49 phospholipase A2 homologues of snake venoms. Cell Biology International. 31: 263-268. ISSN 1065-6995.

[109]   Karthikeyan R.; Karthigayan S.; Sri Balasubashini M.; Vijayalakshmi S.; Somasundaram S.T.; Balasubramanian T. (2007). Inhibition of Cancer Cell Proliferation in vitro and Tumor Growth in vivo by Hydrophis spiralis Sea Snake Venom. International Journal of Cancer Research. 3:186-190. ISSN 1811-9727.

[110]   Wang W.X.; Ji Y.H. (2005). Scorpion venom induces glioma cell apoptosis in-vivo and inhibits glioma tumor growth in-vitro. The Journal of Neuro-Oncology. 73:1-7. ISSN 1573-7373.

[111]   Gao R.; Zhang Y.,;Gopalakrishnakone P. (2008). Purification and N-terminal sequence of a serine proteinase-like protein (BMK-CBP) from the venom of the Chinese scorpion (Buthus martensii Karsch). Toxicon. 52:348-53. ISSN 0041-0101.

[112]   DasGupta S.; Debnath A.; Saha A.; Giri B.; Tripathi G.; Vedasiromoni J.R.; Gomes A.; Gomes A. (2007). Indian black scorpion (*Heterometrus bengalensis Koch*) venom induced antiproliferative and apoptogenic activity against human leukemic cell lines U937 and K562. *Leukemia Research*. 31:817-82. *ISSN 0145-2126.*

[113] DeBin J.A.; Maggio J.E.; Strichartz G.R. (1993). Purification and characterization of chlorotoxin, a chloride channel ligand from the venom of the scorpion. American Journal of Physiology. 264:361–369. ISSN 0363-6119.

[114] Lyons S.A.; O'Neal J.; Sontheimer H. (2002). Chlorotoxin a scorpion-derived peptide, specifically binds to gliomas and tumors of neuroectodermal origin. *Glia* 39:162–173. *ISSN 0894-1491.*

[115] Robey I.F.; Martin N.K. (2011). Bicarbonate and dichloroacetate: Evaluating pH altering therapies in a mouse model for metastatic breast cancer BMC Cancer. 11:235. ISSN 1471-2407.

[116] Robey I.F.; Baggett B. K.; Kirkpatrick N.D.; Roe D.J.; Dosescu J.; Sloane B.F.; Hashim A.I.; Morse D.L.; Raghunand N.; Gatenby R.A.; Gillies R.J.(2009). Bicarbonate Increases Tumor pH and Inhibits Spontaneous Metastases. *Cancer Research.* 69:2260–8. ISSN 0008-5472.

[117] Nilsonne G.; Olm E.; Szulkin A.; Mundt F.; Stein A.; Kocic B.; Rundlöf A.K.; Fernandes A.P.; Björnstedt M.; Dobra K. (2009). Phenotype-dependent apoptosis signalling in mesothelioma cells after selenite exposure. Journal of Experimental & Clinical Cancer Research. 28:92. ISSN 0392-9078.

[118] DeVita V.T.; Chu E. (2008). A History of Cancer Chemotherapy. (AACR Centennial series). *Cancer Research.* 68: 8643-8653. ISSN 0008-5472.

[119] Holland-Frei Cancer Medicine. (2000). 5th edition. E.D. Bast R.C. Jr, Kufe D.W., Pollock R.E., et al., Hamilton (ON): BC Decker. ISBN 1607950146.

[120] Cisplatin Chemistry and Biochemistry of a Leading Anticancer Drug (1999). Ed. B.Lippert, Verlag Helvetica Chimica Acta, Zürich. ISBN 3906390209.

[121] Muggia F.M.; Fojo, T. (2004). Platinums: extending their therapeutic spectrum. Journal of chemotherapy. 16:77-82. ISSN 1120-009X.

[122] Latosińska J.N., Latosińska M. (2011). Towards Understanding Drugs on the Molecular Level to Design Drugs of Desired Profiles. In Drug Discovery and Development - Present and Future, Eds. Kapetanovic I.M. Intech. ISBN 9789533076157.

[123] Sun Y.; Campisi J.; Higano C.; Beer T.M.; Porter P.; Coleman I.; True L.; Nelson P.S. (2012) Treatment-induced damage to the tumor microenvironment promotes prostate cancer therapy resistance through WNT16B. *Nature Medicine.* 18: 1359–1368. ISSN: 1078-8956.

Chapter 3

Drug Interactions, Pharmacogenomics and Cardiovascular Complication

Irina Piatkov, Trudi Jones and Mark McLean

Additional information is available at the end of the chapter

1. Introduction

Early identification of patients who will be at a higher risk for the development of adverse side effects and who will need dosage adjustment has the potential to help the clinician to limit a patient's exposure to drug side effects. When on multiple medications and complex regimens, cardiac patients are at increased risk and particularly vulnerable to drug interactions. A rational and informed approach to drug interactions, based on scientific knowledge, can reduce the chance of adverse effects and improve patient outcomes.

Cardiovascular drugs are used to treat various forms of illnesses, but there are often large differences between individual patients in drug response and dosage requirement. Treatment that has been proven effective for one person can be ineffective or even dangerous for another.

A drug produces its therapeutic effect when it reaches its target concentration in the bloodstream. Whether a steady therapeutic concentration is obtained largely depends on the balance between the dose administered and the rate at which the body metabolises the drug. An individual patient's response to a drug is not totally predictable. Below the target therapeutic range, a drug may be ineffective or, when it is higher, the drug may cause adverse reactions or become toxic. To ensure the safe and effective action of many drugs, the concentration in the bloodstream and their clinical effects are monitored. If necessary, the dose can be adjusted or the medication changed to achieve the best possible outcome.

To avoid unintended and untoward adverse drug reactions, the prescriber should use the fundamental principles of pharmacology and pharmacogenetics. Several drugs are metabolised through the same pathways and knowledge of the potential pathway capacity could help to predict treatment success. Variability in the reaction to medication may be due to age, gender, morbidity, co-medication, food components, smoking and environmental factors. However, polymorphisms present in genes, are responsible for most of the variation. Pharmacogenetic research and candidate gene approaches have succeeded in the identification of several genetic factors influencing treatment response. In particular, associations between variants in CYP enzymes and transporter genes have been repeatedly associated with different response and treatment--associated side effects [1-6]. Knowledge of pharmacogenomics is providing a key to understanding fundamentals of the drug interaction process.

A specific genotype might differ in its frequency in different ethnic populations, leading to differences in drug response. However, gene combination between ethnic groups makes it impossible for the practitioner to simply predict if a drug will be efficient or not. There is no specific genetic definition of ethnicity and ethnicity does not sufficiently separate those for whom a given therapy will be effective.

In contrast, the pharmacogenetics potentially presents a more effective way of identifying responders, nonresponders and potential adverse drug reactions. Pharmacogenetics provides defined clinical biomakers for individualised therapy [7].

Personalised medicine can be defined as a form of medicine that uses information about a person's genes, proteins and environment to prevent, diagnose and treat diseases, including predicting therapeutic response, nonresponse and likelihood of adverse reactions. Diagnostic biomarkers are necessary to successfully select patients for therapy, distinguish likely responders from nonresponders, identify patients at high risk for adverse events, or select an appropriate dose for safe and efficacious use of the therapy.

The human genome consists of approximately 3 billion base pairs (NCBI database) and the sequence of these varies among individuals. These variations can change the function of proteins that interact with a drug and hence, the response to a drug may differ among individuals. Sequence variations in drug-disposition genes can alter the pharmacokinetics of a drug and those in drug-target genes can change the pharmacodynamics of a drug.

When a genetic polymorphism alters the function of a protein that is involved in the absorption, metabolism, distribution and excretion of a drug, the concentrations of the parent drug or its active metabolites may be affected. For example, *CYP2D6**4 polymorphism leads to lower activity of a metabolising enzyme and the plasma concentrations of the parent drug metabolised by cytochrome P-450 isoenzyme 2D6 may increase and concentration of metabolites may decrease (some antidepressants). As a result, it could lead to the development of toxicity. For prodrugs, when metabolites have pharmacologic activity, the genetic polymorphism may reduce the drug response (some analgesics). Genetic polymorphisms that change the activity of the drug target (pharmacodynamics) may also alter the drug response. For example, vitamin K epoxide reductase complex subunit 1 gene polymorphisms influence warfarin response and β_1-adrenergic receptor gene polymorphisms after β-blocker response. Therefore, drugs can compete for binding sites on the receptors or be metabolised by the same enzyme, consequently create dug-drug interaction problem.

The information about pharmacogenetic terms and recourses is presented in the Appendix.

Early identification of patients who will be at a higher risk for the development of adverse side effects and who will need dosage adjustment has the potential to help the clinician to limit a patient's exposure to drug side effects. Characterisation of drug metabolising polymorphisms has been shown to be useful for identifying individuals who are poor drug metabolisers and at risk of developing adverse reactions, and several genotyping methods are already being used in clinical settings (Table1). The evidence provided by pharmacogenetics and pharmacogenomics can be successfully used for drug interaction interpretation.

Drugs	Tests of polymorphisms	Affected WSLHD Population*
Wafarin	CYP2C9	1% - Poor Metabolisers, 15% - Intermediate
Phenytoin		
Warfarin	VKORC1	11% with altered function
Clopidogrel	*CYP2C19*	4% - Poor Metabolisers, 13% - Intermediate, 20% - Ultra fast metabolisers
Carvedilol	CYP2D6	5% - Poor Metabolisers, 27% - Intermidiate, 1% - Ultra fast metabolisers
Metoprolol		
Propafenone		
Propranolol		
Quinidine		
Isosorbide	NAT1, NAT2	10-90%
Hydralazine		
Warfarin	Protein C Deficiencies	1/200 population, 2-5% Patients with Venous Thromboembolism
Atorvastatin	LDLR	1-5% Familial Cholesterolemia Patients
Statins	SINM PhyzioType (50 genes)	10-30% Patients on statin (multi-gene biomarker system manufacture results, no data available)

Table 1. Available Pharmacogenetics tests for cardiovascular medication. (*Western Sydney Population combined data. WSLHD population is a mix of Caucasians, Asians and Africans.)

2. Hypertensive drugs

Hypertension is a common condition associated with increased risk of stroke, heart failure, ischemic heart disease, and chronic renal failure. Thiazide diuretics, β-blockers, ACE inhibitors, angiotensin receptor blockers (ARBs) and calcium channel blockers (CCBs) are a common first line treatment for hypertension [8].

Despite availability of many effective agents, only about 40 percent [9] of treated hypertensive patients have their blood pressure controlled, mostly due to the unpredictable individual responses to treatment. Blood pressure responses to monotherapy vary widely within ethnic and gender subgroups [10].

Numerous studies have tried to establish associations between genetic polymorphisms and response to antihypertensive drugs. New developments in pharmacogenetics and pharmacogenomics already offer in pharmacogenetics and pharmacogenomics already offers the opportunity to provide individualised drug therapy on the basis of a person's genetic make-up for some drugs, despite varied approaches in study designs and methodology. These tests are provided by several laboratories and available at some hospitals; pharmacogenetic methods will not only help to achieve treatment goals and limit adverse effects, but also avoid drug interactions.

2.1. β-blockers

β-blockers through binding to β-adrenergic receptors (BAR) antagonise the binding of endogenous agonists. Variations in the gene encoding the β1-adrenergic receptor probably influence the treatment outcome. Two single nucleotide polymorphism (SNPs), resulting in Ser49Gly and Arg389Gly were identified and these variants demonstrate altered biological function in vitro, including enhanced agonist induced adenylyl cyclase activation by Gly49 compared to Ser49 and by Arg389 compared to Gly389 [11].

Some studies have shown that the Arg389Arg genotype and Ser49/Arg389 haplotype are associated with a greater response to blood pressure-lowering metoprolol [12].

The differential survival of Acute Coronary Syndrome (ACS) patients treated with β-blockers was associated with patients' β-adrenergic receptors 2 variant Gly16Arg and Gln27Glu genotypes; however, β-adrenergic receptors 1 variants showed no significant associations [13, 14].

No significant correlation has been found for outcomes of death, MI or stroke in coronary artery disease patients on atenolol treatment and β-adrenergic receptors variants or haplotypes [15] and β-adrenergic receptors 2 variants in MI and stroke outcomes. However, the case-control study found significant interaction with two SNPs in β-adrenergic receptors variant and cardiovascular complications [16, 17].

Angiotensin-converting enzyme (ACE) genes variations were also associated with β-blockers therapy outcome. In heart failure, patients survival without a transplant, has been associated with the angiotensin-converting enzyme I/D genotype (insertion/deletion).

Patients with the D allele may derive greater benefits from pharmacologic interventions with Beta-blocker treatment, probably through the decrease of sympathetic nervous system activity [18].

The effects of the CYP450 enzyme systems has been studied intensively during the last years and its role in the metabolism of drugs and other endogenous and exogenous chemicals is well defined. Numerous publications confirm the association of these enzymes with drug-drug, drug-toxins and drug-food interactions. Polymorphisms in the gene coding for the CYP2D6 isoenzyme, which catalyses the metabolism of β-blockers such as metoprolol, carvedilol, timolol, and propranolol, may also affect blocker response. It has been demonstrated that the clearance of the R(+) enantiomer of carvedilol was 66% lower and the area under the concentration-versus-time curve 156% higher among poor metabolizers than extensive metabolizers [19-22].

Some studies showed association with other genes. Genes involved in calcium signalling - CACNA1C, CACNB2, and KCNMB1- were found to be associated with myocardial infarction or stroke with β-blockers versus calcium channel blockers [23-25]. Variable stroke risk by genotype was described for an MMP3 promoter polymorphism in patients treated with lisinopril [26] and different treatment-related outcomes with thiazides and β-blockers, but not diltiazem, by NEDD4L (protein reduce renal tubular expression of epithelial Na+ channel) genotype [27].

Finally, the two studies by Schelleman et al reported no β-blocker interactions (for outcomes MI or stroke) variants of angiotensin receptor II type 1 (AGTR1) and ACE [28, 29].

2.2. Diuretics

Diuretics may act at a number of sites, including the proximal tubule, the Loop of Henle, and the distal and collecting tubules. Diuretics are thought to indirectly activate the renin-angiotensin-aldosterone system and block sensitivity of blood vessels to catecholamines. Thiazide diuretics are the drug of choice for initial therapy, but genes responsible for renal sodium reabsorption can affect the patient's responsiveness to diuretic therapy.

Antihypertensive response in black African Americans is found to be associated with locus at chromosome12q15 [30, 31] where the FRS2 gene is located, which is involved in fibroblast growth factor signalling. FRS2 plays a role in vascular smooth muscle cell regulation.

Genome-wide association (GWA) studies are aimed at identifying common genetic variants modulating disease susceptibility, physiological traits and variable drug responses. These studies also provide further evidence for the large effects that single gene variants may exert for some drugs. GWA has explained relatively large proportions of variability compared to studies of traits such as disease susceptibility or physiological measurements. GWAS demonstrated that SNPs in lysozyme and Yeats domain-containing protein 4 (YEATS4) were associated with response to diuretic [30].

Lynch et al. found that C carriers of the NPPA T2238C variant, which codes for the precursor of atrial natriuretic polypeptide, had more favourable clinical outcomes when treated with a diuretic, whereas individuals homozygous for the T allele responded better to a calcium channel blocker [32].

Patients with SNP of T594M gene (epithelial sodium channel) variant responded more favourably to amiloride therapy for BP control than to thiazide-based drugs. In cases of severe hypokalemia, potassium-sparing diuretics such as amiloride or triamterene should be used according to serum sodium and potassium levels [33, 34].

NEDD4L is also a candidate gene with a documented functional SNP, a role in sodium reabsorption, and several studies have found an association between this SNP and blood pressure response with thiazides [27, 35].

A common functional polymorphism resulting in Gly460Trp in the α-adducin gene ADD1 has been associated with response to thiazides. This finding led to the development of a novel antihypertensive drug class targeting adducin [36, 37]. Manunta et al. performed single SNP association analysis and combination analysis on ADD1 (Gly460Trp), NEDD4L, WNK1 in a 4-week diuretic trial. They found ADD1 460Trp carriers had significantly greater BP reduction than Gly460 homozygotes. When considered together, there was a significant trend in decreases of systolic blood pressure (SBP) (ranging from −3.4 mm Hg to −23.2 mm Hg) for different combinations of genotypes [35].The ADD1 Gly460Trp polymorphism has been associated with an increased risk of myocardial infarction or stroke during thiazide diuretic treatment [38] In contrast, these findings were not confirmed by other studies [39, 40].

The 825T allele in the G-protein is probably associated with a sodium-sensitive form of hypertension. Blood pressure declines for both the C/T and T/T genotypes were significantly greater than for the C/C genotype. The study revealed that the decreases in blood pressure varied on the basis of genotype and even after multiple regression analysis, genotype remained a significant predictor of blood pressure lowering [41].

2.3. Renin-angiotensin system inhibitors

Numerous genes from the renin-angiotensin system (RAS) pathway have been shown to play a key role in the regulation of blood pressure and influence the cardiovascular system. Several pharmacogenetic studies of the RAS were conducted. However, due to the complexity of RAS, associations between drug efficiency and polymorphisms are not consistent [42-45].

Angiotensin-converting enzyme (ACE) inhibitors prevent the conversion of angiotensin I to angiotensin II in plasma and tissue and prevent the degradation of bradykinin. Clinically, ACE inhibitors reduce peripheral vascular resistance and pulmonary capillary wedge pressure and increase cardiac output and renal blood flow. Treatment with ACE inhibitors in hypertension has been associated with improvements in vascular compliance, regression of left ventricular hypertrophy, improved systolic and diastolic function, and improvements in insulin sensitivity [46]. One study showed that ACE DD polymorphism is associated with poor collateral circulation (PCC). PCC in patients carrying the D allele may be associated with endothelial dysfunction and elevated blood ACE levels in these patients [47].

The insertion/deletion (I/D) in the angiotensin I-converting enzyme (ACE) gene is one of the candidates for studies. The D allele has been associated with more improvement in coronary endothelial dysfunction with ACE inhibitor therapy than the I allele [48]. Reductions in systolic and diastolic blood pressures were significantly greater for patients with the D/D genotype than for patients with the I/D and I/I genotypes [49].

Diastolic blood pressure tended to decrease more for the ACE I/I genotype than for other ACE genotypes and the I/I genotype was also predictive of greater diastolic blood pressure decline [50]. Decline in renal function during ACE inhibitor treatment tended to be greater in heart failure patients with the ACE I/I genotype [51]. The I/I genotype has also been associated with increased susceptibility to the development of cough during ACE inhibitor therapy. After four weeks of therapy with an ACE inhibitor in healthy volunteers, the threshold for cough was significantly reduced for the I/I genotype but not the D/D genotype [52].

Another gene of interest is the angiotensinogen (AGT) gene. It was reported that the angiotensinogen 235Met/Thr polymorphism is also associated with RAS activity and drug responses. In subjects on ACE inhibitor monotherapy with 235Thr allele the response is higher than in the control group. Systolic and diastolic blood pressures were higher and the likelihood of using two or more antihypertensive medications was 2.1 times higher with the 235Thr polymorphism [53].

An association with polymorphisms in the angiotensin AT1 receptor (AGT1R) gene and ACE inhibitors' efficiency are found in some studies. The AGT1R mediates some negative effects of angiotensin II, such as vasoconstriction, cardiac remodelling, and aldosterone secretion. Angiotensin II blockers bind to angiotensin II receptors, thereby antagonizing the effect of angiotensin II, a potent vasoconstrictor [54]. The 1166C allele of AGT1R has been associated with increased arterial responsiveness to angiotensin II in ischemic heart disease and increased aortic stiffness in hypertension. During ACE inhibitor treatment, reductions in aortic stiffness were reported to be three times greater in carriers of the 1166C allele than in 1166A homozygotes [55, 56]. AGTR1 (C573T) and ACE (ID) association between ACE inhibitor therapy and increased MI risk for carriers of the AGTR1 C573 allele were reported; however, no significant interaction between ACE inhibitor treatment and ACE (ID) alleles for either stroke or MI were found [28]. One research group found no associations between BP response and ACE (ID), AGTR1 (A1166C), CYP11B2 (-344 C/T), AGT (-6 A/G) [57].

After 12 weeks of treatment with irbesartan (Angiotensin II Blocker), plasma concentration of the drug was related to change in systolic BP in TT homozygotes of AGTR1 (C5245T) but not for other genotypes [58].

3. Calcium Channel Blockers (CCBs)

Drugs in this class block voltage-gated calcium channels in the heart and vasculature, thereby reducing intracellular calcium. Calcium channel blockers drugs vary in their effect on cardiac versus vascular calcium channels. CCBs fall into three subclasses: phenylalkylamines, which are selective for the myocardium; dihydropyridines which mostly affecting smooth muscle and benzothiazepines with a broad range.

A few studies describe some association; three SNPs in CACNA1C had significant associations with treatment in a study of BP lowering with calcium channel blockers [59]; between CYP3A5*3 and *6 variants and verapamil treatment for BP and hypertension risk outcomes in blacks and Hispanics [60]; individuals that are homozygous for the T allele of NPPA T2238C had more favourable clinical outcomes when treated with a calcium channel blocker whereas C carriers responded better to a diuretic [32]. Beta Adrenergic Receptor 1 (BAR1) Ser49-Arg389 haplotype carriers had higher death rates than those with other haplotypes when treated with verapamil [15].

4. Anticoagulants

4.1. Warfarin

Warfarin is a widely used anticoagulant in the treatment and prevention of thrombosis. It was initially marketed as a pesticide against rats and mice and is still used for this purpose. It was approved for use as a medication in the early 1950s and is widely prescribed. Despite its common use, warfarin therapy can be associated with significant bleeding complications. Achieving a safe therapeutic response can be difficult because of warfarin's narrow therapeutic index and great individual variability in the dose required, which is mostly a consequence of individual genetic variants. This fact is well known among clinicians and the wide range, from 1 mg/day to 20 mg/day, of warfarin maintenance doses are observed across the population. To maintain a therapeutic level of anti-thrombosis and to minimise the risk of bleeding complications, warfarin therapy requires intensive monitoring via the International Normalized Ratio (INR) to guide its dosing. The INR is used to monitor the effectiveness of warfarin and measures the pathway of blood coagulation. It is used to standardize the results for a prothrombin time. INR is the ratio of a patient's prothrombin time to a control sample, raised to the power of the index value for the analytical system used.

Several factors increase the risk of over-anticoagulation: genetic polymorphisms affecting the metabolising enzymes, impaired liver function, drug interactions, congestive heart failure, diarrhoea, fever, and diets rich in vitamin K [61] [62]. Nevertheless, genetic factors and drug interactions mostly account for the risk of over-anticoagulation. Warfarin metabolism involves primarily the cytochrome P450 (CYP) enzymes. Some loss-of-function CYP2C9 and vitamin K epoxide reductase complex subunit 1 (VKORC1) polymorphisms are known to be associated with decreased enzymatic activity and as a result, with an increased risk of haemorrhage. These are CYP2C9*2 (Cysl44/Ile359), CYP2C9*3 (Argl44/Leu359) and VKORC1 (-1639G>A) [63-65].

Warfarin-induced haemorrhage is an important complication of anticoagulation therapy. A review of many studies shows average yearly rates of warfarin-related bleeding as high as 0.8%, 4.9%, and 15%, for fatal, major and minor bleeding complications respectively [66].

Vitamin K is required by proteins C and S, together with clotting factors II, VII, IX, and X, to allow assembly of the procoagulant enzyme complexes necessary to generate fibrin. Warfarin as an anticoagulant agent has the ability to interfere with the recycling of vitamin K in the liver. The pharmacologic effect of warfarin is mediated by the inhibition of vitamin K epoxide reductase complex subunit 1 (EC 1.1.4.1) [67].

Warfarin consists of (R)- and (S)-warfarin enantiomers. (R)- and (S)-warfarins differ in their relative plasma concentrations, in their antithrombotic potency and in the specific isoenzymes responsible for their metabolism. (S)-warfarin has a 3 to 5 times greater anticoagulant effect than the (R)-enantiomer and accounts for 60% to 70% of warfarin's overall anticoagulant activity. (S)-warfarin is metabolised almost exclusively by CYP2C9 [68-70].

The activity of the CYP2C9 enzyme has a significant impact on the clearance of (S)-warfarin and as a consequence on anticoagulant effect. In the presence of genetic variations where the activity of CYP2C9 is reduced, clearance of (S)-warfarin is also reduced. Activity of CYP2C9 between individuals can vary by more than 20-fold. (R)-warfarin is metabilised by multiple different CYP enzymes [71].

While several single-nucleotide polymorphisms of CYP2C9 have been reported, the CYP2C9*2 (Cysl44/Ile359) and CYP2C9*3 (Argl44/Leu359) polymorphisms have been identified as clinically relevant [72]. Both of these variants are associated with decreased enzymatic activity [24, 73-78].

Homozygous CYP2C9*3 variant genotypes have only 5% to 10% metabolic efficiency compared to the wild-type genotype. As a result, compared to wild-type CYP2C9*1*1 controls, enzyme activity and the median maintenance warfarin dose for CYP2C9*3*1 heterozygotes was reduced by 40%, and by approximately 90% for CYP2C9*3*3 homozygotes [72-74].

Furuya [79] and Steward [75] showed that the CYP2C9*2 variant is also associated with reduced warfarin elimination. Heterozygotes demonstrate 40% and homozygotes 15% of the wild-type enzyme activity, causing dose adjustment for heterozygote CYP2C9*2 individuals down to 20% less than the standard dose.

Margaglione [76] has also demonstrated bleeding rates as high as 27.9 per 100 patient-years in carriers of CYP variants. In this study, findings were adjusted for other common variables associated with increased bleeding risk, such as increased age, drug interactions and abnormal liver function.

Several studies of the *2 and *3 CYP2C9 polymorphisms consistently show that patients with at least one CYP2C9 allele polymorphism have reduced warfarin requirements [76, 80-84]. Freeman [85] reported reduced warfarin weekly dosages for carriers of CYP2C9*2 or CYP2C9*3 alleles compared with patients who were homozygous for the wild-type allele (0.307 mg/kg/wk and 0.397 mg/kg/wk, respectively). Taube [83] compared warfarin maintenance dosages in 683 patients carrying different CYP2C9 genotypes. Mean warfarin maintenance dosages were 86% in patients with CYP2C9*1*2, 79% in patients with CYP2C9*1*3, 82% in compound heterozygotes CYP2C9*2/*3, and 61% in patients homozygous for CYP2C9*2. Furthermore, Aithal [80] warns that even when warfarin dosages are decreased, carriers of CYP2C9 poor metaboliser alleles experience a rate of major bleeding that is 3.68-fold higher than the rate seen in patients with the wild type genotype.

The frequency of CYP2C9 alleles is ethnically related [82, 86]. Approximately 20% of the Caucasian population carries one of the loss-of-function CYP2C9 alleles, and it is estimated that 1% of Caucasian carry two such alleles [71]. The frequency of the CYP2C9*2 allele reportedly ranges from 8-13% in different Caucasian populations. CYP2C9*2 is present in 4% of African-Americans and is rare among Japanese individuals [87, 88]. The frequency of CYP2C9*3 is 6-10% among Caucasian populations and 3.8% in Japanese populations [88, 89]. This data suggests that a substantial fraction of the Caucasian patient population may carry at least one defective CYP2C9 allele. In this group, the usual prescription dosage of warfarin may lead to major or even life-threatening haemorrhage.

Warfarin is commonly prescribed in combination with selective serotonin reuptake inhibitors (SSRIs), as depression often coexists with cardiovascular disease. Case reports suggest that some SSRIs can interact with warfarin to increase the likelihood of bleeding [90]. SSRIs cause adverse effects in isolation [91, 92] and can interact with other medications by inhibiting various isoenzymes of the CYP450 enzyme group [93, 94]. It has been shown that metronidazole and cimetadine increase the prothrombin time in patients on warfarin therapy. Chloramphenicol enhances warfarin's effect by inhibiting the action of the hepatic P450 system [71]. Some authors [95], [96] have warned that antidepressants with a known or predictable interaction with warfarin, such as fluoxetine and fluvoxamine, should be avoided in patients receiving warfarin because of the risk of adverse outcomes.

Drug-drug interaction is a main concern in adverse drug reactions. The primary complication occurring with warfarin treatment is bleeding. SSRIs may increase the risk of bleeding during warfarin therapy by hindering platelet aggregation through depletion of platelet serotonin levels [97-99]. Some SSRIs may also inhibit the oxidative metabolism of warfarin by CYP 2C9 [95].

It has been shown that concurrent use of selective serotonin reuptake inhibitors and warfarin increases the risk of hospitalisation due to haemorrhage [90, 98]. Drugs which affect serotonin may have a detrimental effect on platelet function, as drugs which inhibit the reuptake of serotonin may decrease platelet serotonin levels leading to a reduction in serotonin-mediated platelet aggregation. Potential drug interactions can involve modification in either of these mechanisms and may result in pharmacodynamic interference or enhancement of warfarin's action.

It was shown that major and moderate drug-drug interactions with warfarin are very common in inpatients and are associated with INR results outside the therapeutic range. The most common drugs involved in the increase of anticoagulation effect were enoxaparin, simvastatin, omeprazole and tramadol. Multivariate analysis showed that age, length of hospital stay, exposure to >/=4 major or moderate drug interactions, and refusal of pharmacist recommendations contribute significantly to the patient's INR result >5 [100].

One study demonstrated that acetaminophen, at 2 g/day or 3 g/day, enhanced the anticoagulant effect of warfarin in stable patients, thus requiring close INR monitoring in the clinical setting [101].

4.2. Heparin

One of the preventative treatments of thromboembolic disease in patients is a prescription of heparin. However, heparin induced thrombocytopenia (HIT) is one of the most serious adverse reactions. HIT consequences can include thromboembolic complications and death.

An association between the Fc receptor gene and the risk for HIT has been found in some studies and it was demonstrated that the homozygous 131Arg/Arg genotype occurred significantly more often in patients with HIT than in the healthy volunteers' group [102] [103] ; however, another group have found no association [104]. Results are very preliminary and more evidence are needed before it may be possible to genotype candidates for heparin therapy to identify those at risk for drug-induced thromboembolic complications.

5. Statins

Hydroxymethylglutaryl-coenzyme A reductase inhibitors (statins) have reduced coronary and cerebrovascular events and overall mortality when used for both primary and secondary prevention of ischemic heart disease [105]. Several known gene polymorphisms are associated with the treatment progress [106, 107].

Some studies examined polymorphism in the gene encoding cholesteryl ester transfer protein (CETP), which is involved in the metabolism of high-density lipoprotein (HDL). Pravastatin-treated patients with either the B1/B1 or B1/B2 genotype (B1 presence and B2 absence of polymorphism) had significantly less atherosclerotic progression than patients receiving a placebo. Placebo-treated patients with the B2/B2 genotype had the least progression. However, pravastatin-treated patients with the B2/B2 genotype (16% of the study population) derived no benefit from pravastatin [108, 109].

The substitution (-455G/A) of the fibrinogen gene was found to be associated with an increased risk of myocardial infarction and stroke. During follow-up, placebo-treated patients homozygous for the -455A genotype had the greatest disease progression; although, no association was found with benefit in disease progression in patients on pravastatin therapy [110].

A five year study of pravastatin therapy in patients with a history of myocardial infarction and hypercholesterolemia showed that the largest benefit of pravastatin treatment in reducing these events occurred in patients with the platelet GP IIIa PlA1/A2 genotype who also carried at least one D allele of the ACE gene [111, 112].

An effect of polymorphism in the alloprotein gene was found on simvastatin therapy in a Scandinavian study. Among patients who received the placebo and had at least one apolipoprotein e4 allele, the relative risk of death from all causes was higher than in simastatin patients with the same polymorphism [113]. This study demonstrates the potential clinical value of the alloprotein APOE genotype as a robust marker for low-density lipoprotein (LDL) responses to statin drugs, which might contribute to the identification of a particularly drug-resistant subgroup of patients [114].

Genetic variants in CYP3A4, which metabolises simvastatin, atorvastatin and lovastatin, have been associated with variability in statin efficacy. Both a nonsynonymous polymorphism (M445T) as well the CYP3A4*4 haplotype have been associated with lower LDL cholesterol levels with atorvastatin. However, in carriers of either a CYP3A4 promoter polymorphism (A290G) or the CYP3A4*1G haplotype the lipid-lowering effect of statins is not demonstrated [115-117].

Variation in Hydroxymethylglutaryl-coenzyme A reductase (HMGCR) and low-density lipoprotein receptor (LDLR) genes are associated with the LDL-lowering effect of statins. The H7 haplotype within HMGCR, defined by the presence of three intronic SNPs, has been associated with an 11% to 19% reduction in LDL cholesterol with statin treatment in multiple independent populations as well as ethnically diverse population-based cohorts [107, 114, 118]. The H7 haplotype has been shown to interact with other genetic variants, including a second HMGCR haplotype, H2, as well as the LDLR L5 haplotype, defined by six SNPs within the LDLR 3' untranslated region. Ethnic variations in LDL cholesterol-lowering with statin treatment is also demonstrated in African-Americans who carry multiple copies of these haplotypes versus any haplotype alone [106, 118, 119].

Statin-related myotoxicity, especially rhabdomyolysis, is the subject of medical concerns as it requires changes in medications and treatment discontinuation. It was found that variants in CYP3A5 and solute carrier organic anion transporter family (SLCO1B1) gene can be potential predictors of myotoxicity [120-123].

Increased risk of coronary artery disease, coronary heart disease and myocardial infarction are associated in some studies with a missense SNP, Trp719Arg, in the KIF6 gene (kinesin family member 6). Statin treatment significantly reduce coronary events in carriers of Trp719Arg, and SNPs in high linkage disequilibrium with it, whereas no benefit of statin treatment is reported in noncarriers [124].

The differences in drug-drug interaction profiles among available statins offer the possibility of reducing the risk of myotoxicity among high-risk patients. The risk of developing the rhabdomyolysis condition with statin therapy increases at higher therapeutic doses. This effect is increased by combination with certain other medications due to drug-drug interactions. Co-administration of drugs that inhibit the cytochrome P450 (CYP) enzymes responsible for metabolizing statins, or that interact with the organic anion-transporting polypeptides (OATPs) responsible for statin uptake into hepatocytes, substantially increases the risk of developing myotoxicity. Pitavastatin, a novel statin approved for the treatment of hypercholesterolemia and combined (mixed) dyslipidemia, is not catabolized by CYP3A4, unlike other lipophilic statins, and may be less dependent on the OATP1B1 transporter for its uptake into hepatocytes before clearance [125].

6. Antiarrhythmic

Many antiarrhythmic agents have antagonistic effects on sodium ion and potassium ion channels in the heart. A risk of proarrhythmic effects of antiarrhythmic drugs and its mechanism is associated with genetic variations. Some evidence indicates that polymorphisms in genes encoding components of cardiac ion channels have been associated with congenital arrhythmia syndromes, such as long-QT and idiopathic ventricular fibrillation syndromes [126].

The fact that the risk of drug-induced arrhythmia usually increases with increasing drug concentrations also indicates the involvement of liver enzyme polymorphisms. The CYP2D6 gene regulates cytochrome P450 metabolic pathways and some evidence shows an association between poor metaboliser phenotype and antiarrhythmic drug toxicity {127}.

A number of polymorphisms in the N-acetyltransferace 2 gene contribute to different acetylator phenotypes. Rapid acetylators have increased conversion of procainamide by N-acetyltransferase 2 to N-acetylprocainamide (NAPA) consequently leading to the QT-interval prolongation, and life-threatening ventricular arrhythmias. Slow acetylators will attain an increased concentration of procainamide levels with normal procainamide dosages, which can lead to a procainamide- induced lupus-like syndrome [128].

Sotalol, dofetilide and quinidine increase the chances of QT interval prolongation, polymorphic ventricular tachycardia and torsades de pointes. Several genes encoding ion channels or function-modifying subunits were associated with these syndromes [129],[130-132].

One study suggested that a NOS1AP variant in the gene encoding an accessory protein for neuronal nitric oxide synthase, was associated with total and cardiovascular mortality during treatment with dihydropyridine calcium channel blockers. Variants in NOS1AP also have been reported to modulate the risk of arrhythmias, at equivalent QT interval durations, in patients with the congenital long QT syndrome and to modulate risk for sudden death in the general population [133-135].

7. Antiplatelet agents

7.1. Aspirin

Pharmacogenetic studies of aspirin response to date have found associations with a few genes. It was reported that PLA2 (Leu59Pro) carriers, the variant in platelet glycoprotein IIIa, have impaired aspirin responses. After seven days of aspirin therapy in healthy volunteers, plasma prothrombin fragment concentrations in bleeding-time wounds were reduced in 23 of 25 PLA1 homozygotes, compared with 9 of 15 PLA2 carriers [136]. A meta-analysis [137] of 50 polymorphisms in 11 genes reported in 31 studies with a combined sample size of 2834 subjects suggested that the common PLA1/2 polymorphism does confer aspirin resistance (odds ratio in healthy subjects=2.36; P=0.009); however, when combining both healthy subjects and those with cardiovascular disease, the odds ratio was 1.14 (P=0.40). The PLA2 allele occurs with a frequency of approximately 15% in humans and has been associated with increased platelet activation and aggregation in vitro [138].

Associations between the PLA polymorphisms and subacute thrombosis after coronary intervention have been described in some reports [139-141] and it was shown that an increased risk of subacute thrombosis is associated with the PLA2 allele. In one study, the risk of subacute thrombosis after coronary angioplasty and stent placement was five times greater in coronary artery disease patients with the PLA2 polymorphism than in patients homozygous for the PLA1 allele, despite similar antiplatelet therapy and similar clinical, angiographic and procedural characteristics [139].

7.2. Clopidogrel

The obvious candidates for pharmacogenetic analysis are genes involved in clopidogrel metabolism. Clopidogrel is a prodrug and its active form, thiol, is formed during the biotransformation in the liver. CYP2C19, CYP3A4/5, CYP1A2, and CYP2B6 are involved in this process [142].

P2Y12 belongs to the G protein-coupled purinergic receptor for adenosine diphosphate (ADP). The P2Y12 protein is found mainly, but not exclusively, on the surface of blood platelets, and is an important regulator in blood clotting. The active clopidogrel metabolite irreversibly binds to platelet ADP P2Y12 receptors. ADP P2Y12 receptors and loss-of-function CYP2C19*2 was identified as the single major genetic determinant of biochemical response to clopidogrel, accounting for approximately 12% of the variation in ADP-stimulated platelet aggregation during drug treatment [143]. CYP2C19*2 carriers treated with clopidogrel have an increased risk for major adverse cardiovascular events compared to noncarriers and increased risks of stent thrombosis [144].

Loss-of-function CYP2C19*2 allele has been reproducibly shown to be associated with a decreased conversion of clopidogrel into its active metabolite, reduced antiplatelet effect and increased risk for cardiovascular events in patients using clopidogrel [4, 145].

The frequency of CYP2C19*2 polymorphism varies in different populations: in Caucasian, African American, and Mexicans it presence is 18% to 33% (2%–3% homozygotes) and the allele frequency is higher in Asians. The loss-of-function *3 variant is also associated with poorer response and is highly prevalent in Asians [146, 147].

P-glycoprotein, also known as multidrug resistance protein 1 (MDR1) or ATP-binding cassette sub-family B member 1 (ABCB1) or cluster of differentiation 243 (CD243), is a glycoprotein that in humans is encoded by the ABCB1 gene. ABC transporters are transmembrane proteins that utilize the energy of adenosine triphosphate hydrolysis to carry out certain biological processes including translocation of various substrates across membranes and non-transport-related processes such as translation of RNA and DNA repair. Contradicting results have been reported for variants in ABCB1 and Gln192Arg allele in paraoxonase 1, which have been implicated in clopidogrel responsiveness. These associations need further confirmation [148-150].

8. Conclusion

Adverse drug reactions (ADRs) have been reported to be the cause for drug withdrawal after marketing, hospital admissions, death in hospitalised patients and to be the fourth leading cause of death in developed countries. The costs associated with ADRs may radically escalate the cost for healthcare.

There is an increasing use of multiple medications to treat patients with chronic illnesses. Drug-drug interactions are common and growing in frequency due to increasing numbers of medications available and the number of patients on multiple medications. The knowledge of the pharmacodynamics and pharmacokinetics of the drugs helps to avoid unintended and problematic drug interactions. Several web sites, books, and cards are available for the clinician. The web sites are updated on a regular basis and are useful tools for prescribers.

The necessity to understand drug combination pharmacokinetics and pharmacodinamics in drug interactions is illustrated by the following example: a patient who is taking a drug equally cleared by CYP2D6 and CYP3A. That patient may not be at substantial risk for toxicity when treated with either a CYP2D6 or CYP3A inhibitor alone, but may be if treated with both inhibitors at the same time [151]. Pharmacodynamic or pharmacokinetic drug interaction is a complex process and includes understanding of individual variations in drug metabolism.

Pharmacogenetics has a potential role in reducing ADRs at the pre-marketing and post-marketing stages of drug development and in clinical care. A priori identification of individuals at risk of developing ADRs for a given drug will help develop strategies to reduce the risk for ADRs in these patients. It can also be used to identify individuals at risk of developing serious ADRs and to treat these individuals with alternative therapy, thus converting ADRs that are traditionally considered unavoidable to avoidable ADRs.

Although pharmacogenetics is a highly complex and ever-evolving science, it has amassed knowledge that can readily be used to provide efficient care to patients. It has been shown that gene variants that play a role in drug metabolism pathways can alter a patient's response or increase toxicity at normal dosage range, especially in combinational drug treatments. Pharmacogenetics seeks to understand the nature of variable drug responses. Several pharmacogenetics tests are already available for cardiovascular medications in biomedical laboratories (Table 1).

Pharmacogenetic findings may help to explain ethnic differences in drug response. The accumulated facts of ethnic differences in cardiovascular drug responses and the fact that many genetic polymorphisms differ in frequency on the basis of ethnicity (example in the Western Sydney population, Fig. 1) will undoubtedly support future development of pharmacogenetics in patient care and in drug interaction interpretation.

It is possible that use of genetic and other patient-specific information, including environmental factors will help guide drug therapy decisions for certain drugs and drug combinations.

Prevalence of clinically relevant polymorphisms with altered enzyme activity, Western Sydney Population Data

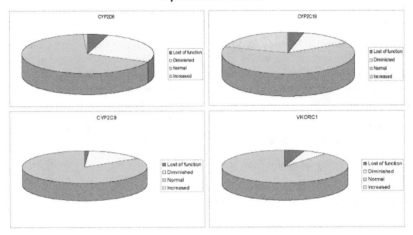

Distribution of CYP2D6 Poor Metabolisers and Ultra Extensive Metabolisers in different ethnic groups (combined data)

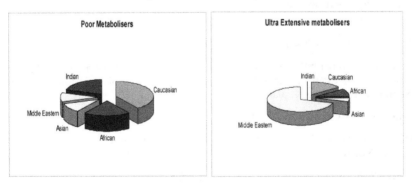

Figure 1. Example of diversity in prevalence of clinically relevant polymorphisms. (*Western Sydney Population combined data. WSLHD population is a mix of Caucasians, Asians and Africans.)

Appendix

Glossary of some Pharmacogenetic Terms

- **Allele:** An alternative form of a gene at a given locus.

- **Genetic polymorphism:** Minor allele frequency of ≥1% in the population.

- **Genome:** The complete DNA sequence of an organism. Sum total of the genetic material included in every cell of the human body, apart from the red blood cells.

- **Genomewide association study (GWAS):** A genetic association study in which the density of genetic markers and the extent of linkage disequilibrium are sufficient to capture a large proportion of the common variation in the human genome in the population under study, and the number of specimens genotyped provides sufficient power to detect variants of modest effect.

- **Genotype:** The alleles at a specific locus an individual carries. The genetic constitution of an individual, i.e. the specific allelic makeup of an individual.

- **Haplotype:** A group of alleles from two or more loci on a chromosome; inherited as a unit.

- **Heterozygote:** A person who has two copies of an allele that are different.

- **Homozygote:** A person who has two copies of an allele that are the same.

- **Pharmacogenetics:** A study of genetic causes of individual variations in drug response. In this review, the term "pharmacogenetics" is interchangeable with "pharmacogenomics."

- **Pharmacogenomics:** Genomewide analysis of the genetic determinants of drug efficacy and toxicity. Pharmacogenetics focuses on a single gene while pharmacogenomics studies multiple genes.

- **Phenotype:** Observable expression of a particular gene or genes.

- **Single nucleotide polymorphism (SNP):** is a DNA sequence variation occurring when a single nucleotide in the genome differs between members of a biological species or paired chromosomes in an individual.

Useful Internet Resources and databases:

- OMIM (Online Mendelian Inheritance in Man), National Centre for Biotechnology Information (NCBI): www.ncbi.nlm.nih.gov/sites/entrez?db=omim

- PharmGKB (The Pharmacogenetics and Pharmacogenomics Knowledge Base): www.pharmgkb.org/#public

- NCBI, Individual SNP information, such as genetic location, nucleotide and amino acid changes, and allele frequencies in diverse populations, can be obtained from dbSNP: www.ncbi.nlm.nih.gov/sites/entrez?db=snp

- Databases: ensembl (www.ensembl.org/index.html) and HapMap (www.hapmap.org/cgi-perl/gbrowse/hapmap_B35)

- FDA: http://www.fda.gov/Drugs/ScienceResearch/ResearchAreas/Pharmacogenetics

- FDA: Table of Pharmacogenomic Biomarkers in Drug Labels: http://www.fda.gov/Drugs/ScienceResearch/ResearchAreas/Pharmacogenetics/ucm083378.htm

Author details

Irina Piatkov*, Trudi Jones and Mark McLean

*Address all correspondence to: irina.piatkov@swahs.health.nsw.gov.au

University of Western Sydney, Blacktown Clinical School and Research Centre,, Blacktown Hospital, Western Sydney Local Health District, Blacktown, Australia

References

[1] Verschuren JJ, Trompet S, Wessels JA, Guchelaar HJ, de Maat MP, Simoons ML, Jukema JW (2012) A systematic review on pharmacogenetics in cardiovascular disease: is it ready for clinical application? Eur Heart J 33:165-175

[2] Scheen AJ (2011) Cytochrome P450-mediated cardiovascular drug interactions. Expert Opin Drug Metab Toxicol 7:1065-1082

[3] Rodriguez Arcas MJ, Garcia-Jimenez E, Martinez-Martinez F, Conesa-Zamora P (2011) Role of CYP450 in pharmacokinetics and pharmacogenetics of antihypertensive drugs. Farm Hosp 35:84-92

[4] Roden DM, Johnson JA, Kimmel SE, Krauss RM, Medina MW, Shuldiner A, Wilke RA (2011) Cardiovascular pharmacogenomics. Circ Res 109:807-820

[5] Masca N, Sheehan NA, Tobin MD (2011) Pharmacogenetic interactions and their potential effects on genetic analyses of blood pressure. Stat Med 30:769-783

[6] Howe LA (2011) Pharmacogenomics and management of cardiovascular disease. Nursing 41 Suppl:1-7

[7] PharmGKB d (2011) http://www.pharmgkb.org/. Stanford University

[8] Chobanian AV, Bakris GL, Black HR, Cushman WC, Green LA, Izzo JL, Jr., Jones DW, Materson BJ, Oparil S, Wright JT, Jr., Roccella EJ (2003) The Seventh Report of the Joint National Committee on Prevention, Detection, Evaluation, and Treatment of High Blood Pressure: the JNC 7 report. Jama 289:2560-2572

[9] Egan BM, Zhao Y, Axon RN (2010) US trends in prevalence, awareness, treatment, and control of hypertension, 1988-2008. Jama 303:2043-2050

[10] AHA (2008) Heart Disease and Stroke Statistics - 2008 Update. American Heart Association

[11] Brodde OE (2008) Beta-1 and beta-2 adrenoceptor polymorphisms: functional importance, impact on cardiovascular diseases and drug responses. Pharmacol Ther 117:1-29

[12] Liu J, Liu ZQ, Tan ZR, Chen XP, Wang LS, Zhou G, Zhou HH (2003) Gly389Arg polymorphism of beta1-adrenergic receptor is associated with the cardiovascular response to metoprolol. Clin Pharmacol Ther 74:372-379

[13] Lanfear DE, Jones PG, Marsh S, Cresci S, McLeod HL, Spertus JA (2005) Beta2-adrenergic receptor genotype and survival among patients receiving beta-blocker therapy after an acute coronary syndrome. Jama 294:1526-1533

[14] Lanfear DE, Spertus JA, McLeod HL (2006) Beta2-adrenergic receptor genotype predicts survival: implications and future directions. J Cardiovasc Nurs 21:474-477

[15] Pacanowski MA, Gong Y, Cooper-Dehoff RM, Schork NJ, Shriver MD, Langaee TY, Pepine CJ, Johnson JA (2008) beta-adrenergic receptor gene polymorphisms and beta-blocker treatment outcomes in hypertension. Clin Pharmacol Ther 84:715-721

[16] Lemaitre RN, Heckbert SR, Sotoodehnia N, Bis JC, Smith NL, Marciante KD, Hindorff LA, Lange LA, Lumley TS, Rice KM, Wiggins KL, Psaty BM (2008) beta1- and beta2-adrenergic receptor gene variation, beta-blocker use and risk of myocardial infarction and stroke. Am J Hypertens 21:290-296

[17] Lemaitre RN, Siscovick DS, Psaty BM, Pearce RM, Raghunathan TE, Whitsel EA, Weinmann SA, Anderson GD, Lin D (2002) Inhaled beta-2 adrenergic receptor agonists and primary cardiac arrest. Am J Med 113:711-716

[18] Hunt SA, Baker DW, Chin MH, Cinquegrani MP, Feldman AM, Francis GS, Ganiats TG, Goldstein S, Gregoratos G, Jessup ML, Noble RJ, Packer M, Silver MA, Stevenson LW, Gibbons RJ, Antman EM, Alpert JS, Faxon DP, Fuster V, Jacobs AK, Hiratzka LF, Russell RO, Smith SC, Jr. (2001) ACC/AHA guidelines for the evaluation and management of chronic heart failure in the adult: executive summary. A report of the American College of Cardiology/American Heart Association Task Force on Practice Guidelines (Committee to revise the 1995 Guidelines for the Evaluation and Management of Heart Failure). J Am Coll Cardiol 38:2101-2113

[19] Marez D, Legrand M, Sabbagh N, Lo Guidice JM, Spire C, Lafitte JJ, Meyer UA, Broly F (1997) Polymorphism of the cytochrome P450 CYP2D6 gene in a European population: characterization of 48 mutations and 53 alleles, their frequencies and evolution. Pharmacogenetics 7:193-202

[20] Relling MV, Cherrie J, Schell MJ, Petros WP, Meyer WH, Evans WE (1991) Lower prevalence of the debrisoquin oxidative poor metabolizer phenotype in American black versus white subjects. Clin Pharmacol Ther 50:308-313

[21] Zhou HH, Wood AJ (1995) Stereoselective disposition of carvedilol is determined by CYP2D6. Clin Pharmacol Ther 57:518-524

[22] Wang B, Wang J, Huang SQ, Su HH, Zhou SF (2009) Genetic Polymorphism of the Human Cytochrome P450 2C9 Gene and Its Clinical Significance. Curr Drug Metab 10:781-834

[23] Beitelshees AL, Gong Y, Wang D, Schork NJ, Cooper-Dehoff RM, Langaee TY, Shriver MD, Sadee W, Knot HJ, Pepine CJ, Johnson JA (2007) KCNMB1 genotype influences response to verapamil SR and adverse outcomes in the INternational VErapamil SR/Trandolapril STudy (INVEST). Pharmacogenet Genomics 17:719-729

[24] Beitelshees AL, Navare H, Wang D, Gong Y, Wessel J, Moss JI, Langaee TY, Cooper-DeHoff RM, Sadee W, Pepine CJ, Schork NJ, Johnson JA (2009) CACNA1C gene polymorphisms, cardiovascular disease outcomes, and treatment response. Circ Cardiovasc Genet 2:362-370

[25] Niu Y, Gong Y, Langaee TY, Davis HM, Elewa H, Beitelshees AL, Moss JI, Cooper-Dehoff RM, Pepine CJ, Johnson JA (2010) Genetic variation in the beta2 subunit of the voltage-gated calcium channel and pharmacogenetic association with adverse cardiovascular outcomes in the INternational VErapamil SR-Trandolapril STudy GENEtic Substudy (INVEST-GENES). Circ Cardiovasc Genet 3:548-555

[26] Sherva R, Ford CE, Eckfeldt JH, Davis BR, Boerwinkle E, Arnett DK (2011) Pharmacogenetic effect of the stromelysin (MMP3) polymorphism on stroke risk in relation to antihypertensive treatment: the genetics of hypertension associated treatment study. Stroke 42:330-335

[27] Svensson-Farbom P, Wahlstrand B, Almgren P, Dahlberg J, Fava C, Kjeldsen S, Hedner T, Melander O (2011) A functional variant of the NEDD4L gene is associated with beneficial treatment response with beta-blockers and diuretics in hypertensive patients. J Hypertens 29:388-395

[28] Schelleman H, Klungel OH, Witteman JC, Breteler MM, Hofman A, van Duijn CM, de Boer A, Stricker BH (2008) Interaction between polymorphisms in the renin-angiotensin-system and angiotensin-converting enzyme inhibitor or beta-blocker use and the risk of myocardial infarction and stroke. Pharmacogenomics J 8:400-407

[29] Schelleman H, Klungel OH, Witteman JC, Breteler MM, Yazdanpanah M, Danser AH, Hofman A, van Duijn CM, de Boer A, Stricker BH (2007) Angiotensinogen M235T polymorphism and the risk of myocardial infarction and stroke among hypertensive patients on ACE-inhibitors or beta-blockers. Eur J Hum Genet 15:478-484

[30] Turner ST, Bailey KR, Fridley BL, Chapman AB, Schwartz GL, Chai HS, Sicotte H, Kocher JP, Rodin AS, Boerwinkle E (2008) Genomic association analysis suggests

chromosome 12 locus influencing antihypertensive response to thiazide diuretic. Hypertension 52:359-365

[31] Duarte JD, Turner ST, Tran B, Chapman AB, Bailey KR, Gong Y, Gums JG, Langaee TY, Beitelshees AL, Cooper-Dehoff RM, Boerwinkle E, Johnson JA (2012) Association of chromosome 12 locus with antihypertensive response to hydrochlorothiazide may involve differential YEATS4 expression. Pharmacogenomics J

[32] Lynch AI, Boerwinkle E, Davis BR, Ford CE, Eckfeldt JH, Leiendecker-Foster C, Arnett DK (2008) Pharmacogenetic association of the NPPA T2238C genetic variant with cardiovascular disease outcomes in patients with hypertension. Jama 299:296-307

[33] Hollier JM, Martin DF, Bell DM, Li JL, Chirachanchai MG, Menon DV, Leonard D, Wu X, Cooper RS, McKenzie C, Victor RG, Auchus RJ (2006) Epithelial sodium channel allele T594M is not associated with blood pressure or blood pressure response to amiloride. Hypertension 47:428-433

[34] Swift PA, Macgregor GA (2004) Genetic variation in the epithelial sodium channel: a risk factor for hypertension in people of African origin. Adv Ren Replace Ther 11:76-86

[35] Manunta P, Lavery G, Lanzani C, Braund PS, Simonini M, Bodycote C, Zagato L, Delli Carpini S, Tantardini C, Brioni E, Bianchi G, Samani NJ (2008) Physiological interaction between alpha-adducin and WNK1-NEDD4L pathways on sodium-related blood pressure regulation. Hypertension 52:366-372

[36] Lanzani C, Citterio L, Glorioso N, Manunta P, Tripodi G, Salvi E, Carpini SD, Ferrandi M, Messaggio E, Staessen JA, Cusi D, Macciardi F, Argiolas G, Valentini G, Ferrari P, Bianchi G Adducin- and ouabain-related gene variants predict the antihypertensive activity of rostafuroxin, part 2: clinical studies. Sci Transl Med 2:59ra87

[37] Vormfelde SV, Sehrt D, Bolte D, Pahl S, Tzvetkov M, Brockmoller J (2006) Hydrochlorothiazide efficacy and polymorphisms in ACE, ADD1 and GNB3 in healthy, male volunteers. Eur J Clin Pharmacol 62:195-201

[38] Psaty BM, Smith NL, Heckbert SR, Vos HL, Lemaitre RN, Reiner AP, Siscovick DS, Bis J, Lumley T, Longstreth WT, Jr., Rosendaal FR (2002) Diuretic therapy, the alpha-adducin gene variant, and the risk of myocardial infarction or stroke in persons with treated hypertension. Jama 287:1680-1689

[39] Davis BR, Arnett DK, Boerwinkle E, Ford CE, Leiendecker-Foster C, Miller MB, Black H, Eckfeldt JH (2007) Antihypertensive therapy, the alpha-adducin polymorphism, and cardiovascular disease in high-risk hypertensive persons: the Genetics of Hypertension-Associated Treatment Study. Pharmacogenomics J 7:112-122

[40] Gerhard T, Gong Y, Beitelshees AL, Mao X, Lobmeyer MT, Cooper-DeHoff RM, Langaee TY, Schork NJ, Shriver MD, Pepine CJ, Johnson JA (2008) Alpha-adducin polymorphism associated with increased risk of adverse cardiovascular outcomes: results

from GENEtic Substudy of the INternational VErapamil SR-trandolapril STudy (IN-VEST-GENES). Am Heart J 156:397-404

[41] Poch E, Gonzalez-Nunez D, Compte M, De la Sierra A (2002) G-protein beta3-subu-nit gene variant, blood pressure and erythrocyte sodium/lithium countertransport in essential hypertension. Br J Biomed Sci 59:101-104

[42] Brugts JJ, Isaacs A, de Maat MP, Boersma E, van Duijn CM, Akkerhuis KM, Uitterlin-den AG, Witteman JC, Cambien F, Ceconi C, Remme W, Bertrand M, Ninomiya T, Harrap S, Chalmers J, Macmahon S, Fox K, Ferrari R, Simoons ML, Danser AJ (2011) A pharmacogenetic analysis of determinants of hypertension and blood pressure re-sponse to angiotensin-converting enzyme inhibitor therapy in patients with vascular disease and healthy individuals. J Hypertens 29:509-519

[43] He J, Gu D, Kelly TN, Hixson JE, Rao DC, Jaquish CE, Chen J, Zhao Q, Gu C, Huang J, Shimmin LC, Chen JC, Mu J, Ji X, Liu DP, Whelton PK (2011) Genetic variants in the renin-angiotensin-aldosterone system and blood pressure responses to potassium intake. J Hypertens 29:1719-1730

[44] Katsuya T, Iwashima Y, Sugimoto K, Motone M, Asai T, Fukuda M, Fu Y, Hatanaka Y, Ohishi M, Rakugi H, Higaki J, Ogihara T (2001) Effects of antihypertensive drugs and gene variants in the renin-angiotensin system. Hypertens Res 24:463-467

[45] Konoshita T (2011) Do genetic variants of the Renin-Angiotensin system predict blood pressure response to Renin-Angiotensin system-blocking drugs?: a systematic review of pharmacogenomics in the Renin-Angiotensin system. Curr Hypertens Rep 13:356-361

[46] Kraja AT, Hunt SC, Rao DC, Davila-Roman VG, Arnett DK, Province MA (2011) Ge-netics of hypertension and cardiovascular disease and their interconnected path-ways: lessons from large studies. Curr Hypertens Rep 13:46-54

[47] Ceyhan K, Kadi H, Celik A, Burucu T, Koc F, Sogut E, Sahin S, Onalan O (2012) An-giotensin-converting enzyme DD polymorphism is associated with poor coronary collateral circulation in patients with coronary artery disease. J Investig Med 60:49-55

[48] Prasad A, Narayanan S, Husain S, Padder F, Waclawiw M, Epstein N, Quyyumi AA (2000) Insertion-deletion polymorphism of the ACE gene modulates reversibility of endothelial dysfunction with ACE inhibition. Circulation 102:35-41

[49] Stavroulakis GA, Makris TK, Krespi PG, Hatzizacharias AN, Gialeraki AE, Anasta-siadis G, Triposkiadis P, Kyriakidis M (2000) Predicting response to chronic antihy-pertensive treatment with fosinopril: the role of angiotensin-converting enzyme gene polymorphism. Cardiovasc Drugs Ther 14:427-432

[50] Ohmichi N, Iwai N, Uchida Y, Shichiri G, Nakamura Y, Kinoshita M (1997) Relation-ship between the response to the angiotensin converting enzyme inhibitor imidapril and the angiotensin converting enzyme genotype. Am J Hypertens 10:951-955

[51] O'Toole L, Stewart M, Padfield P, Channer K (1998) Effect of the insertion/deletion polymorphism of the angiotensin-converting enzyme gene on response to angiotensin-converting enzyme inhibitors in patients with heart failure. J Cardiovasc Pharmacol 32:988-994

[52] Takahashi T, Yamaguchi E, Furuya K, Kawakami Y (2001) The ACE gene polymorphism and cough threshold for capsaicin after cilazapril usage. Respir Med 95:130-135

[53] Schunkert H, Hense HW, Gimenez-Roqueplo AP, Stieber J, Keil U, Riegger GA, Jeunemaitre X (1997) The angiotensinogen T235 variant and the use of antihypertensive drugs in a population-based cohort. Hypertension 29:628-633

[54] van Geel PP, Pinto YM, Zwinderman AH, Henning RH, van Boven AJ, Jukema JW, Bruschke AV, Kastelein JJ, van Gilst WH (2001) Increased risk for ischaemic events is related to combined RAS polymorphism. Heart 85:458-462

[55] Benetos A, Topouchian J, Ricard S, Gautier S, Bonnardeaux A, Asmar R, Poirier O, Soubrier F, Safar M, Cambien F (1995) Influence of angiotensin II type 1 receptor polymorphism on aortic stiffness in never-treated hypertensive patients. Hypertension 26:44-47

[56] Benetos A, Cambien F, Gautier S, Ricard S, Safar M, Laurent S, Lacolley P, Poirier O, Topouchian J, Asmar R (1996) Influence of the angiotensin II type 1 receptor gene polymorphism on the effects of perindopril and nitrendipine on arterial stiffness in hypertensive individuals. Hypertension 28:1081-1084

[57] Filigheddu F, Argiolas G, Bulla E, Troffa C, Bulla P, Fadda S, Zaninello R, Degortes S, Frau F, Pitzoi S, Glorioso N (2008) Clinical variables, not RAAS polymorphisms, predict blood pressure response to ACE inhibitors in Sardinians. Pharmacogenomics 9:1419-1427

[58] Kurland L, Melhus H, Karlsson J, Kahan T, Malmqvist K, Ohman KP, Nystrom F, Hagg A, Lind L (2001) Angiotensin converting enzyme gene polymorphism predicts blood pressure response to angiotensin II receptor type 1 antagonist treatment in hypertensive patients. J Hypertens 19:1783-1787

[59] Bremer T, Man A, Kask K, Diamond C (2006) CACNA1C polymorphisms are associated with the efficacy of calcium channel blockers in the treatment of hypertension. Pharmacogenomics 7:271-279

[60] Langaee TY, Gong Y, Yarandi HN, Katz DA, Cooper-DeHoff RM, Pepine CJ, Johnson JA (2007) Association of CYP3A5 polymorphisms with hypertension and antihypertensive response to verapamil. Clin Pharmacol Ther 81:386-391

[61] Makris M, van Veen JJ, Maclean R (2010) Warfarin anticoagulation reversal: management of the asymptomatic and bleeding patient. J Thromb Thrombolysis 29:171-181

[62] Watson HG, Baglin T, Laidlaw SL, Makris M, Preston FE (2001) A comparison of the efficacy and rate of response to oral and intravenous Vitamin K in reversal of over-anticoagulation with warfarin. Br J Haematol 115:145-149

[63] Horne BD, Lenzini PA, Wadelius M, Jorgensen AL, Kimmel SE, Ridker PM, Eriksson N, Anderson JL, Pirmohamed M, Limdi NA, Pendleton RC, McMillin GA, Burmester JK, Kurnik D, Stein CM, Caldwell MD, Eby CS, Rane A, Lindh JD, Shin JG, Kim HS, Angchaisuksiri P, Glynn RJ, Kronquist KE, Carlquist JF, Grice GR, Barrack RL, Li J, Gage BF (2012) Pharmacogenetic warfarin dose refinements remain significantly influenced by genetic factors after one week of therapy. Thromb Haemost 107:232-240

[64] Johnson JA, Gong L, Whirl-Carrillo M, Gage BF, Scott SA, Stein CM, Anderson JL, Kimmel SE, Lee MT, Pirmohamed M, Wadelius M, Klein TE, Altman RB (2011) Clinical Pharmacogenetics Implementation Consortium Guidelines for CYP2C9 and VKORC1 genotypes and warfarin dosing. Clinical pharmacology and therapeutics 90:625-629

[65] Limdi NA, Wadelius M, Cavallari L, Eriksson N, Crawford DC, Lee MT, Chen CH, Motsinger-Reif A, Sagreiya H, Liu N, Wu AH, Gage BF, Jorgensen A, Pirmohamed M, Shin JG, Suarez-Kurtz G, Kimmel SE, Johnson JA, Klein TE, Wagner MJ (2010) Warfarin pharmacogenetics: a single VKORC1 polymorphism is predictive of dose across 3 racial groups. Blood 115:3827-3834

[66] Palareti G, Leali N, Coccheri S, Poggi M, Manotti C, D'Angelo A, Pengo V, Erba N, Moia M, Ciavarella N, Devoto G, Berretini M, Musolesi S (1997) [Hemorrhagic complications of oral anticoagulant therapy: results of a prospective multicenter study IS-COAT (Italian Study on Complications of Oral Anticoagulant Therapy)]. G Ital Cardiol 27:231-243

[67] Hirsh J, Bates SM (2001) Clinical trials that have influenced the treatment of venous thromboembolism: a historical perspective. Ann Intern Med 134:409-417

[68] Jones DR, Kim SY, Guderyon M, Yun CH, Moran JH, Miller GP (2010) Hydroxywarfarin metabolites potently inhibit CYP2C9 metabolism of S-warfarin. Chem Res Toxicol 23:939-945

[69] Kamali F, Wynne H (2010) Pharmacogenetics of warfarin. Annu Rev Med 61:63-75

[70] Kaminsky LS, Zhang ZY (1997) Human P450 metabolism of warfarin. Pharmacol Ther 73:67-74

[71] Adcock DM, Koftan C, Crisan D, Kiechle FL (2004) Effect of polymorphisms in the cytochrome P450 CYP2C9 gene on warfarin anticoagulation. Arch Pathol Lab Med 128:1360-1363

[72] Takahashi H, Echizen H (2001) Pharmacogenetics of warfarin elimination and its clinical implications. Clin Pharmacokinet 40:587-603

[73] Rettie AE, Wienkers LC, Gonzalez FJ, Trager WF, Korzekwa KR (1994) Impaired (S)-warfarin metabolism catalysed by the R144C allelic variant of CYP2C9. Pharmacogenetics 4:39-42

[74] Haining RL, Hunter AP, Veronese ME, Trager WF, Rettie AE (1996) Allelic variants of human cytochrome P450 2C9: baculovirus-mediated expression, purification, structural characterization, substrate stereoselectivity, and prochiral selectivity of the wild-type and I359L mutant forms. Arch Biochem Biophys 333:447-458

[75] Steward DJ, Haining RL, Henne KR, Davis G, Rushmore TH, Trager WF, Rettie AE (1997) Genetic association between sensitivity to warfarin and expression of CYP2C9*3. Pharmacogenetics 7:361-367

[76] Margaglione M, Colaizzo D, D'Andrea G, Brancaccio V, Ciampa A, Grandone E, Di Minno G (2000) Genetic modulation of oral anticoagulation with warfarin. Thromb Haemost 84:775-778

[77] Scordo MG, Pengo V, Spina E, Dahl ML, Gusella M, Padrini R (2002) Influence of CYP2C9 and CYP2C19 genetic polymorphisms on warfarin maintenance dose and metabolic clearance. Clin Pharmacol Ther 72:702-710

[78] Visser LE, van Vliet M, van Schaik RH, Kasbergen AA, De Smet PA, Vulto AG, Hofman A, van Duijn CM, Stricker BH (2004) The risk of overanticoagulation in patients with cytochrome P450 CYP2C9*2 or CYP2C9*3 alleles on acenocoumarol or phenprocoumon. Pharmacogenetics 14:27-33

[79] Furuya H, Fernandez-Salguero P, Gregory W, Taber H, Steward A, Gonzalez FJ, Idle JR (1995) Genetic polymorphism of CYP2C9 and its effect on warfarin maintenance dose requirement in patients undergoing anticoagulation therapy. Pharmacogenetics 5:389-392

[80] Aithal GP, Day CP, Kesteven PJ, Daly AK (1999) Association of polymorphisms in the cytochrome P450 CYP2C9 with warfarin dose requirement and risk of bleeding complications. Lancet 353:717-719

[81] Higashi MK, Veenstra DL, Kondo LM, Wittkowsky AK, Srinouanprachanh SL, Farin FM, Rettie AE (2002) Association between CYP2C9 genetic variants and anticoagulation-related outcomes during warfarin therapy. Jama 287:1690-1698

[82] Tabrizi AR, Zehnbauer BA, Borecki IB, McGrath SD, Buchman TG, Freeman BD (2002) The frequency and effects of cytochrome P450 (CYP) 2C9 polymorphisms in patients receiving warfarin. J Am Coll Surg 194:267-273

[83] Taube J, Halsall D, Baglin T (2000) Influence of cytochrome P-450 CYP2C9 polymorphisms on warfarin sensitivity and risk of over-anticoagulation in patients on long-term treatment. Blood 96:1816-1819

[84] Wadelius M, Sorlin K, Wallerman O, Karlsson J, Yue QY, Magnusson PK, Wadelius C, Melhus H (2004) Warfarin sensitivity related to CYP2C9, CYP3A5, ABCB1 (MDR1) and other factors. Pharmacogenomics J 4:40-48

[85] Freeman BD, Zehnbauer BA, McGrath S, Borecki I, Buchman TG (2000) Cytochrome P450 polymorphisms are associated with reduced warfarin dose. Surgery 128:281-285

[86] Takahashi H, Echizen H (2003) Pharmacogenetics of CYP2C9 and interindividual variability in anticoagulant response to warfarin. Pharmacogenomics J 3:202-214

[87] London SJ, Daly AK, Leathart JB, Navidi WC, Idle JR (1996) Lung cancer risk in relation to the CYP2C9*1/CYP2C9*2 genetic polymorphism among African-Americans and Caucasians in Los Angeles County, California. Pharmacogenetics 6:527-533

[88] Nasu K, Kubota T, Ishizaki T (1997) Genetic analysis of CYP2C9 polymorphism in a Japanese population. Pharmacogenetics 7:405-409

[89] Bhasker CR, Miners JO, Coulter S, Birkett DJ (1997) Allelic and functional variability of cytochrome P4502C9. Pharmacogenetics 7:51-58

[90] Schalekamp T, Klungel OH, Souverein PC, de Boer A (2008) Increased bleeding risk with concurrent use of selective serotonin reuptake inhibitors and coumarins. Arch Intern Med 168:180-185

[91] Dalton SO, Sorensen HT, Johansen C (2006) SSRIs and upper gastrointestinal bleeding: what is known and how should it influence prescribing? CNS Drugs 20:143-151

[92] Meijer WE, Heerdink ER, Leufkens HG, Herings RM, Egberts AC, Nolen WA (2004) Incidence and determinants of long-term use of antidepressants. Eur J Clin Pharmacol 60:57-61

[93] Greenblatt DJ, von Moltke LL, Harmatz JS, Shader RI (1998) Drug interactions with newer antidepressants: role of human cytochromes P450. J Clin Psychiatry 59 Suppl 15:19-27

[94] DeVane CL (1998) Differential pharmacology of newer antidepressants. J Clin Psychiatry 59 Suppl 20:85-93

[95] Duncan D, Sayal K, McConnell H, Taylor D (1998) Antidepressant interactions with warfarin. Int Clin Psychopharmacol 13:87-94

[96] Sayal KS, Duncan-McConnell DA, McConnell HW, Taylor DM (2000) Psychotropic interactions with warfarin. Acta Psychiatr Scand 102:250-255

[97] Hauta-Aho M, Tirkkonen T, Vahlberg T, Laine K (2009) The effect of drug interactions on bleeding risk associated with warfarin therapy in hospitalized patients. Ann Med 41:619-628

[98] Wallerstedt SM, Gleerup H, Sundstrom A, Stigendal L, Ny L (2009) Risk of clinically relevant bleeding in warfarin-treated patients--influence of SSRI treatment. Pharmacoepidemiol Drug Saf 18:412-416

[99] Wessinger S, Kaplan M, Choi L, Williams M, Lau C, Sharp L, Crowell MD, Keshavarzian A, Jones MP (2006) Increased use of selective serotonin reuptake inhibitors in

patients admitted with gastrointestinal haemorrhage: a multicentre retrospective analysis. Aliment Pharmacol Ther 23:937-944

[100] Castro TA, Heineck I (2012) Interventions to Improve Anticoagulation With Warfarin. Ther Drug Monit 34:209-216

[101] Zhang Q, Bal-dit-Sollier C, Drouet L, Simoneau G, Alvarez JC, Pruvot S, Aubourg R, Berge N, Bergmann JF, Mouly S, Mahe I (2011) Interaction between acetaminophen and warfarin in adults receiving long-term oral anticoagulants: a randomized controlled trial. Eur J Clin Pharmacol 67:309-314

[102] Burgess JK, Lindeman R, Chesterman CN, Chong BH (1995) Single amino acid mutation of Fc gamma receptor is associated with the development of heparin-induced thrombocytopenia. Br J Haematol 91:761-766

[103] Carlsson LE, Santoso S, Baurichter G, Kroll H, Papenberg S, Eichler P, Westerdaal NA, Kiefel V, van de Winkel JG, Greinacher A (1998) Heparin-induced thrombocytopenia: new insights into the impact of the FcgammaRIIa-R-H131 polymorphism. Blood 92:1526-1531

[104] Arepally G, McKenzie SE, Jiang XM, Poncz M, Cines DB (1997) Fc gamma RIIA H/R 131 polymorphism, subclass-specific IgG anti-heparin/platelet factor 4 antibodies and clinical course in patients with heparin-induced thrombocytopenia and thrombosis. Blood 89:370-375

[105] Waters DD (2001) What do the statin trials tell us? Am J Manag Care 7:S138-143

[106] Poduri A, Khullar M, Bahl A, Sehrawat BS, Sharma Y, Talwar KK (2010) Common variants of HMGCR, CETP, APOAI, ABCB1, CYP3A4, and CYP7A1 genes as predictors of lipid-lowering response to atorvastatin therapy. DNA Cell Biol 29:629-637

[107] Chasman DI, Posada D, Subrahmanyan L, Cook NR, Stanton VP, Jr., Ridker PM (2004) Pharmacogenetic study of statin therapy and cholesterol reduction. Jama 291:2821-2827

[108] Boekholdt SM, Kuivenhoven JA, Hovingh GK, Jukema JW, Kastelein JJ, van Tol A (2004) CETP gene variation: relation to lipid parameters and cardiovascular risk. Curr Opin Lipidol 15:393-398

[109] Kuivenhoven JA, Hovingh GK, van Tol A, Jauhiainen M, Ehnholm C, Fruchart JC, Brinton EA, Otvos JD, Smelt AH, Brownlee A, Zwinderman AH, Hayden MR, Kastelein JJ (2003) Heterozygosity for ABCA1 gene mutations: effects on enzymes, apolipoproteins and lipoprotein particle size. Atherosclerosis 171:311-319

[110] de Maat MP, Kastelein JJ, Jukema JW, Zwinderman AH, Jansen H, Groenemeier B, Bruschke AV, Kluft C (1998) -455G/A polymorphism of the beta-fibrinogen gene is associated with the progression of coronary atherosclerosis in symptomatic men: proposed role for an acute-phase reaction pattern of fibrinogen. REGRESS group. Arterioscler Thromb Vasc Biol 18:265-271

[111] Bray PF, Cannon CP, Goldschmidt-Clermont P, Moye LA, Pfeffer MA, Sacks FM, Braunwald E (2001) The platelet Pl(A2) and angiotensin-converting enzyme (ACE) D allele polymorphisms and the risk of recurrent events after acute myocardial infarction. Am J Cardiol 88:347-352

[112] Sacks FM, Pfeffer MA, Moye LA, Rouleau JL, Rutherford JD, Cole TG, Brown L, Warnica JW, Arnold JM, Wun CC, Davis BR, Braunwald E (1996) The effect of pravastatin on coronary events after myocardial infarction in patients with average cholesterol levels. Cholesterol and Recurrent Events Trial investigators. N Engl J Med 335:1001-1009

[113] Gerdes LU, Gerdes C, Kervinen K, Savolainen M, Klausen IC, Hansen PS, Kesaniemi YA, Faergeman O (2000) The apolipoprotein epsilon4 allele determines prognosis and the effect on prognosis of simvastatin in survivors of myocardial infarction : a substudy of the Scandinavian simvastatin survival study. Circulation 101:1366-1371

[114] Donnelly LA, Doney AS, Dannfald J, Whitley AL, Lang CC, Morris AD, Donnan PT, Palmer CN (2008) A paucimorphic variant in the HMG-CoA reductase gene is associated with lipid-lowering response to statin treatment in diabetes: a GoDARTS study. Pharmacogenet Genomics 18:1021-1026

[115] Kajinami K, Brousseau ME, Ordovas JM, Schaefer EJ (2004) CYP3A4 genotypes and plasma lipoprotein levels before and after treatment with atorvastatin in primary hypercholesterolemia. Am J Cardiol 93:104-107

[116] Wang A, Yu BN, Luo CH, Tan ZR, Zhou G, Wang LS, Zhang W, Li Z, Liu J, Zhou HH (2005) Ile118Val genetic polymorphism of CYP3A4 and its effects on lipid-lowering efficacy of simvastatin in Chinese hyperlipidemic patients. Eur J Clin Pharmacol 60:843-848

[117] Gao Y, Zhang LR, Fu Q (2008) CYP3A4*1G polymorphism is associated with lipid-lowering efficacy of atorvastatin but not of simvastatin. Eur J Clin Pharmacol 64:877-882

[118] Krauss RM, Mangravite LM, Smith JD, Medina MW, Wang D, Guo X, Rieder MJ, Simon JA, Hulley SB, Waters D, Saad M, Williams PT, Taylor KD, Yang H, Nickerson DA, Rotter JI (2008) Variation in the 3-hydroxyl-3-methylglutaryl coenzyme a reductase gene is associated with racial differences in low-density lipoprotein cholesterol response to simvastatin treatment. Circulation 117:1537-1544

[119] Mangravite LM, Wilke RA, Zhang J, Krauss RM (2008) Pharmacogenomics of statin response. Curr Opin Mol Ther 10:555-561

[120] Wilke RA, Moore JH, Burmester JK (2005) Relative impact of CYP3A genotype and concomitant medication on the severity of atorvastatin-induced muscle damage. Pharmacogenet Genomics 15:415-421

[121] Pasanen MK, Neuvonen M, Neuvonen PJ, Niemi M (2006) SLCO1B1 polymorphism markedly affects the pharmacokinetics of simvastatin acid. Pharmacogenet Genomics 16:873-879

[122] Voora D, Shah SH, Spasojevic I, Ali S, Reed CR, Salisbury BA, Ginsburg GS (2009) The SLCO1B1*5 genetic variant is associated with statin-induced side effects. J Am Coll Cardiol 54:1609-1616

[123] Donnelly LA, Doney AS, Tavendale R, Lang CC, Pearson ER, Colhoun HM, McCarthy MI, Hattersley AT, Morris AD, Palmer CN (2011) Common nonsynonymous substitutions in SLCO1B1 predispose to statin intolerance in routinely treated individuals with type 2 diabetes: a go-DARTS study. Clin Pharmacol Ther 89:210-216

[124] Li Y, Sabatine MS, Tong CH, Ford I, Kirchgessner TG, Packard CJ, Robertson M, Rowland CM, Bare LA, Shepherd J, Devlin JJ, Iakoubova OA (2011) Genetic variants in the KIF6 region and coronary event reduction from statin therapy. Hum Genet 129:17-23

[125] Catapano AL (2012) Statin-induced myotoxicity: pharmacokinetic differences among statins and the risk of rhabdomyolysis, with particular reference to pitavastatin. Curr Vasc Pharmacol 10:257-267

[126] Priori SG, Barhanin J, Hauer RN, Haverkamp W, Jongsma HJ, Kleber AG, McKenna WJ, Roden DM, Rudy Y, Schwartz K, Schwartz PJ, Towbin JA, Wilde AM (1999) Genetic and molecular basis of cardiac arrhythmias: impact on clinical management parts I and II. Circulation 99:518-528

[127] Thorn HA, Lundahl A, Schrickx JA, Dickinson PA, Lennernas H (2011) Drug metabolism of CYP3A4, CYP2C9 and CYP2D6 substrates in pigs and humans. Eur J Pharm Sci 43:89-98

[128] Ylitalo P, Ruosteenoja R, Leskinen O, Metsa-Ketela T (1983) Significance of acetylator phenotype in pharmacokinetics and adverse effects of procainamide. Eur J Clin Pharmacol 25:791-795

[129] Roden DM (2006) Long QT syndrome: reduced repolarization reserve and the genetic link. J Intern Med 259:59-69

[130] Paulussen AD, Gilissen RA, Armstrong M, Doevendans PA, Verhasselt P, Smeets HJ, Schulze-Bahr E, Haverkamp W, Breithardt G, Cohen N, Aerssens J (2004) Genetic variations of KCNQ1, KCNH2, SCN5A, KCNE1, and KCNE2 in drug-induced long QT syndrome patients. J Mol Med (Berl) 82:182-188

[131] Yang P, Kanki H, Drolet B, Yang T, Wei J, Viswanathan PC, Hohnloser SH, Shimizu W, Schwartz PJ, Stanton M, Murray KT, Norris K, George AL, Jr., Roden DM (2002) Allelic variants in long-QT disease genes in patients with drug-associated torsades de pointes. Circulation 105:1943-1948

[132] Itoh H, Sakaguchi T, Ding WG, Watanabe E, Watanabe I, Nishio Y, Makiyama T, Ohno S, Akao M, Higashi Y, Zenda N, Kubota T, Mori C, Okajima K, Haruna T, Miya-

moto A, Kawamura M, Ishida K, Nagaoka I, Oka Y, Nakazawa Y, Yao T, Jo H, Sugimoto Y, Ashihara T, Hayashi H, Ito M, Imoto K, Matsuura H, Horie M (2009) Latent genetic backgrounds and molecular pathogenesis in drug-induced long-QT syndrome. Circ Arrhythm Electrophysiol 2:511-523

[133] Becker ML, Visser LE, Newton-Cheh C, Hofman A, Uitterlinden AG, Witteman JC, Stricker BH (2009) A common NOS1AP genetic polymorphism is associated with increased cardiovascular mortality in users of dihydropyridine calcium channel blockers. Br J Clin Pharmacol 67:61-67

[134] Crotti L, Monti MC, Insolia R, Peljto A, Goosen A, Brink PA, Greenberg DA, Schwartz PJ, George AL, Jr. (2009) NOS1AP is a genetic modifier of the long-QT syndrome. Circulation 120:1657-1663

[135] Tomas M, Napolitano C, De Giuli L, Bloise R, Subirana I, Malovini A, Bellazzi R, Arking DE, Marban E, Chakravarti A, Spooner PM, Priori SG (2010) Polymorphisms in the NOS1AP gene modulate QT interval duration and risk of arrhythmias in the long QT syndrome. J Am Coll Cardiol 55:2745-2752

[136] Undas A, Sanak M, Musial J, Szczeklik A (1999) Platelet glycoprotein IIIa polymorphism, aspirin, and thrombin generation. Lancet 353:982-983

[137] Goodman T, Ferro A, Sharma P (2008) Pharmacogenetics of aspirin resistance: a comprehensive systematic review. Br J Clin Pharmacol 66:222-232

[138] Goodall AH, Curzen N, Panesar M, Hurd C, Knight CJ, Ouwehand WH, Fox KM (1999) Increased binding of fibrinogen to glycoprotein IIIa-proline33 (HPA-1b, PlA2, Zwb) positive platelets in patients with cardiovascular disease. Eur Heart J 20:742-747

[139] Walter DH, Schachinger V, Elsner M, Dimmeler S, Zeiher AM (1997) Platelet glycoprotein IIIa polymorphisms and risk of coronary stent thrombosis. Lancet 350:1217-1219

[140] Kastrati A, Koch W, Gawaz M, Mehilli J, Bottiger C, Schomig K, von Beckerath N, Schomig A (2000) PlA polymorphism of glycoprotein IIIa and risk of adverse events after coronary stent placement. J Am Coll Cardiol 36:84-89

[141] Abbate R, Marcucci R, Camacho-Vanegas O, Pepe G, Gori AM, Capanni M, Simonetti I, Prisco D, Gensini GF (1998) Role of platelet glycoprotein PL(A1/A2) polymorphism in restenosis after percutaneous transluminal coronary angioplasty. Am J Cardiol 82:524-525

[142] Savi P, Nurden P, Nurden AT, Levy-Toledano S, Herbert JM (1998) Clopidogrel: a review of its mechanism of action. Platelets 9:251-255

[143] Shuldiner AR, O'Connell JR, Bliden KP, Gandhi A, Ryan K, Horenstein RB, Damcott CM, Pakyz R, Tantry US, Gibson Q, Pollin TI, Post W, Parsa A, Mitchell BD, Faraday N, Herzog W, Gurbel PA (2009) Association of cytochrome P450 2C19 genotype with the antiplatelet effect and clinical efficacy of clopidogrel therapy. Jama 302:849-857

[144] Mega JL, Simon T, Collet JP, Anderson JL, Antman EM, Bliden K, Cannon CP, Danchin N, Giusti B, Gurbel P, Horne BD, Hulot JS, Kastrati A, Montalescot G, Neumann FJ, Shen L, Sibbing D, Steg PG, Trenk D, Wiviott SD, Sabatine MS (2010) Reduced-function CYP2C19 genotype and risk of adverse clinical outcomes among patients treated with clopidogrel predominantly for PCI: a meta-analysis. Jama 304:1821-1830

[145] Roden DM, Stein CM (2009) Clopidogrel and the concept of high-risk pharmacokinetics. Circulation 119:2127-2130

[146] Santos PC, Soares RA, Santos DB, Nascimento RM, Coelho GL, Nicolau JC, Mill JG, Krieger JE, Pereira AC (2011) CYP2C19 and ABCB1 gene polymorphisms are differently distributed according to ethnicity in the Brazilian general population. BMC Med Genet 12:13

[147] Solus JF, Arietta BJ, Harris JR, Sexton DP, Steward JQ, McMunn C, Ihrie P, Mehall JM, Edwards TL, Dawson EP (2004) Genetic variation in eleven phase I drug metabolism genes in an ethnically diverse population. Pharmacogenomics 5:895-931

[148] Jaitner J, Morath T, Byrne RA, Braun S, Gebhard D, Bernlochner I, Schulz S, Mehilli J, Schomig A, Koch W, Kastrati A, Sibbing D (2012) No association of ABCB1 C3435T genotype with clopidogrel response or risk of stent thrombosis in patients undergoing coronary stenting. Circ Cardiovasc Interv 5:82-88, S81-82

[149] Kubica A, Kozinski M, Grzesk G, Fabiszak T, Navarese EP, Goch A (2011) Genetic determinants of platelet response to clopidogrel. J Thromb Thrombolysis 32:459-466

[150] Luo M, Li J, Xu X, Sun X, Sheng W (2011) ABCB1 C3435T polymorphism and risk of adverse clinical events in clopidogrel treated patients: A meta-analysis. Thromb Res

[151] Preskorn SH (2003) Relating clinical trials to psychiatric practice: part I: the case of a 13-year old on aripiprazole and fluoxetine. J Psychiatr Pract 9:307-313

Chapter 4

Small Molecule Screens to Identify Inhibitors of Infectious Disease

Elizabeth Hong-Geller and Sofiya Micheva-Viteva

Additional information is available at the end of the chapter

1. Introduction

In the 1940's, the development of penicillin as a potent broad-range antibiotic revolutionized the treatment of infectious disease and ushered in a prolific discovery period of natural small molecules produced by microorganisms that were antagonistic towards the growth of other bacteria. Antibiotics have generally been classified by their mechanism of action. For example, the β-lactam compounds, penicillin and cephalosporins, disrupt the synthesis of the peptidoglycan layer of the bacterial cell wall, whereas protein synthesis inhibitors, such as tetracycline and some aminoglycosides, bind to the 30S ribosomal subunit and block addition of amino acids to the growing peptide chain. By the 1960's, the majority of all antibiotics in use today had been isolated and developed for public consumption, leading the U.S. Surgeon General to declare in 1968 that the war on infectious disease had been won.

Unfortunately, nature has found a way to thwart mankind's effort to contain infectious disease. Under the selective pressure of antibiotics that target different cell processes, bacteria have evolved to become resistant to the lethal effects of many classes of antibiotics. One stark example that has emerged as a major public health threat is methicillin-resistant *Staphylococcus aureus* (MRSA), which is estimated to cause ~19,000 deaths in the US annually [1]. MRSA has become resistant to β-lactam antibiotics by acquiring the resistance gene *mecA*, which encodes for a unique penicillin binding protein PBP2A that can function as a surrogate for native staphylococcal PBPs normally inactivated by β-lactam antibiotics. In the last decades of the 20th century, MRSA has continued to evolve in response to a continually changing human environment, from a primary agent of hospital-acquired infections to a multi-drug resistant strain that has also acquired Tn1546 transposon-based vancomycin resistance. Furthermore, the appearance of MRSA strains in a community setting may be a stepping stone to the evolution of a completely drug-resistant strain.

There is no question that new strategies that target different aspects of pathogen function are urgently needed to combat multi-drug resistant bacteria. However, very few new scaffolds for drug discovery developed after the 1960s have been found to be effective [2]. To date, only four new classes of antibiotics, including mutilins and lipopeptides, have been introduced, but none of these have proven to be as effective as the panel of classic antibiotics. Instead, established scaffolds have been modified or re-purposed to develop successive generations of effective antibiotics. For example, the core structure of cephalosporins have been left intact to preserve activity, but the peripheral chemical groups have been modified to impart the molecule with the ability to penetrate the bacterial membrane more efficiently or be more resistant to β-lactamase [3]. Modifications of four classic antibiotics, cephalosporin, penicillin, quinolone, and macrolide, account for ~73% of the "new" antibiotics filed between 1981 and 2005 [4]. It is also important to note that small compounds need to exhibit not only anti-microbial activity, but also minimized cytotoxic properties to widen their therapeutic window.

Although advances in organic synthesis have extended the lifetime of classic antibiotics through synthetic modifications, new scaffolds are also needed. Recent efforts to search for new modalities amongst previously-overlooked natural sources, such as unmined bacterial taxa and ecological niches, have started to bear fruit. The increasingly rapid data acquisition and low cost of ultra high-throughput sequencing has provided rich coverage of bacterial genomes and transcriptomes. For example, genomic analyses of a vancomycin-resistant strain of *Amycolatopsis orientalis* revealed the presence of genetic loci that encode for at least 10 other secondary metabolites. One compound, ECO-0501, exhibited strong anti-bacterial properties against Gram-positive pathogens, including several strains of MRSA [5]. Mass spectroscopy (MS) is another primary methodology used to identify small molecule metabolites with potential anti-microbial properties. The polycyclic small molecule, abyssomicin C, from the marine actinomycete *Verrucosispora* was characterized as an inhibitor of *p*-aminobenzoate biosynthesis by MS and also exhibited antimicrobial properties against MRSA strains [6].

2. Methodology for high-throughput screens (HTS) using small molecule libraries

The workhorse platform for anti-bacterial drug discovery is a chemical genetics HTS approach using small molecule compound libraries to identify candidates that inhibit bacterial growth or the function of key bacterial enzymes. Small molecules, generally <500 molecular weight, have the potential to enter cells and selectively perturb specific protein activity, thus functioning as therapeutic agents against disease. In general, the precise mechanism of inhibitor activity remains unknown in the initial screen. Subsequent identification of the molecular targets of small molecules will have to be performed to implicate the specific bacterial functions that were inactivated in the screen. Thus, HTS can sample a large unbiased collection of structurally diverse molecules to select compounds that perturb the defined cell phenotype of interest. (Fig. 1)

Various chemical compound libraries are now available through commercial and public re-
sources that include FDA-approved bioactive compounds, therapeutic agents, and natural
products. To maximize the structural complexity and diversity of small molecule libraries,
scientists have also employed diversity-oriented synthesis,

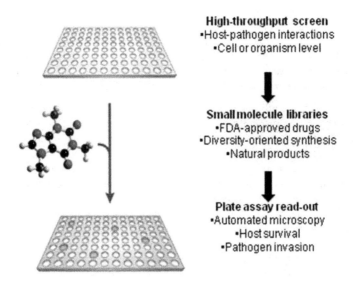

High-throughput screen
•Host-pathogen interactions
•Cell or organism level

Small molecule libraries
•FDA-approved drugs
•Diversity-oriented synthesis
•Natural products

Plate assay read-out
•Automated microscopy
•Host survival
•Pathogen invasion

Figure 1. General flowchart of high-throughput methodology to screen small molecule libraries for inhibitors of host-pathogen interactions

in which different scaffolds are modified with highly diverse functional groups. [7, 8]. To
bolster academic research in chemical biology efforts for HTS-driven identification of bioactive compounds, the NIH launched the Molecular Libraries Program in 2005 to offer ac-
cess to ten large-scale automated HTS centers in the Molecular Libraries Probe Production
Centers Network, including diverse compound libraries through the Small Molecule Repo-
sitory and information on biological activities of small molecules in the PubChem BioAssay public database.

A variety of different molecular and cellular methods have been developed for HTS using
small molecule libraries. Automated microscopy has been utilized for high-content, image-
based screens of cells exposed to small molecules. Acquired cell images can be analyzed by
automated image analysis software to quantitate physiological changes at the single-cell level, including phenotypes such as morphology and cell toxicity. Small molecule microarrays,
in which ~10,000 small molecules are covalently bound to a glass slide, has been generated
to detect high affinity binding to a protein of interest, as a potential inhibitor of function.
Binding of the protein of interest to specific compounds on the microarray was then detected with fluorescent antibodies [9].

3. Disruption of host-pathogen interactions for novel drug discovery

Given the innovation gap in the discovery of novel antibiotics post-1960, strategies to inhibit novel targets are greatly needed to combat infectious disease. Multiple studies have identified small molecule inhibitors that target gene expression of pathogen TTSS components in *P. aeruginosa*, enteropathogenic *E. coli*, and *Y. pestis* [10, 11, 12]. The small molecule virstatin, 4-[N1,8-naphthalimide)]-n-butyric acid, was identified as an inhibitor of the transcriptional regulator ToxT in *Vibrio cholerae* [13]. The small molecule, 2-imino-5-arylidene thiazolidinone, which blocks TTSS-dependent functions in *S. typhimurium*, was also found to inhibit virulence in *Yersinia, Pseudomonas,* and *Francisella* strains, indicating that compounds can be identified that target common processes in multiple pathogens [14].

Research efforts have recently begun to focus on disruption of host-pathogen interactions as a new approach to identify potential targets for drug discovery, rather than solely on specific pathogen targets or processes. In particular, the screening of small molecule libraries to identify inhibitors that block pathogen infection of the host, using such phenotypes as pathogen invasion, host morphology, and pathogen replication in the host, is a powerful approach for therapeutic development that may uncover fundamental mechanisms of pathogenesis and potentially lead to discovery of new classes of anti-infective agents. Here, we describe case studies of the use of small molecules in host infection screens to identify novel inhibitors against infectious disease, including bacterial, viral, parasitic, and fungal infections. We will discuss these studies in the context of re-purposing known drugs, inhibitor specificity, and discovery of basic mechanisms of host-pathogen interactions. The screen results are summarized in Table 1.

Screening for inhibitors of intracellular infection

Intracellular pathogens, including viruses, parasites, and some bacteria, manipulate specific host factors in order to downregulate the host immune response or modulate host actin cytoskeleton rearrangements to induce phagocytic uptake of the pathogen. *L. monocytogenes,* an intracellular Gram-positive bacteria, infects the human host primarily through ingestion of contaminated foods and causes gastrointestinal infection. In 2011, *Listeria* contamination of cantaloupes led to at least 30 deaths and ~150 illnesses in 28 states. Following internalization of *L. monocytogenes* in host membrane-bound vacuoles, the pore-forming cytolysin, listeriolysin O (LLO) and a phosphatidylinositol-specific phospholipase C (PI-PLC) mediates lysis of the vacuoles to release the pathogen into the host cell cytosol. *L. monocytogenes* then polymerizes host actin to propel itself into adjacent host cells to continue the infection process. To identify compounds that inhibited *L. monocytogenes* intracellular infection, a screen of 480 small molecules from the Biomol ICCB Known Bioactives library was performed using automated microscopy and image analysis [15]. Murine bone marrow-derived macrophages were infected with a GFP-expressing *L. monocytogenes* strain to assess efficiency of invasion, survival, and replication in the host. Twenty-one compounds, affecting cell functions such as actin polymerization, calcium signaling, and apoptosis, were identified that markedly decreased *Listeria monocytogenes* infection efficiency. In particular, the FDA-approved anti-psychotic drug pimozide, used to treat Tourette's syndrome and schizophrenia, was shown to

decrease internalization of not just *L. monocytogenes,* but other bacterial species as well, including *Bacillus subtilis, Salmonella typhimurium,* and *E. coli.* Furthermore, pimozide decreased vacuole escape and cell-to-cell spread of *L. monocytogenes* in the host. Thus, pimozide is an example of a small molecule that can be re-purposed to treat infectious disease with potential for broad spectrum anti-microbial applications.

Parasites also employ a life cycle of host cell invasion, replication, and host cell lysis during onset of infection. *Taxoplasma gondii* is the protozoan intracellular human parasite of the phylum Apicomplexa and is related to *Plasmodium* and *Cryptosporidium,* the causative agents of malaria and diarrheal disease, respectively. To discover inhibitors of *T. gondii* invasion, a high-throughput

Pathogen	#Compounds	#Hits	Assay and methods	Ref
Bacteria				
L. monocytogenes	480	21	Host cell invasion, automated microscopy	15
P. aeruginosa	50,000	88	ExoU-,edoated host cytotoxicity	18
	56,280	6	Cytotoxicity in yeast model	19
Y. pseudotuberculosis	100,000	45	Translocation of Yops into the host	20
B. anthracis	70,094	30	Lethal factor entry into host	21
	10,000	24	Interaction between edema factor and CaM	22
P. syringae	~200	3	Bleaching of *Arabidopsis* seedlings	23
	80	1	Bleaching of *Arabidopsis* seedlings	24
Parasite				
T. gondii	12,160	24	Host cell invasion, motility, adhesins	16
Virus				
HIV	~200,000	27	Induction of viral latency	49

Table 1 Small molecule screens using host-pathogen systems

microscopy assay was developed to distinguish between extracellular and intracellular parasites in a BS-C-1 epithelial cell model, using differential labeling with fluorescent dyes [16]. Out of a 12,160 structurally-diverse small molecule library, 24 non-cytotoxic inhibitors were identified that reduced parasite invasion to <20% compared to control wells. These molecules inhibited different aspects of the infection process, including gliding motility and secretion of host cell adhesins. One of these inhibitors, tachypleginA, was found to post-translationally modify TgMLC1, a myosin light chain component of the *T. gondii* myosin motor complex, which drives host cell penetration and parasite mobility [17]. TgMLC1 exposed to the small molecule exhibited a rapid and irreversible change in electrophoretic mobility on SDS-PAGE gels. Although the exact nature of the modification remains unclear, the modification has been mapped to amino acids V46-R59 by mass spectroscopy. These studies provide key mechanistic information on the importance of *T. gondii* motility in pathogenesis and illustrate the potential for small molecules to form covalent interactions with target proteins.

Targeting virulence toxin mechanisms of infection

Many Gram-negative bacteria, including *Pseudomonas* and *Yersinia,* utilize the TTSS as a primary mechanism of virulence to inject effector proteins into the host cytosol to downregulate the host immune response. A host cytotoxicity assay was designed to screen for small molecule inhibitors of *Pseudomonas aeruginosa,* a leading cause of hospital-acquired infections in cystic fibrosis patients. *P. aeruginosa* ExoU, a TTSS effector protein, is a member of the patatin family of phospholipase A_2 (PLA_2) that can lyse host cell membranes during infection. A high-throughput screen of 50,000 compounds from the Chembridge Microformat Library E was performed using a colorimetric live/dead assay to identify small molecules that protected Chinese hamster ovary (CHO) cells from cytotoxicity mediated by *P. aeruginosa* expressing ExoU as the sole TTSS effector [18]. A primary list of 88 compounds exhibited rescue of CHO cells from ExoU-mediated cytotoxicity. The most effective compound, pseudolipasin A, inhibited ExoU function downstream of TTSS delivery into the host. In addition to inhibition of CHO cytotoxicity, pseudolipasin A also protected the amoeba *Dictyolstelium discoideum* from ExoU-mediated killing by *P. aeruginosa* and inhibited cytotoxicity in the yeast *Saccharomyces cerevisiae* expressing ExoU. Interestingly, pseudolipasin A did not affect eukaryotic PLA_2, suggesting that this small molecule may specifically target bacterial PLA_2. Pseudolipasin A is representative of small molecules that do not kill or inhibit the growth of pathogens, but instead attenuate their virulence.

Inhibitors of *P. aeruginosa* virulence have also been identified using a cell-based yeast phenotypic assay in combination with a large-scale small molecule screen. A total of 505 *P. aeruginosa* virulence factors and essential genes were individually overexpressed in *S. cerevisae* to downselect genes that inhibited yeast growth [19]. Nine genes strongly or partially impaired yeast growth, including three TTSS effectors, ExoS, ExoT, and ExoY. ExoS has been previously shown to ADP-ribosylate multiple downstream targets, including vimentin, the Ras family of small GTP-binding proteins, and cyclophilin A. Given that ExoS is a critical mediator of *P. aeruginosa* chronic infections, a library of 56,280 compounds was screened to find inhibitors of ExoS ADP-ribosylation activity that rescued cytotoxicity in yeast. Six compounds were identified that restored yeast growth. The most promising compound, exosin, was found to modulate ExoS enzymatic activity *in vitro* and exhibited a protective effect against *P. aeruginosa* infection in mammalian CHO cells. This study demonstrates the effective use of a simple eukaryotic host, baker's yeast, as a tool for drug screening for applications in controlling infectious disease in humans.

Another pathogen family that employs the TTSS is *Yersinia,* which secrete Yop effectors into the host cell. There are three *Yersinia* human pathogens, *Y. pestis,* the etiological agent of plague via intradermal fleabites or inhalation, and *Y. pseudotuberculosis* and *Y. enterocolitica,* which cause mild and self-limiting enteric disease by the oral route. HTS strategies have been developed to identify small molecules that inhibit translocation of the Yops into host cells. A recombinant *Y. pseudotuberculosis* strain was constructed to express a chimeric protein containing the first 100 amino acids of YopE, which contains the proper translocation signals to inject into the host, fused to a fragment of β-lactamase. [20]. This bacterial strain was used to infect HEp-2 host cells treated with a non-membrane-permeating, non-fluorescent dye CCF2-AM, which fluoresces green at 520nm, as a result of intramolecular FRET between the 7-hydroxycoumarin and fluorescein molecules, conjugated by a lactam ring. Upon cellular uptake, CCF2-AM is modified by cytoplasmic esterases and is trapped in the host cell. If the YopE-β-lactamase fusion is introduced into the host, the β-lactamase will cleave the lactam ring in CCF2-AM and liberate the fluorescein, leaving the coumarin to fluoresce blue at 447nm. Using this differential fluorescence assay, 100,000 compounds from a number of sources, including the ChemDiv 2, ChemDiv 3, ChemDiv 4, Maybridge 3, Maybridge 4, and Biomol ICCB libraries, were screened for low ratios of blue-to-green fluorescence. In total, 200 compounds were deemed potential hits, and 45 were assessed further using secondary assays, including rounded host morphology in response to *Yersinia* infection. Finally, 6 compounds were found that inhibited translocation of effectors into the host without affecting expression and function of TTSS components. Several of these compounds also inhibited host cell rounding when induced by *Pseudomonas* effectors, suggesting that these compounds may have a broad-spectrum anti-infective effect.

A screen to identify small molecule inhibitors of *B. anthracis* also employed the CCF2-AM FRET assay. *B. anthracis*, the Gram-positive causative agent of anthrax, secretes three major toxins during infection, lethal factor (LF), protective antigen (PA), and edema factor (EF). A fusion protein between LF and β-lactamase was introduced into host cells by PA-directed endocytosis to hydrolyze the CCF2-AM fluorogenic substrate [21]. Out of 70,094 compounds tested, 1170 initial hits exhibited concentration-dependent inhibition of β-lactamase activity. Thirty compounds with known biological activities and/or were high confidence hits were selected for further analysis. Three compounds, NCGC00084148-01, diphyllin, and niclosamide, exhibited protective effects from anthrax LF, a LF fusion to *Pseudomonas* exotoxin, and diphtheria toxin in RAW264.7 murine macrophages and CHO cells, and are thought to interfere with toxin internalization in the host.

The interaction between *B. anthracis* EF and its cellular activator, calmodulin (CaM), became the basis of a two-step tandem screen to identify small molecule inhibitors of anthrax infection. A library of 10,000 compounds (Chembridge, Library # ET350-1) in pools of 8 was screened to identify small molecules that blocked an EF-induced flat to round morphology change in Y1 murine adrenocortical cells [22]. Twenty-four initial hits were then individually tested using surface plasmon resonance (SPR) to identify molecules that block interactions between EF and immobilized CaM. One compound, (4-[4-(3,4-cichlorophenyl)-thiazolylamino]-benzenesulfonamide) 10506-2A, efficiently inhibited EF-CaM binding in a dose-dependent manner, and was found to specifically target the CaM binding region of EF by fluorescence spectroscopy. Since this compound was found to be toxic in cultured mammalian cells, a series of structurally-related compounds was synthesized, and a new inhibitory compound with reduced toxicity was subsequently identified.

Small molecule discovery in plant-pathogen interactions

Discovery of small molecule inhibitors has also been extended to plant pathogen systems as an approach to develop commercially-relevant chemicals to protect crops assets from disease. The Gram-negative pathogen *Pseudomonas syringae* expresses a TTSS, enters plant tissues through the stomata or wounds, and infects a wide range of plant species. A major challenge in the application of small molecule screens to plant-pathogen interactions is the development of high-throughput methodology with a plant model system. A high-throughput liquid assay was developed based on *P. syringae*-induced bleaching of *Arabidopsis thali-*

ana cotyledon seedlings, which signifies a loss of chlorophyll from plant tissues and is indicative of bacterial pathogenesis [23]. A screen of ~200 small molecules active in *Arabidopsis* (LATCA, Library of Active Compounds in Arabidopsis) identified several sulfanilamide compounds, including sulfamethoxazole, sulfadiazine, and sulfapyridine, that prevented cotyledon bleaching upon *P. syringae* infection. The most potent compound, sulfamethoxazole, also inhibited *P. syringae* growth in mature soil-grown plants. A similar assay was used to implicate the same compound, sulfamethoxazole, and the indole alkaloid gramine as inhibitors of *Fusarium graminearum* fungal infection in *Arabidopsis* and wheat, indicating that this strategy represents a relevant surrogate system for identification of compounds that can prevent agriculturally-important infectious disease [24].

Combinational antiviral therapies for HIV

Given that viral pathogens are absolutely dependent on the host for propagation, even more so than bacterial pathogens, research in host-directed anti-virals has advanced at a faster pace than that for anti-bacterial agents. Human Immunodeficiency virus type 1 (HIV-1), a lentivirus of the retroviral family and the causative agent of AIDS, is the most-widely studied viral pathogen to date. HIV-1 infection causes a dramatic decline in host CD4+ T cell numbers and a progressive failure of the immune response, which makes the host susceptible to opportunistic infections and cancer. The highly glycosylated HIV-1 envelope, in combination with the extreme diversity of circulating viral strains, have presented daunting challenges for development of an effective vaccine. Furthermore, the virus establishes chronic infection that resists the highly active antiretroviral therapy (HAART). Conventional HAART for HIV-1 infection combines three main classes of anti-viral drugs:

1. nucleoside reverse transcriptase inhibitors (NRTIs),

2. non-nucleoside RT inhibitors (NNRTIs), which target the non-catalytic domain of RT, and

3. protease inhibitors (PIs).

HAART is usually patient-specific, and its formulation is determined by the viral load and drug resistance. A traditional HAART consists of two NRTIs and a NNRTI or a PI [25]. More advanced combination therapies include a fourth class of antiretroviral drugs, HIV entry inhibitors. HIV-1 entry into human cells is dependent on several sequential steps that include binding of viral envelope protein gp120 to the CD4 receptor, and conformational change in gp120 that increases its affinity to the chemokine co-receptors (CCR5 or CXCR4) and exposes gp41, an HIV envelope protein that executes the fusion of HIV and host cell membranes.

Currently, there are two approved inhibitors of HIV-1 entry:

1. enfuvirtide, a peptide fusion inhibitor that binds to gp41 and

2. maraviroc, a small molecule entry inhibitor that prevents interaction between gp120 and CCR5.

The β-chemokine receptor CCR5 was found to act as a major co-receptor for the macrophage-tropic HIV-1 R5 strains, predominant in the early asymptomatic stages of virus infection, whereas the T-cell-tropic strains (using the CXCR4 co-receptor) become prevalent in the symptomatic stages concomitant with the decline of CD4+ T-cells [26]. CCR5 is an attractive target for development of HIV-1 entry inhibitors, given the discovery that HIV-1 non-progressors, individuals homozygous for a 32-bp deletion in the coding region of CCR5 gene (CCR5Δ32) were naturally resistant to infection with R5 HIV-1 [27]. Natural and synthetic CCR5 ligands such as RANTES, AOP-RANTES, Mip-1α, Mip-1β, and Met-RANTES were found to efficiently protect against R5 HIV-1 infection [28, 29]. Thus, the first published high throughput screen (HTS) for discovery of non- peptide inhibitors of HIV-1 entry was performed in a virus-free cell-based system using [^{125}I]-labeled RANTES. A strong inhibitor of RANTES binding to CCR5 stably expressed on the surface of CHO cells was identified from the library of Takeda Chemical Industries. Further chemical modifications of the lead compound designated TAK-779 produced a potent (IC50 1.4 nM in CHO/CCR cells) and selective CCR5 antagonist capable of blocking R5 HIV-1 infection *in vitro* [30].

The number of CCR5 inhibitors has significantly grown since the discovery of TAK-779, but very few compounds have entered clinical trials, and only maraviroc has been approved for clinical use [31]. A radiolabeled-chemokine binding assay similar to one applied for the identification of TAK-779 was used in a HTS of a small molecule library at Pfizer for the discovery of UK-107,543, which had become a scaffold for intensive medicinal chemistry, producing ~1,000 analog compounds, from which maraviroc (UK-427,857) was selected for its excellent preclinical pharmacokinetics (90% inhibitory concentration of 2 nM in pool of PBMCs from various donors) [32]. Despite its proven efficacy against HIV-1 R5 infection, maraviroc is vulnerable to gp120 escape mutations [33]. Site-directed mutagenesis and molecular modeling studies have identified a common binding pocket on CCR5 that is shared by various small-molecule CCR5 inhibitors [34, 35, 36]. Emerging details on gp120 and CCR5 points of interaction and binding thermodynamics provide valuable information that can be applied in developing tools for rational design of novel HIV-1 entry inhibitors [37, 38]. Efficient block of HIV entry into host cells is essential to curtail virus dissemination and is a key step towards eradication of HIV infection. The current HAART regiment can reduce HIV replication to very low levels (below 50 copies/ml plasma) and can lead to recovery of CD4$^+$ T-cell counts but not cure the infection. Patients that have been successfully treated with HAART for years have experienced a rapid virus rebound upon termination of the therapeutic regiment [39, 40]. Such clinical cases present evidence that HIV establishes a chronic infection that resists current HAART designed to target actively replicating virus. A deliberate and controllable induction of HIV-1 replication from its latent reservoirs in combination with HAART is a novel and actively pursued approach that aims to eliminate both active and latent viral pools [41].

Researchers often seek new anti-infective agents amongst small molecules that have previously been approved for the treatment of cancer and neurological diseases, since they have well-established pharmacokinetics and in most cases, known molecular mechanisms of action. One example of this is the histone deacetylase (HDAC) inhibitor, valproic acid (VA), which had previously been approved for treatment of neurological and psychiatric disorders. HIV-1 has been shown to enter dormancy using epigenetic silencing via deaceylation

of histones in the vicinity of the integrated viral genome [42]. Thus, VA was tested as a potential agent to disrupt HIV-1 latent infection. However, years of VA treatment in combination with HAART showed no clearance of the latent HIV reservoir [43]. A more potent
HDAC inhibitor, suberoylanilide hydroxamic acid (SAHA), approved for treatment of cutaneous T-cell lymphoma, was subsequently tested as a potential agent that could 'flush out'
HIV-1 from latently infected cells, based on its superior effect to VA in cell culture models
[44, 45]. A substantial effort has also been invested in the design and synthesis of bryostatin
chemical analogs, small molecules that activate protein kinase C (PKC) with single nanomo-
lar concentration [46]. PKC activation leads to phosphorylation of nuclear factor κB (NFκB),
a key transcription factor regulator of HIV-1 gene expression [47]. However, modulation of
NFκB activity requires great caution, since abnormal NFκB signaling has been related to the
pathophysiology of inflammatory diseases and neurodegenerative disorders [48].

A HTS of a small molecule library recently identified novel HIV latency activators [49]. The
screen was performed using a lymphoma CD4+ T-cell line (SupT1) harboring latent recombinant HIV-1 and two reporters that reflect early and late virus gene expression incorporated
in the HIV-1 genome [50]. A luminescent assay based on secreted alkaline phosphatase
(SEAP) activity, incorporated in the late virus gene transcripts, was applied to screen a
chemical library of ~200,000 compounds. Validation of 27 hits with diverse chemical structures demonstrated induction of latent virus from various cell models. Compounds with a
selective index (CC_{50}/EC_{50}) above 25 were chosen for downstream medicinal chemistry modifications. Moreover, the lead compounds were shown to reactivate latent HIV from primary
resting CD4+ T-cells with no induction of cell proliferation. Small molecule activators of latent HIV that act in concert using different mechanisms have a better chance of purging the
virus out of infected cells [49]. Such pre-clinical data strongly suggests that successful treatment of HIV infection can be achieved only through combinational therapy consisting of diverse class of antiviral drugs.

4. Whole animal small molecule screens using *C. elegans*

In vitro high-throughput screens have several limitations for the discovery of therapeutic inhibitors with high efficacy. Synthetic compound libraries often contain toxic compounds
with poor pharmacokinetic properties, and many *in vitro* assays are not physiologically-rele-
vant in the context of which a specific drug is expected to function. In a previous section, we
had described the use of a HTS whole organism-based assay based on *Arabidopsis* seedlings
as the host system. Here, we detail the use of a whole animal model, the nematode worm *C.
elegans*, in chemical screens that permit simultaneous assessment of the immunomodulatory
effects, potential toxicity of compounds, and drug efficacy in a host with a functioning immune system. The results of these screens are summarized in Table 2. Whole animal screens
have the distinct advantage of being able to directly discard compounds that induce organismal toxicity and can identify compounds that target host-pathogen interactions in a relevant physiological context.

C. elegans, a hermaphroditic nematode normally found in soil, is a versatile, more ethically-acceptable whole animal system for high-throughput analysis of host response to pathogen infection. *C. elegans* contains a fully sequenced genome that facilitates both genetic and genomic analysis, offering an ideal compromise between organismal complexity and experimental tractability. *C. elegans* offers other experimental advantages, including a rapid 2-3 week life span, simple growth conditions, target-selected gene inactivation, and a relatively low cost of maintenance compared to other whole animal systems. A wealth of experimental data has demonstrated that many developmental, neurological, and biochemical processes have been highly conserved between *C. elegans* and mammals. For example, cellular functions as diverse as innate immunity, the first line of defense against pathogen infection, and RNA interference to downregulate gene expression via double-stranded RNA, are found in both *C. elegans* and higher eukaryotes, suggesting the existence of a common ancestor of these diverse species. Thus, anti-infective compounds identified using a *C. elegans* infection model may also be translatable in humans.

C. elegans as a model host system has been well-studied for numerous bacterial pathogens, including the Gram-positive *S. aureus*, *S. pneumoniae*, and *B. thuringiensis*, and the Gram-negative *B. pseudomallei*, *P. aeruginosa*, and *S. marcescens*. In general, different types of bacteria are fed to *C. elegans* in place of their normal *E. coli* food source to provoke detectable symptoms of illness, such as locomotion dysregulation, intestinal cell lysis, and shortened life span.

Small molecule inhibitors of bacterial infection

A small manual screen of 6000 synthetic compounds and 1136 natural extracts were analyzed in an immunocompromised mutant of *C. elegans* infected with *Enterococcus faecalis* to identify compounds that promoted host survival. [51]. A total of 16 compounds and 9 extracts were identified that either modulated bacterial growth *in vitro*, impaired pathogen virulence, or boosted host innate immunity. Furthermore, 15 out the 16 compounds did not kill *C. elegans* or mammalian erythrocytes, indicating that the compounds are not toxic.

The development of automated sorting and handling of *C. elegans* rapidly enabled high-throughput screening of small chemical libraries to identify compounds that enhanced survival of *C. elegans* in response to bacterial infection. This methodology was enabled by the Complex Object Parametric Analyzer and Sorter (COPAS) BioSort worm sorter (Union Biometrica) to dispense a defined number of living worms into multi-well plates, which were then imaged using automated microscopy to quantify worm survival. A library of 37,200 compounds and natural product extracts was screened using the same *C. elegans-E. faecalis* infection system described above [52]. Twenty-eight compounds and extracts were identified that enhanced survival of infected *C. elegans*. Six structural classes of identified compounds did not affect the growth of *E. faecalis* itself, suggesting that the small molecules inhibited a specific aspect of the host-pathogen interaction. Interestingly, two structural classes are similar to compounds previously identified in a high-throughput screen to identify inhibitors of *P. aeruginosa* biofilm development, indicating the presence of common molecular targets across multiple bacterial species for drug discovery [53].

A *P. aeruginosa* infection model of *C. elegans* has also been developed to screen for novel anti-infective compounds. The high-throughput assay was based on *P. aeruginosa*-induced slow killing of *C. elegans* in the presence of 1300 bioactive extracts produced by endophytic fungi associated with medicinal plants [54]. The screen identified 36 extracts that promoted the survival of the infected worms, while 4 extracts were found to inhibit *P. aeruginosa* growth using a disc diffusion assay. Given that these extracts contain a mixture of metabolites, the specific compound against *P. aeruginosa* remains to be determined. Nevertheless, this study illustrates the rich reservoir of small molecules in natural symbiotic organisms with antibacterial activity.

Pathogen	#Compounds	#Hits	Assay and methods	Ref
E. faecalis	7136	25	Host survival	51
	37,214	28	HTS, automated microscopy of host survival	52
P. aeruginosa	1300	40	Host survival	54
C. albicans	1266	15	Host survival, inhibition of *C. albicans* filamentation	55
	3228	19	HTS, co-inoculation of worms with *C. albicans*	58

Table 2 Small molecule screens using *C. elegans* as host model for infection

Discovery of novel antifungal agents

The *C. elegans* infection model was also used to screen for compounds that prolonged host survival following infection with the human pathogenic fungus *Candida albicans*. [55]. Given that most compounds that have antifungal activity are also toxic to the human host, high-throughput methods can greatly increase the likelihood of discovering specific antifungal inhibitors. From a screen of 1266 compounds with known pharmaceutical activities, 15 small molecules were identified that increased survival of *C. albicans*-infected nematodes and inhibited *in vivo* filamentation of *C. albicans*, a mechanism of pathogenesis seen during mammalian infection. Two compounds, caffeic acid phenethyl ester (CAPE), a natural component of honeybee propolis, and the fluoroquinolone agent enoxacin, were further shown to exhibit antifungal activity in a mouse model, validating the use of a *C. elegans* model for potential targets in a mammalian system. Interestingly, CAPE is known to inhibit the mammalian transcription factor NF-κB and to induce immunomodulatory effects in mice [56, 57]. Since *C. elegans* does not express a NF-κB homolog, it may be the case that CAPE affects alternative targets to achieve antifungal activity.

An automated high-throughput screen using the COPAS Biosort was also applied to *C. albicans* infection of *C. elegans* to assess a library of 3,228 compounds consisting of 1948 bioactive compounds and 1280 small molecules derived from diversity-oriented synthesis [58]. In total, 19 compounds were identified that increased *C. elegans* survival in response to *C. albicans* infection, 7 of which are currently used antifungal agents. Several immunosuppressant agents identified in this screen, including ascomycin, cyclosporin A, and FK-506, were previously found to exhibit weak antifungal activity against *Cryptococcus* and *Aspergillus*, in addition to *C. albicans* [59, 60]. Other hits were predicted to affect an array of biological activities, such as dequalinium chloride, a potent anti-tumor and protein kinase C inhibitor, and triadimefon, an inhibitor of ergosterol biosynthesis.

5. Conclusion

Chemical library screens are a potent and valuable molecular tool for HTS identification of potential inhibitors of infectious disease. The long-standing paradigm to treat pathogen infection with small molecules that specifically target pathogen growth or metabolism has led to our current dilemma of microbial drug resistance and re-emergence of once-contained infectious diseases. Thus, new approaches to target pathogen virulence or host response factors rather than essential pathogen functions have become increasingly more attractive strategies that are less likely to induce microbial resistance. Some compounds, such as the FDA-approved anti-psychotic, pimozide, exhibited inhibitory properties against infection by several pathogens, suggesting that small molecules can potentially be developed as broad-spectrum anti-infectives. Although the molecular mechanism of inhibition by small molecules remains unknown in most cases, it may be possible to make an educated guess if targeted pathogens share a common virulence strategy, such as the Type III secretion system in Gram-negative bacteria. In other cases, identification of an inhibitor can lead to a molecular understanding of the infection mechanism. For example, the small molecule, tachyplegi-nA, was found to post-translationally modify TgMLC1, a myosin light chain component, to drive host cell penetration by the parasite *T. gondii* [17].

From the various studies detailed in this review, it is apparent that the library screens represent a first step on the road of drug discovery. There has been a growing realization that fundamental discovery of biological mechanisms oftentimes reaches a 'valley of death', in which potential translation avenues into clinical therapies and diagnostics for disease treatment comes to a standstill and is lost. NIH is addressing this widening gap between basic and clinical research with the establishment of Clinical and Translational Science Centers across the country. The research community will have to remain pro-active to move promising leads from the initial screen stage into downstream validation and development modes in a timely manner. As with any drug development strategy, there still remain multiple technical challenges that need to be overcome before small molecule inhibitors can successfully transition into the clinic. Researchers will need to assess such parameters as compound toxicity, pharmacokinetics and pharmacodynamics, and validation in animal models. However, FDA-approved small molecule libraries can be applied to HTS as a cost-effective method to identify existing licensed drugs for repurposing from diseases unrelated to microbial infection. Furthermore, the development of the *C. elegans* whole organism model for small molecule screening provides a novel methodology to simultaneously assess compound toxicity and host response to pathogen infection. It would be informative to determine whether small molecules identified from conventional host cell culture studies can also inhibit pathogen infection in the *C. elegans* model. Future anti-infective treatments will most likely be comprised of combination therapies that produce additive or synergistic effects to target key processes in both the pathogen and the host. The overall promise of discovering novel anti-infective compounds has generated great hope in the biomedical community for discovery of new countermeasures against infectious disease.

Acknowledgements

The writing of this review was supported by a Los Alamos National Laboratory LDRD-DR grant to study development of novel inhibitors that block host-pathogen interactions.

Author details

Elizabeth Hong-Geller* and Sofiya Micheva-Viteva

*Address all correspondence to: ehong@lanl.gov

Bioscience Division, Los Alamos National Laboratory, Bioscience Division, Los Alamos, NM, USA

References

[1] Klevens, R. M., Morrison, M. A., Nadle, J., Petit, S., Gershman, K., Ray, S., Harrison, L. H., Lynfield, R., Dumyati, G., Townes, J. M., Craig, A. S., Zell, E. R., Fosheim, G. E., Mc Dougal, L. K., Carey, R. B., & Fridkin, S. K. (2007). Invasive methicillin-resistant Staphylococcus aureus infections in the United States. *JAMA*, 298, 1763-71.

[2] Fischbach, M. A., & Walsh, C. T. (2009). Antibiotics for emerging pathogens. *Science*, 325, 1089-93.

[3] Neu, H. C., & Fu, K. P. (1978). Cefuroxime, a beta-lactamase-resistant cephalosporin with a broad spectrum of gram-positive and-negative activity. *Antimicrob Agents Chemother*, 13, 657-64.

[4] Newman, D. J., & Cragg, G. M. (2007). Natural products as sources of new drugs over the last 25 years. *J Nat Prod*, 70, 461-77.

[5] Banskota, A. H., Mc Alpine, J. B., Sorensen, D., Ibrahim, A., Aouidate, M., Piraee, M., Alarco, A. M., Farnet, C. M., & Zazopoulos, E. (2006). Genomic analyses lead to novel secondary metabolites. *Part 3. ECO-0501, a novel antibacterial of a new class. J Antibiot (Tokyo)*, 59, 533-42.

[6] Bister, B., Bischoff, D., Strobele, M., Riedlinger, J., Reicke, A., Wolter, F., Bull, A. T., Zahner, H., Fiedler, H. P., & Sussmuth, R. D. (2004). Abyssomicin C-A polycyclic antibiotic from a marine Verrucosispora strain as an inhibitor of the p-aminobenzoic acid/tetrahydrofolate biosynthesis pathway. *Angew Chem Int Ed Engl*, 43, 2574-6.

[7]   Schreiber, S. L. (2000). Target-oriented and diversity-oriented organic synthesis in drug discovery. *Science*, 287, 1964-9.

[8]   Tan, D. S. (2005). Diversity-oriented synthesis: exploring the intersections between chemistry and biology. *Nat Chem Biol*, 1, 74-84.

[9]   Kuruvilla, F. G., Shamji, A. F., Sternson, S. M., Hergenrother, P. J., & Schreiber, S. L. (2002). Dissecting glucose signalling with diversity-oriented synthesis and small-molecule microarrays. *Nature*, 416, 653-7.

[10] Aiello, D., Williams, J. D., Majgier-Baranowska, H., Patel, I., Peet, N. P., Huang, J., Lory, S., Bowlin, T. L., & Moir, D. T. (2010). Discovery and characterization of inhibitors of Pseudomonas aeruginosa type III secretion. *Antimicrob Agents Chemother*, 54, 1988-99.

[11] Gauthier, A., Robertson, M. L., Lowden, M., Ibarra, J. A., Puente, J. L., & Finlay, B. B. (2005). Transcriptional inhibitor of virulence factors in enteropathogenic Escherichia coli. Antimicrob Agents Chemother , 49, 4101-9.

[12] Pan, N. J., Brady, M. J., Leong, J. M., & Goguen, J. D. (2009). Targeting type III secretion in Yersinia pestis. *Antimicrob Agents Chemother*, 53, 385-92.

[13] Hung, D. T., Shakhnovich, E. A., Pierson, E., & Mekalanos, J. J. (2005). Small-molecule inhibitor of Vibrio cholerae virulence and intestinal colonization. *Science*, 310, 670-4.

[14] Felise, H. B., Nguyen, H. V., Pfuetzner, R. A., Barry, K. C., Jackson, S. R., Blanc, M. P., Bronstein, P. A., Kline, T., & Miller, S. I. (2008). An inhibitor of gram-negative bacterial virulence protein secretion. *Cell Host Microbe*, 4, 325-36.

[15] Lieberman, L. A., & Higgins, D. E. (2009). A small-molecule screen identifies the antipsychotic drug pimozide as an inhibitor of Listeria monocytogenes infection. *Antimicrob Agents Chemother*, 53, 756-64.

[16] Carey, K. L., Westwood, N. J., Mitchison, T. J., & Ward, G. E. (2004). A small-molecule approach to studying invasive mechanisms of Toxoplasma gondii. *Proc Natl Acad Sci U S A*, 101, 7433-8.

[17] Heaslip, A. T., Leung, J. M., Carey, K. L., Catti, F., Warshaw, D. M., Westwood, N. J., Ballif, BA, & Ward, G. E. (2010). A small-molecule inhibitor of T. gondii motility induces the posttranslational modification of myosin light chain-1 and inhibits myosin motor activity. *PLoS Pathog*, 6, e1000720.

[18] Lee, V. T., Pukatzki, S., Sato, H., Kikawada, E., Kazimirova, AA, Huang, J., Li, X., Arm, J. P., Frank, D. W., & Lory, S. (2007). Pseudolipasin A is a specific inhibitor for phospholipase A2 activity of Pseudomonas aeruginosa cytotoxin ExoU. *Infect Immun*, 75, 1089-98.

[19] Arnoldo, A., Curak, J., Kittanakom, S., Chevelev, I., Lee, V. T., Sahebol-Amri, M., Koscik, B., Ljuma, L., Roy, P. J., Bedalov, A., Giaever, G., Nislow, C., Merrill, A. R., Lory,

S., & Stagljar, I. (2008). Identification of small molecule inhibitors of Pseudomonas aeruginosa exoenzyme S using a yeast phenotypic screen. *PLoS Genet*, 4, e1000005.

[20] Harmon, D. E., Davis, A. J., Castillo, C., & Mecsas, J. (2010). Identification and characterization of small-molecule inhibitors of Yop translocation in Yersinia pseudotuberculosis. *Antimicrob Agents Chemother*, 54, 3241-54.

[21] Zhu, P. J., Hobson, J. P., Southall, N., Qiu, C., Thomas, C. J., Lu, J., Inglese, J., Zheng, W., Leppla, S. H., Bugge, T. H., Austin, CP, & Liu, S. (2009). Quantitative high-throughput screening identifies inhibitors of anthrax-induced cell death. *Bioorg Med Chem*, 17, 5139-45.

[22] Lee, Y. S., Bergson, P., He, W. S., Mrksich, M., & Tang, W. J. (2004). Discovery of a small molecule that inhibits the interaction of anthrax edema factor with its cellular activator, calmodulin. *Chem Biol*, 11, 1139-46.

[23] Schreiber, K., Ckurshumova, W., Peek, J., & Desveaux, D. (2008). A high-throughput chemical screen for resistance to Pseudomonas syringae in Arabidopsis. *Plant J*, 54, 522-31.

[24] Schreiber, K. J., Nasmith, C. G., Allard, G., Singh, J., Subramaniam, R., & Desveaux, D. (2011). Found in translation: high-throughput chemical screening in Arabidopsis thaliana identifies small molecules that reduce Fusarium head blight disease in wheat. *Mol Plant Microbe Interact*, 24, 640-8.

[25] Hammer, S. M., Eron, J. J. Jr, Reiss, P., Schooley, R. T., Thompson, M. A., Walmsley, S., Cahn, P., Fischl, M. A., Gatell, J. M., Hirsch, M. S., Jacobsen, D. M., Montaner, J. S., Richman, D. D., Yeni, P. G., & Volberding, P. A. (2008). Antiretroviral treatment of adult HIV infection: 2008 recommendations of the International AIDS Society-USA panel. *JAMA*, 300, 555-70.

[26] Berger, E. A., Murphy, P. M., & Farber, J. M. (1999). Chemokine receptors as HIV-1 coreceptors: roles in viral entry, tropism, and disease. *Annu Rev Immunol*, 17, 657-700.

[27] Liu, R., Paxton, W. A., Choe, S., Ceradini, D., Martin, S. R., Horuk, R., Mac Donald., ME, Stuhlmann, H., Koup, R. A., & Landau, N. R. (1996). Homozygous defect in HIV-1 coreceptor accounts for resistance of some multiply-exposed individuals to HIV-1 infection. *Cell*, 86, 367-77.

[28] Alkhatib, G., Combadiere, C., Broder, C. C., Feng, Y., Kennedy, P. E., Murphy, P. M., & Berger, E. A. (1996). CC CKR5: a RANTES, MIP-1alpha, MIP-1beta receptor as a fusion cofactor for macrophage-tropic HIV-1. *Science*, 272, 1955-8.

[29] Simmons, G., Clapham, P. R., Picard, L., Offord, R. E., Rosenkilde, MM, Schwartz, T. W., Buser, R., Wells, T. N., & Proudfoot, A. E. (1997). Potent inhibition of HIV-1 infectivity in macrophages and lymphocytes by a novel CCR5 antagonist. *Science*, 276, 276-9.

[30] Baba, M., Nishimura, O., Kanzaki, N., Okamoto, M., Sawada, H., Iizawa, Y., Shiraishi, M., Aramaki, Y., Okonogi, K., Ogawa, Y., Meguro, K., & Fujino, M. (1999). A

small-molecule, nonpeptide CCR5 antagonist with highly potent and selective anti-HIV-1 activity. *Proc Natl Acad Sci U S A*, 96, 5698-703.

[31] Kuhmann, S. E., & Hartley, O. (2008). Targeting chemokine receptors in HIV: a status report. *Annu Rev Pharmacol Toxicol*, 48, 425-61.

[32] Dorr, P., Westby, M., Dobbs, S., Griffin, P., Irvine, B., Macartney, M., Mori, J., Rickett, G., Smith-Burchnell, C., Napier, C., Webster, R., Armour, D., Price, D., Stammen, B., Wood, A., & Perros, M. (2005). Maraviroc (UK-427,857), a potent, orally bioavailable, and selective small-molecule inhibitor of chemokine receptor CCR5 with broad-spectrum anti-human immunodeficiency virus type 1 activity. *Antimicrob Agents Chemother*, 49, 4721-32.

[33] Roche, M., Jakobsen, M. R., Sterjovski, J., Ellett, A., Posta, F., Lee, B., Jubb, B., Westby, M., Lewin, S. R., Ramsland, P. A., Churchill, MJ, & Gorry, P. R. (2011). HIV-1 escape from the CCR5 antagonist maraviroc associated with an altered and less-efficient mechanism of gp120-CCR5 engagement that attenuates macrophage tropism. *J Virol*, 85, 4330-42.

[34] Dragic, T., Trkola, A., Thompson, D. A., Cormier, E. G., Kajumo, F. A., Maxwell, E., Lin, S. W., Ying, W., Smith, S. O., Sakmar, T. P., & Moore, J. P. (2000). A binding pocket for a small molecule inhibitor of HIV-1 entry within the transmembrane helices of CCR5. *Proc Natl Acad Sci U S A*, 97, 5639-44.

[35] Nishikawa, M., Takashima, K., Nishi, T., Furuta, R. A., Kanzaki, N., Yamamoto, Y., & Fujisawa, J. (2005). Analysis of binding sites for the new small-molecule CCR5 antagonist TAK-220 on human CCR5. *Antimicrob Agents Chemother*, 49, 4708-15.

[36] Maeda, K., Das, D., Ogata-Aoki, H., Nakata, H., Miyakawa, T., Tojo, Y., Norman, R., Takaoka, Y., Ding, J., Arnold, G. F., Arnold, E., & Mitsuya, H. (2006). Structural and molecular interactions of CCR5 inhibitors with CCR5. *J Biol Chem*, 281, 12688-98.

[37] Huang, C. C., Lam, S. N., Acharya, P., Tang, M., Xiang, S. H., Hussan, S. S., Stanfield, R. L., Robinson, J., Sodroski, J., Wilson, I. A., Wyatt, R., Bewley, C. A., & Kwong, P. D. (2007). Structures of the CCR5 N terminus and of a tyrosine-sulfated antibody with HIV-1 gp120 and CD4. *Science*, 317, 1930-4.

[38] Brower, E. T., Schon, A., Klein, J. C., & Freire, E. (2009). Binding thermodynamics of the N-terminal peptide of the CCR5 coreceptor to HIV-1 envelope glycoprotein gp120. *Biochemistry*, 48, 779-85.

[39] Chun, T. W., Davey, R. T. Jr, Ostrowski, M., Shawn, Justement. J., Engel, D., Mullins, J. I., & Fauci, AS. (2000). Relationship between pre-existing viral reservoirs and the re-emergence of plasma viremia after discontinuation of highly active anti-retroviral therapy. *Nat Med*, 6, 757-61.

[40] Brooks, D. G., Hamer, D. H., Arlen, P. A., Gao, L., Bristol, G., Kitchen, C. M., Berger, E. A., & Zack, J. A. (2003). Molecular characterization, reactivation, and depletion of latent HIV. *Immunity*, 19, 413-23.

[41] Richman, D. D., Margolis, D. M., Delaney, M., Greene, W. C., Hazuda, D., & Pomerantz, R. J. (2009). The challenge of finding a cure for HIV infection. *Science*, 323, 1304-7.

[42] Lehrman, G., Hogue, I. B., Palmer, S., Jennings, C., Spina, CA, Wiegand, A., Landay, A. L., Coombs, R. W., Richman, D. D., Mellors, J. W., Coffin, J. M., Bosch, R. J., & Margolis, D. M. (2005). Depletion of latent HIV-1 infection in vivo: a proof-of-concept study. *Lancet*, 366, 549-55.

[43] Siliciano, J. D., Lai, J., Callender, M., Pitt, E., Zhang, H., Margolick, J. B., Gallant, J. E., Cofrancesco, J. Jr, Moore, R. D., Gange, S. J., & Siliciano, R. F. (2007). Stability of the latent reservoir for HIV-1 in patients receiving valproic acid. *J Infect Dis*, 195, 833-6.

[44] Edelstein, L. C., Micheva-Viteva, S., Phelan, B. D., & Dougherty, J. P. (2009). Short communication: activation of latent HIV type 1 gene expression by suberoylanilide hydroxamic acid (SAHA), an HDAC inhibitor approved for use to treat cutaneous T cell lymphoma. *AIDS Res Hum Retroviruses*, 25, 883-7.

[45] Archin, N. M., Espeseth, A., Parker, D., Cheema, M., Hazuda, D., & Margolis, D. M. (2009). Expression of latent HIV induced by the potent HDAC inhibitor suberoylanilide hydroxamic acid. *AIDS Res Hum Retroviruses*, 25, 207-12.

[46] De Christopher, B. A., Loy, B., Marsden, M., Schrier, A. J., Zack, J. A., & Wender, P. A. (2012). Designed, synthetically accessible bryostatin analogues potently induce activation of latent HIV reservoirs in vitro. *Nat Chem; In Press*.

[47] Williams, S. A., Chen, L. F., Kwon, H., Fenard, D., Bisgrove, D., Verdin, E., & Greene, W. C. (2004). Prostratin antagonizes HIV latency by activating NF-kappaB. *J Biol Chem*, 279, 42008-17.

[48] Pikarsky, E., Porat, R. M., Stein, I., Abramovitch, R., Amit, S., Kasem, S., Gutkovich-Pyest, E., Urieli-Shoval, S., Galun, E., & Ben-Neriah, Y. (2004). NF-kappaB functions as a tumour promoter in inflammation-associated cancer. *Nature*, 431, 461-6.

[49] Micheva-Viteva, S., Kobayashi, Y., Edelstein, L. C., Pacchia, A. L., Lee, H. L., Graci, J. D., Breslin, J., Phelan, B. D., Miller, L. K., Colacino, J. M., Gu, Z., Ron, Y., Peltz, S. W., & Dougherty, J. P. (2011). High-throughput screening uncovers a compound that activates latent HIV-1 and acts cooperatively with a histone deacetylase (HDAC) inhibitor. *J Biol Chem*, 286, 21083-91.

[50] Micheva-Viteva, S., Pacchia, A. L., Ron, Y., Peltz, S. W., & Dougherty, J. P. (2005). Human immunodeficiency virus type 1 latency model for high-throughput screening. *Antimicrob Agents Chemother*, 49, 5185-8.

[51] Moy, T. I., Ball, A. R., Anklesaria, Z., Casadei, G., Lewis, K., & Ausubel, F. M. (2006). Identification of novel antimicrobials using a live-animal infection model. *Proc Natl Acad Sci U S A*, 103, 10414-9.

[52] Moy, T. I., Conery, A. L., Larkins-Ford, J., Wu, G., Mazitschek, R., Casadei, G., Lewis, K., Carpenter, A. E., & Ausubel, F. M. (2009). High-throughput screen for novel anti-microbials using a whole animal infection model. *ACS Chem Biol*, 4, 527-33.

[53] Junker, L. M., & Clardy, J. (2007). High-throughput screens for small-molecule inhibitors of Pseudomonas aeruginosa biofilm development. *Antimicrob Agents Chemother*, 51, 3582-90.

[54] Zhou, Y. M., Shao, L., Li, J. A., Han, L. Z., Cai, W. J., Zhu, C. B., & Chen, D. J. (2011). An efficient and novel screening model for assessing the bioactivity of extracts against multidrug-resistant Pseudomonas aeruginosa using Caenorhabditis elegans. Biosci Biotechnol Biochem , 75, 1746-51.

[55] Breger, J., Fuchs, B. B., Aperis, G., Moy, T. I., Ausubel, F. M., & Mylonakis, E. (2007). Antifungal chemical compounds identified using a C. elegans pathogenicity assay. *PLoS Pathog*, 3, e18.

[56] Watabe, M., Hishikawa, K., Takayanagi, A., Shimizu, N., & Nakaki, T. (2004). Caffeic acid phenethyl ester induces apoptosis by inhibition of NFkappaB and activation of Fas in human breast cancer MCF-7 cells. *J Biol Chem*, 279, 6017-26.

[57] Park, J. H., Lee, J. K., Kim, H. S., Chung, S. T., Eom, J. H., Kim, K. A., Chung, S. J., Paik, S. Y., & Oh, H. Y. (2004). Immunomodulatory effect of caffeic acid phenethyl ester in Balb/c mice. *Int Immunopharmacol*, 4, 429-36.

[58] Okoli, I., Coleman, J. J., Tampakakis, E., An, W. F., Holson, E., Wagner, F., Conery, A. L., Larkins-Ford, J., Wu, G., Stern, A., Ausubel, F. M., & Mylonakis, E. (2009). Identification of antifungal compounds active against Candida albicans using an improved high-throughput Caenorhabditis elegans assay. *PLoS One*, 4, e7025.

[59] Fox, D. S., Cruz, M. C., Sia, R. A., Ke, H., Cox, G. M., Cardenas, M. E., & Heitman, J. (2001). Calcineurin regulatory subunit is essential for virulence and mediates interactions with FKBP12-FK506 in Cryptococcus neoformans. *Mol Microbiol*, 39, 835-49.

[60] Steinbach, W. J., Schell, W. A., Blankenship, J. R., Onyewu, C., Heitman, J., & Perfect, J. R. (2004). In vitro interactions between antifungals and immunosuppressants against Aspergillus fumigatus. Antimicrob Agents Chemother , 48, 1664-9.

Chapter 5

Fruit/Vegetable-Drug Interactions: Effects on Drug Metabolizing Enzymes and Drug Transporters

Lourdes Rodríguez-Fragoso and
Jorge Reyes-Esparza

Additional information is available at the end of the chapter

1. Introduction

Dietary habits are an important modifiable environmental factor influencing human health and disease. Epidemiologic evidence suggests that regular consumption of fruits and vegetables may reduce risk of some diseases, including cancer [1]. These properties have been attributed to foods that are rich sources of numerous bioactive compounds such as phytochemicals [2]. Modifying the intake of specific foods and/or their bioactive components seems to be a prudent, noninvasive, and cost-effective strategy for preventing some diseases in people who appear to be "healthy" [3]. As will be discussed in this chapter, potential problems occur when patients taking medicines regularly also consume certain fruits or vegetables.

Thousands of drugs are commercially available and a great percentage of the population takes at least one pharmacologically active agent on a regular basis. Given this magnitude of use and variability in individual nutritional status, dietary habits and food composition, there is a high potential for drug-nutrient interactions. However, there is a relatively short list of documented fruit-drug or vegetable-drug interactions, necessitating further and extensive clinical evaluation. Healthcare providers, such as physicians, pharmacists, nurses, and dietitians, have to be aware of important food-drug interactions in order to optimize the therapeutic efficacy of prescribed and over-the-counter drugs. Here, we review some of the most widely consumed fruits and vegetables to inform healthcare providers of possible nutrient-drug interactions and their potential clinical significance.

There are numerous patients who encounter increased risks of adverse events associated with drug-nutrient interactions. These include elderly patients, patients with cancer and/ or malnutrition, gastrointestinal tract dysfunctions, acquired immunodeficiency syndrome and chronic diseases that require the use of multiple drugs, as well as those receiving enteral nutrition or transplants. Therefore, the main reason for devoting a major review to nutrient-drug interactions is the enormous importance of fruits and vegetables used for their beneficial effects as nutrients and as components in folk medicine. There are currently few studies that combine a nutrient-based and detailed pharmacological approach [4], or studies that systematically explore the risk and benefits of fruit and vegetables [5-7].

2. Food-drug interactions

A drug-nutrient interaction is defined as the result of a physical, chemical, physiological, or pathophysiological relationship between a drug and a nutrient [8,9]. An interaction is considered significant from a clinical perspective if it alters the therapeutic response. Food-drug interactions can result in two main clinical effects: the decreased bioavailability of a drug, which predisposes to treatment failure, or an increased bioavailability, which increases the risk of adverse events and may even precipitate toxicities (See Figure 1) [4, 10,11].

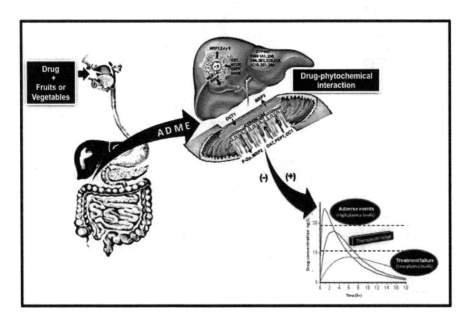

Figure 1. Drug-fruit/vegetable interaction and effects on bioavailability of drugs. During the consumption of drugs with fruits or vegetables the **ADME** properties of drug (**A**bsorption, **D**istribution, **M**etabolism and **E**xcretion) can be modified by drug-phytochemical interaction. As a result of this interaction can be increased or decreased plasma concentrations of a drug which can lead to the presence of adverse events or treatment failure

Nutritional status and diet can affect drug action by altering metabolism and function. In addition, various dietary components can have pharmacological activity under certain circumstances [12]. For healthy-treatment intervention, it is necessary to understand how these drug-food interactions can induce a beneficial result or lead to detrimental therapeutic conditions (less therapeutic action or more toxicity). Drug-drug interactions are widely recognized and evaluated as part of the drug-approval process, whether pharmaceutical, pharmacokinetic, or pharmacodynamic in nature. Equal attention must be paid to food-drug interactions (Figure 2).

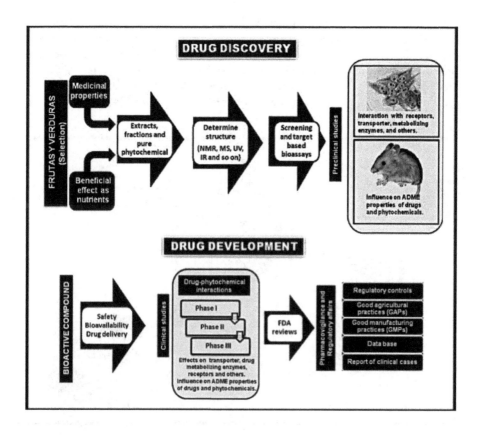

Figure 2. Bioassay models for studying drug-phytochemical interaction.

There are four types of accepted drug-food interactions based on their nature and mechanisms.

• Type I are *ex vivo* bioinactivations, which refer to interactions between the drug and the nutritional element or formulation through biochemical or physical reactions, such as hydrolysis, oxidation, neutralization, precipitation or complexation. These interactions usually occur in the delivery device.

• Type II interactions affect absorption. They cause either an increase or decrease in the oral bioavailability of a drug. The precipitant agent may modify the function of enzymes or transport mechanisms that are responsible for biotransformation.

• Type III interactions affect the systemic or physiologic disposition and occur after the drug or the nutritional element has been absorbed from the gastrointestinal tract and entered the systemic circulation. Changes in the cellular or tissue distribution, systemic transport, or penetration to specific organs or tissues can occur.

• Type IV interactions refer to the elimination or clearance of drugs or nutrients, which may involve the antagonism, impairment or modulation of renal and/or enterohepatic elimination [13].

Drug metabolizing enzymes and drug transporters play important roles in modulating drug absorption, distribution, metabolism, and elimination. Acting alone or in concert with each other, they can affect the pharmacokinetics and pharmacodynamics of a drug. The interplay between drug metabolizing enzymes and transporters is one of the confounding factors that have been recently shown to contribute to potential complex drug interactions [14].

3. Food and drug transporters

The oral administration of drugs to patients is convenient, practical, and preferred for many reasons. Oral administration of drugs, however, may lead to limited and variable oral bioavailability because of absorption across the intestinal barrier [15,16]. Drug absorption across the gastrointestinal tract is highly dependent on affinity for membrane transporters as well as lipophilicity [17]. On the other hand, the liver plays a key role in the clearance and excretion of many drugs. Hepatic transporters are membrane proteins that primarily facilitate nutrient and endogenous substrate transport into the cell via uptake transporters, or protect the cell by pumping out toxic chemicals via canalicular transporters [18]. Consequently, drug transporters in both the gut and the liver are important in determining oral drug disposition by controlling absorption and bioavailability [19]

The major uptake transporters responsible for nutrient and xenobiotic transport, both uptake and efflux transporters, belong to the two solute carrier (SLC and SLCO) superfamilies [20]. The SLC superfamily encompasses a variety of transporters, including the organic anion transporters (OAT, SLC22A), the organic cation transporters (OCT, SLC22A), the electroneutral organic cation transporters (OCTN, SLC22A), the equilibrative nucleoside transporters (ENT, SLC29), the concentrative nucleoside transporters (CNT, SLC28), the apical Na^+–dependent bile salt transporter (ASBT, SLC10), the monocarboxylate transporters (MCT, SLC16), and the peptide transporters (PEPT, SLC15) [21]. The SLCO family is made up of the organic anion transporting polypeptides (OATP) [22]. Efflux transporters expressed in the intestine and liver include P-glycoprotein (Pgp, ABCB1), bile salt export pump (BSEP, ABCB11), multidrug resistance proteins (MRP1- 6, ABCC1-6), and breast cancer resistance protein (BCRP, ABCG2), all members of the ATP-Binding Cassette superfamily (ABC transporters) [23]. Members of this superfamily use ATP as an energy source, allowing them to pump substrates against a concentration gradient. In the liver, uptake transporters are mainly expressed in the sinusoid, and excretion transporters are mainly expressed on the lateral and canalicular membranes. There are transporters on the lateral membrane the primary function of which is pumping drugs back into the blood circulation from the hepatocytes. Nowadays, a large amount of work has identified and characterized intestinal and hepatic transporters in regards to tissue expression profiles, regulation, mechanisms of transport, substrate and inhibitor profiles, species differences, and genetic polymorphisms. Given the circumstances outlined above, there is no doubt of the overall relevance of drug transport for clinical pharmacokinetics.

Until recently, little regard was given to the possibility that food and food components could cause significant changes to the extent of drug absorption via effects on intestinal and liver transporters. It is now well known that drug-food interactions might affect the pharmacokinetics of prescribed drugs when co-administered with food [24]. Common foods, such as fruits and vegetables, contain a large variety of secondary metabolites known as phytochemicals (Tabla 1), many of which have been associated with health benefits [25]. However, we know little about the processes through which these phytochemicals (and/or their metabolites) are absorbed into the body, reach their biological target, and are eliminated. Recent studies show that some of these phytochemicals are substrates and modulators of specific members of the superfamily of ABC transporting proteins [26]. Indeed, *in vitro* and preclinical data in rats suggest that a variety of foodstuffs [27,28], including herbal teas [29,30] and vegetables and herbs [31,32] can modulate the activity of drug transporters. It is not yet known whether these effects are predictive of what will be observed clinically.

4. Foods and drug-metabolizing enzyme

It has been shown that, before reaching the systemic circulation, the metabolism of orally ingested drugs ('first-pass metabolism' or 'presystemic clearance') has clinically relevant influences on the potency and efficacy of drugs. Both the intestine and liver account for the presystemic metabolism in humans. Drug metabolism reactions are generally grouped into 2 phases. Phase I reactions involve changes such as oxidation, reduction, and hydrolysis and are primarily mediated by the cytochrome P450 (CYP) family of enzymes. Phase II reactions use an endogenous compound such as glucuronic acid, glutathione, or sulfate, to conjugate with the drug or its phase I–derived metabolite to produce a more polar end product that can be more readily excreted [33].

The CYP enzymes involved in drug metabolism in humans are expressed predominantly in the liver. However, they are also present in the large and small intestine, lungs and brain [34]. CYP proteins are categorized into families and subfamilies and can metabolize almost any organic xenobiotic [35]. CYP enzymes combined with drug transport proteins constitute the first-pass effect of orally administered drugs [33]. On the other hand, the Phase II drug metabolizing or conjugating enzymes consist of many enzyme superfamilies, including sulfotransferases (SULT), UDP-glucuronosyltransferases (UGT), DT-diaphorase or NAD(P)H:quinone oxidoreductase (NQO) or NAD(P)H: menadione reductase (NMO), epoxide hydrolases (EPH), glutathione S-transferases (GST) and N-acetyltransferases (NAT). The conjugation reactions by Phase II drug-metabolizing enzymes increase hydrophilicity and thereby enhance excretion in the bile and/or the urine and consequently affect detoxification [36].

The metabolism of a drug can be altered by foreign chemicals and such interactions can often be clinically significant [37]. The most common form of drug interactions entail a foreign chemical acting either as an inhibitor or an inducer of the CYP enzyme isoform responsible for metabolizing an administered medicinal drug, subsequently leading to an unusually slow or fast clearance of said drug [38,39]. Inhibition of drug metabolism will result in a concentration elevation in tissues, leading to various adverse reactions, particularly for drugs with a low therapeutic index.

Often, influence on drug metabolism by compounds that occur in the environment, most remarkably foodstuffs, is bypassed. Dietary changes can alter the expression and activity of hepatic drug metabolizing enzymes. Although this can lead to alterations in the systemic elimination kinetics of drugs metabolized by these enzymes, the magnitude of the change is generally small [8, 40]. Metabolic food-drug interactions occur when a certain food alters the activity of a drug-metabolizing enzyme, leading to a modulation of the pharmacokinetics of drugs metabolized by the enzyme [12]. Foods, such as fruits, vegetables, alcoholic beverages, teas, and herbs, which consist of complex chemical mixtures, can inhibit or induce the activity of drug-metabolizing enzymes [41].

The observed induction and inhibition of CYP enzymes by natural products in the presence of a prescribed drug has (among other reasons) led to the general acceptance that natural therapies can have adverse effects, contrary to popular beliefs in countries with active ethnomedicinal practices. Herbal medicines such as St. John's wort, garlic, piperine, ginseng, and gingko, which are freely available over the counter, have given rise to serious clinical interactions when co-administered with prescription medicines [42]. Such adversities have spurred various pre-clinical and *in vitro* investigations on a series of other herbal remedies, with their clinical relevance yet to be established. The CYP3A4-related interaction based on food component is the best known; it might be related to the high level of expression of CYP3A4 in the small intestine, as well as its broad substrate specificity. If we consider that CYP3A4 is responsible for the metabolism of more than 50% of clinical pharmaceuticals, all nutrient-drug interactions should be considered clinically relevant, in which case all clinical studies of drugs should include a food-drug interaction screening [43].

5. Nutrient-drug interactions: examples with clinical relevance

Fruits and vegetables are known to be important components in a healthy diet, since they have low energy density and are sources of micronutrients, fiber, and other components with functional properties, called phytochemicals (See Figure 2). Increased fruit and vegetable consumption can also help displace food high in saturated fats, sugar or salt. Low fruit and vegetable intake is among the top 10 risk factors contributing to mortality. According to the World Health Organization (WHO), increased daily fruit and vegetable intake could help prevent major chronic non-communicable diseases [44]. Evidence is emerging that specific combinations of phytochemicals may be far more effective in protecting against some diseases than isolated compounds (Table 1 and 2). Observed drug-phytochemical interactions, in addition to interactions among dietary micronutrients, indicate possibilities for improved therapeutic strategies. However, several reports have examined the effects of plant foods and herbal medicines on drug bioavailability. As shown in Tables 3 and 4 and as discussed below, we have surveyed the literature to identify reports suggesting important food and phytochemical modulation of drug-metabolizing enzymes and drug transporters leading to potential important nutrient-drug interactions.

Fruit	Phytochemicals	Traditional Uses
Grapefruit *Citrus paradisi, Citrus reticulata*	Bergamottin, flavonoids (nobiletin, tangeretin, quercetin, diosmin, naringenin, naringin and kaempferol), and furanocoumarins.	Insomnia, and anxiety or nervousness
Orange *Citrus sinensis, Citrus aurantium*	Flavonoids as tangeretin, nobiletin, diosmin and hesperetin.	Inflammatory ailments in respiratory tract, Arthritis, gastrointestinal tract ailments and others
Tangerine *Citrus reticulata, Citrus deliciosa*	Flavonoids as diosmin, tangeritin, nobilein and quercetin.	Inflammatory ailments in respiratory tract, arthritis, gastrointestinal tract ailments and others
Grapes *Vitis vinifera*	Stilbens (resverestrol, viniferin), and flavonoids.	Antianemic, Inflammatory ailments in respiratory tract and others
Cranberry *Vaccinium macrocarpon Vaccinium myrtillus*	Flavonoids as anthocyanidin (cyaniding and poenidin) and flavonols (quercetin), and carotenoids.	Genitourinary ailments, nephrolithiasis, wound healing and others
Pomegranate *Punica granatum*	Phenolic acids (punicalagin and tannins), flavonoids (anthocyanins) and pectin.	Inflammatory ailments in respiratory tract and others Gastrointestinal tract ailments and others
Apple *Malus domestica*	Phenolic acids (tannins), flavonoids (including quercetin), glycosylated xanthones and Saponins.	Diuretic, genitourinary ailments, inflammatory ailments in respiratory tract and others
Mango *Mangifera indica*	Phenolic acids (tannins), flavonoids (anthocyanins), carotenoids, essential oils, fatty acids, lectins, phenols, saponins, alkaloids, and triterpenes.	Recommended to combat heart disease. It is also a laxative, and diuretic
Black raspberry *Rubus coreanus, Rubus idaeus, Rubus fruticosus*	Phenolic acids (ellagic acid, gallic acid), flavonoids (quercetin, anthocyanins, pelargonidins, Kaempferol and cyanidins), catechins and salicylic acid.	Antianemic, anti-infectious, inflammatory ailments in respiratory tract, gastrointestinal tract ailments and others
Black mulberry *Morus nigra*	2-arylbenzofuran derivative: flavones (mornigrol D, mornigrol G, mornigrol H, and norartocarpetin), flavonol (dihydrokaempferol), albanin A, albanin E, stilbenes (moracin M), and albafuran.	Genitourinary ailments, Inflammatory ailments in respiratory tract, gastrointestinal tract ailments and others
Guava *Psidium guajava*	Flavonoid as quercetin and phloretin.	Genitourinary ailments, hypertension
Papaya (*Carican papaya L.*)	beta-cryptoxanthin and benzyl isothiocyanates	Abdominal discomfort, pain, malaria, diabetes, obesity, infections and oral drug poisonings

Data from: [26,52,53,55, 82, 111, 112]

Table 1. Commonly Consumed Fruits

Vegetable	Phytochemicals	Traditional Uses
Broccoli *Brassica oleracea var. italica*	Isothiocyanate sulforaphane, glucosinolate glucoraphanin, glucosinolates, phenolic acid, indol and dithiolthiones.	Antioxidant, Anti-cancer, Antiseptic, anti-ulcerous, hypoglycemic, anti-anemic, Gastrointestinal tract ailments and others
Cauliflower *Brassica oleracea var. botrytis*	Isothiocyanate, glucosinolate, indole-3-Carbinol, sulforaphane, indol,	Antioxidant
Spinach *Spinacia oleracea*	Flavonoids and p-coumaric acid derivatives, α-lipoic acid, poliphenols, lutein, zeaxantin, betaine	Diuretic, inflammatory ailments, gastrointestinal tract ailments, Inflammatory ailments in respiratory tract and others.
Watercress *Nasturtium officinale*	phenylethyl isothiocyanate (PEITC) and methylsulphinylalkyl isothiocyanates (MEITCs), flavonoids such as quercetin, hydroxycinnamic acids, and carotenoids such as β-carotene and lutein	Antioxidants, diuretic, gastrointestinal tract ailments, Inflammatory ailments in respiratory tract and others.
Tomato *Lycopersicum esculentum*	Carotenoids phytofluene, phytoene, neurosporene, γ-carotene, and ζ-carotene lycopene, phytoene, phytofluene, quercetin, polyphenols, kaempferol	Antioxidant, hydratant, hypocholesterolemic
Carrot *Dactus carrota*	Polyphenols, α and β-carotene, quercetin, myrecetin and panaxynol	Constipation
Avocado *Persea americana*	Persin, carotenoids (zeaxanthin, α-carotene, and β-carotene), lutein, β-sitosterol, glutathione	Genitourinary ailments, inflammatory ailments in respiratory tract, gastrointestinal tract ailments and others
Red pepper *(Capsicum annuum L.)*	Capsaisin, lycopene, anthocyanins	Scarlatina, putrid sore throat, hoarseness, dyspepsia, yellow fiber, peals and snakebite

Data from: [26,105,114,126, 151]

Table 2. Commonly Consumed Vegetables

Fruit	Molecular Target	Drug Interactions in Humans and Others
Grapefruit	Inhibits CYP3A4, CYP1A2, MRP2, OATP-B and P-glycoprotein, [29, 45, 50, 53, 54, 65]	In humans: reports of more than 40 drug interactions: calcium channel antagonists [57], central nervous system modulators [58], HMG-CoA reductase [59], immunosuppressants [60], anti-virals [61], phosphodiesterases-5 inhibitor [62], antihistamines [63], antiarrythmics [62], and antibiotics [64]
Sevilla orange	Inhibits CYP3A4, P-glycoprotein, OATP-A, OATP-B [11, 29, 5469, 117]	In vitro system: vinblastine [55], fexofenadine [29], glibenclamida [53] In humans: atenolol, ciprofloxacine, ciclosporine, celiprolol, levofloxacin and pravastatin [54, 72]
Tangerine	Stimulates CYP3A4 activity and inhibits P-glycoprotein [52]	In vitro system: nifedipine [74], digoxina [52]
Grapes	Inhibits CYP3A4 and CYP2E1 [13]	In humans: cyclosporine [78]
Cranberry	Inhibits CYP3A and CYP2C9 [31, 81, 83]	In humans: Warfarin [81, 82] In vitro system: Diclofenac [83]
Pomegranate	Inhibits CYP3A and phenol sulfotransferase activity [56,89]	Animals: carbamacepine [56]
Mango	Inhibits CYP1A1, CYP1A2, CYP 3A1, CYP2C6, CYP2E1, P-glycoprotein (ABCB1) [97]	In vitro system: midazolam, diclofenac, chlorzoxazone [95, 96], Verapamil [97]
Guava	Inhibits P- glycoprotein [23]	Not documented
Black raspberry	Inhibits CYP3A [49]	In vitro system: midazolam
Black mulberry	Inhibits CYP3A and OATP-B [49]	In vitro system: midazolam; glibenclamida [53]
Apple	Inhibits CYP1A1, OATP family (Oatp-1, Oatp-3 and NTCP) [63, 110]	In vitro system: fexofenadine [63]
Papaya	Inhibits CYP3A4 [114]	No documented

Table 3. Fruit-Drug Interactions

Vegetable	Molecular target	Drug Interactions in Humans and Others.
Broccoli	Inhibits: CYP1A1, CYP2B1/2, CYP3A 4, CYP2E1, hGSTA1/2, MRP-1, MRP-2, BCRP, UDP, Glucorosytransferases, Sulfotransferases, Quincne reductases phenolsulfotransferases [26, 120,121] Induces: UDPglucuronosyltransferases, (UGTs), sulfotransferases, (SULTs) and quinone reductases (QRs) [26]	Not documented
Cauliflower	Inhibits: CYP1A1, CYP2B1/2, CYP3A 4, CYP2E1, hGSTA1/2, MRP-1, MRP-2, BCRP, UDP, Glucorosytransferases, Sulfotransferases, Quincne reductases phenolsulfotransferases [26,120, 121] Induces: UDPglucuronosyltransferases, (UGTs), sulfotransferases, (SULTs) and quinone reductases (QRs) [26]	Not documented
Watercress	Inhibits: CYP2E1, P-glycoprotein, MRP1, MRP2 and BCRP [26, 126]	In humans: Chlorzoxazone
Spinach	Possible inhibition of CYP1A2 [1132]	In vitro system: heterocyclic aromatic amines
Tomato	Inhibits: CYP1A1, CYP1B1, UGP, [138] Increases: UGT and CYP2E1, [139]	In vitro system: diethylnitrosamine, N-methyl-N-nitrosourea, and 1,2-dimethylhydrazine
Carrot	Induces: phenolsulfotransferases and ethoxycoumarin O-deethylase ECD [123, 143] Inhibits: CPY2E1 [122]	Not documented
Avocado	Unknown	Humans: Warfarin
Red pepper	Inhibits CYP 1A2, 2A2, 3A1, 2C11, 2B1, 2B2 and 2C6 [154,155]	In vitro and in vivo

Table 4. Vegetable-Drug Intractions

5.1. Grapefruit (*Citrus paradisi*)

The interaction of grapefruit with certain drugs was unintentionally discovered two decades ago [45]. Since then, there have been numerous reports on the effects of grapefruit and its components on CYP450 drug oxidation and transportation [46,47]. Several findings showed that grapefruit juice had a major effect on the intestinal CYP system with a minor effect at the hepatic level [48]. The predominant mechanism for this interaction is the inhibition of cytochrome *P*-450 3A4 in the small intestine, which results in a significant reduction of drug presystemic metabolism. Grapefruit juice intake has been found to decrease CYP3A4 mRNA activity through a post transcriptional activity, possibly by facilitating degradation of the enzyme [49]. An additional mechanism may be the inhibition of P-glycoprotein and MRP2-mediated drug efflux, transporters that carry drugs from enterocytes back to the gut lumen, all of which results in a further increase in the fraction of drug absorbed and increased systemic drug bioavailability [50-52]. It has also been reported that the major constituents of grapefruit significantly inhibit the OATP-B function *in vitro* [53,54].

The interaction between grapefruit juice and drugs has been potentially ascribed to a number of constituents [27]. It has been suggested that flavonoids such as naringin, naringenin, quercetin, and kaempferol, major components in grapefruit, are responsible for drug interaction. Some of these chemicals are also found in other fruit juices. Pomegranate, for example, shares certain properties with grapefruit, suggesting that both could modify the bioavailability of drugs [55,56]. Another group of compounds that has been detected in grapefruit juice are the furanocoumarins (psoralens), which are known to be mechanism-based inactivators of CYP450. The major furanocoumarin present in grapefruit is bergamottin, which demonstrated a time- and concentration-dependent inactivation of CYP enzymes *in vitro* [49]. One interesting characteristic of this interaction is that grapefruit juice does not need to be taken simultaneously with the medication in order to produce the interaction. The bioavailability of drugs has been reported to be doubled by grapefruit juice, even when taken 12 h after ingestion. Colored grapefruit juice and white grapefruit juice are equally effective in producing drug interactions.

This inhibitory interaction should be kept in mind when prescribing drugs metabolized by CYP3A4. Examples of drugs affected by grapefruit or its components include: calcium channel antagonists such as felodipine, nisoldipine, amlodipines, verapamil, and diltiazem [57]; central nervous system modulators, including diazepam, triazolam, midazolam, alprazolam, carbamazepine, buspurone and sertraline [58]; HMG-CoA reductase inhibitors, such as simvastatin, lovastatin, atorvastatin, and pravastatin [59]; immunosuppressants such as cyclosporine [60]; anti-virals such as saquinavir [61]; a phosphodiesterases-5 inhibitor such as sildenafil [62]; antihistamines, including as terfenadine and fexofenadine [63]; antiarhythmics such as amiodarone [62]; and antibiotics such as eritromicine [64].

Epidemiologic studies reveal that approximately 2% of the population in the United States consumes at least one glass of regular strength grapefruit juice per day. This becomes pertinent if we consider that many people suffer from chronic metabolic diseases (including hypertension, hyperlipidemia, and cardiovascular diseases) and receive calcium channel antagonis therapy and HMG-CoA reductase inhibitors. Patients with mental disorders also chronically receive central nervous system modulators. In the case of many drugs, an increase in serum drug concentration has been associated with increased frequency of dose-dependent adverse effects [65-67]. In light of the wide ranging effects of grapefruit juice on the pharmacokinetics of various drugs, physicians need to be aware of these interactions and should make an attempt to warn and educate patients regarding the potential consequences of concomitant ingestion of these agents.

5.2. Orange (*Citrus sinensis*)

Consumption of most types of orange juice does not appear to alter CYP3A4 activity *in vivo* [55]. However, orange juice made from Seville oranges appears to be somewhat similar to grapefruit juice and can affect the pharmacokinetics of CYP3A4 substrates [68]. It has been previously shown that consumption of a single 240 mL serving of Sevilla orange juice resulted in a 76% increase in felodipine exposure, comparable to what is observed after grapefruit juice consumption [11]. Presumably, the mechanism of this effect is similar to that of grapefruit juice-mediated interactions, because Sevilla orange contains significant concentrations of flavonoids, mainly bergamottin and 6',7'-dihydroxybergamottin [69]. Orange juice has also been shown to exert inhibitory effects on P-glycoprotein (P-gp)-mediated drug efflux. Takanaga and others showed that 3,3',4',5,6,7,8-heptamethoxyflavon and tangeretin were the major P-gp inhibitors present in orange juice and showed that another component, nobiletin, was also a P-gp inhibitor [55]. Therefore, the intake of orange juice might inhibit the efflux transporters by P-gp, which could enhance the bioavailability of drugs and thus lead to an increase in the risk of adverse events [52].

It has also been observed that components of orange juice -naringin in particular- are *in vitro* inhibitors of OATP transport activity [70]. Dresser et al., have previously reported that orange juice inhibits the function of human OATP-A (OATP1A2, gene symbol *SLC21A3/ SLCO1A2*) *in vitro* [29]. OATP-A, however, is predominantly expressed in the brain, but not in the intestine. On the other hand, Satoh et al. reported that OATP-B-mediated uptake of glibenclamide as well as estrone-3-sulfate was significantly inhibited by 5% orange juice [53]. Orange juice might reduce the intestinal absorption of substrates of OATP-B (e.g., digoxin, benzylpenicillin, and hormone conjugates), resulting in a decrease in concentration in the blood.

Previous studies in humans using fexofenadine as a probe showed that oral coadministration with orange juice decreased the oral bioavailability of fexofenadine [63]. Orange juice and its constituents were shown to interact with members of the OATP transporter family by reducing their activities. The functional consequences of such an interaction are reflected in a significant reduction in the oral bioavailability of fexofenadine, possibly by preferential direct inhibition of intestinal OATP activity. Other reports indicate that orange juice slightly reduced the absorption of ciprofloxacin, levofloxacin and celiprolol [65] A study of an interaction between orange juice and pravastatin showed an increase in AUC [54].Orange juice also moderately reduces the bioavailability of atenolol, which may necessitate a dose adjustment [71,72].

5.3. Tangerine (*Citrus reticulata*)

Early studies demonstrated the influence of tangeretin, a flavonoid found in high levels in tangerine juice, on drug metabolizing liver enzymes. It was demonstrated that tangeretin inhibits P450 1A2 and P450 3A4 activity in human liver microsomes [73]. Tangeretin is a potent regioselective stimulator of midazolam 1'-hydroxylation by human liver microsomes CYP3A4. Although, clinical studies have shown no influence on midazolam pharmacokinetics *in vivo*, further studies are needed to evaluate its effects on other drugs [74]. Diosmin is one of the main components of citrus fruits, such as tangerine. Diosmin may increase the absorption or bioavailability of co-administered drugs able to serve as P-gp substrates. As a result, some caution may be required with its clinical use [52].

5.4. Grapes (*Vitis vinifera*)

Grapes are one of the most valued conventional fruits worldwide. The grape is considered a source of unique and potentially useful medicinal natural products; they are also used in the manufacturing of various industrial products [75,76](Yadav and others 2009; Vislocky and Fernandez 2010). The main biologically active and well-characterized constituent from the grape is resveratrol, which is known for various medicinal properties in treating human diseases [75](Yadav and others 2009). Resveratrol was shown to be an irreversible (mechanism-based) inhibitor of CYP3A4 and a non-competitive reversible inhibitor for CYP2E1 in microsomes from rat liver and human liver cells containing cDNA-expressed CYPs [77,78] (Chan and Delucchi 2000; Piver and others 2001). Resveratrol is an electron-rich molecule with two aromatic benzene rings linked by an ethylene bridge. CYP3A-mediated aromatic hydroxylation and epoxidation of resveratrol are possible, resulting in a reactive p-benzo-quinone methide metabolite which is capable of binding covalently to CYP3A4, leading to inactivation and potential drug interactions.

5.5. Cranberry (*Vaccinium macrocarpon*)

American cranberry is a fruit used as a prophylactic agent against urinary tract infections [79]. Drug interactions with cranberry juice might be related to the fact that the juice is rich in flavonol glycosides, anthocyanins, proanthocyanidins, and organic and phenolic acids [80]. Izzo [81] described a total of eight cases of interaction between cranberry juice and warfarin, leading to changes in international normalized ratio (INR) values and bleeding. The mechanism behind this interaction might be the inhibition by cranberry flavonoids of CYP3A4 and/or CYP2C9 enzymes, which are responsible for warfarin metabolism [31,82].

It has also been shown that cranberry juice inhibits diclofenac metabolism in human liver microsomes, but this has not been demonstrated clinically in human subjects [83]. Cranberry juice may increase the bioavailability of CYP3A4 substrates (e.g., calcium antagonists or calcineurin inhibitors) as was discussed [61]. Uesawa and Mohri have demonstrated that nifedipine metabolism in rat intestinal and human hepatic microsomes are inhibited by preincubation with cranberry juice. Furthermore, cranberry juice increased the nifedipine concentration in rat plasma. These findings suggest that cranberry juice might affect the plasma concentration of nifedipine in humans as well [84].

5.6. Pomegranate (*Punica granatum*)

Pomegranate is commonly eaten around the world and has been used in folk medicine for a wide variety of therapeutic purposes [85-86]. Pomegranate is a rich source of several chemicals such as pectin, tannins, flavonoids, and anthocyanins. It has been have reported that pomegranate juice influenced the pharmacokinetics of carbamazepine in rats by inhibiting enteric CYP3A activity. Such inhibition of the enteric CYP3A activity by a single exposure to pomegranate juice appears to last for approximately 3 days [56]. Nagata and others [88] found that pomegranate juice inhibited human CYP2C9 activity and increased tolbutamide bioavailability in rats. Recently, pomegranate juice was shown to potently inhibit the sulfo-conjugation of 1-naphthol in Caco-2 cells. It has been suggested that some constituents of pomegranate juice, most probably punicalagin, may impair the metabolic functions of the intestine (specifically sulfoconjugation) and therefore might have effects upon the bioavailability of drugs [89].

5.7. Mango (*Mangifera indica*)

The beneficial effects of mango include anti-inflammatory and antimicrobial activities [90,91] Preliminary phytochemical screening revealed the presence of flavonoids, including quercetin and glycosylated xanthones such as mangiferin [92,93] Quercetin has been shown to possess antioxidant, antimicrobial, antitumor, antihypertensive, antiatherosclerosis, and anti-inflammatory properties [94]. In a series of studies, Rodeiro and others have shown the effects of mango on drug metabolizing enzymes and drug transporters [95, 96] They found that exposure of hepatocytes to mango extract produced a significant reduction (60%) in 7-methoxyresorufin-O-demethylase (MROD; CYP1A2) activity and an increase (50%) in 7-penthoxyresorufin-O-depentylase (PROD; CYP2B1) activity. This group also studied the effect of mangiferin on CYP enzymes and found that mangiferin reduced the activities of five P450s: POD (CYP1A2), midazolam 1'-hydroxylation (M1OH; CYP3A1), diclofenac 4'-hydroxylation (D4OH; CYP2C6), S-mephenytoin 4'-hydroxylation (SM4OH), and chlorzoxazone 6-hydroxyaltion (C6OH; CYP2E1). Recently, mango and mango-derived polyphenols have been shown to potentially affect the activity of the multidrug transporter P-gp ABCB1 [97]. These findings suggest that mango and its components inhibit the major human P450 enzymes involved in drug metabolism and some transporters. The potential for drug interactions with mango fruit should therefore be considered.

5.8. Guava (*Psidium guajava* L)

Guava is an important food crop and medicinal plant in tropical and subtropical countries; it is widely used as food and in folk medicine around the world [98, 99]. A number of metabolites such as phenolics, flavonoid, carotenoid, terpenoid and triterpene have been found in this fruit. Extracts and metabolites of this plant, particularly those from the leaves and fruit, possess useful pharmacological activities [100]. There is only one report about the effect of guava extracts on drug transport: guava extract showed a potent inhibitory effect on P-gp mediated efflux in Caco-2 cells. It was also found to inhibit efflux transport from serosal to mucosal surfaces in the rat ileum [101]. This means that guava could interact with P-gp substrates such as digoxin, fexofenadine, indinavir, vincristine, colchicine, topotecan, and paclitaxel in the small intestine. For this reason, this fruit should be consumed with caution by patients taking medicines.

5.9. Raspberry (*Rubus* spp.)

Berries have been shown to have a positive impact on several chronic conditions including obesity, cancer, and cardiovascular and neurodegenerative diseases [102-104]. Like other fruits, raspberries contain micro- and macronutrients such as vitamins, minerals, and fiber. Their biological properties, however, have been largely attributed to high levels of various phenolic compounds, as well as the interactive synergies among their natural phytochemical components (e.g., ellagic acid, quercetin, gallic acid, anthocyanins, cyanidins, pelargonidins, catechins, kaempferol and salicylic acid). Raspberry or raspberry constituents have antioxidant and anti-inflammatory properties, and inhibit cancer cell growth [105-107]. Black raspberries (*Rubus coreanus*) have been called the "king of berries" for their superior health benefits, whereas black mulberry (*Morus nigra*) is most commonly used for its antioxidants properties and for its high bioactive content of phenolics, anthocyanins, and gallic acid. It has been shown that black raspberry and black mulberry are able to inhibit the human

CYP3A-catalyzed midazolam 1-hydroxylation activity in liver microsomes, and the inhibitory effects are somewhat greater than those of pomegranate [49, 56]. It has also been reported that black mulberry extract potently inhibits OATP-B function at concentrations that seem to be physiologically relevant *in vitro* [53]. These results suggest that black raspberry and black mulberry may decrease the plasma concentrations of concomitantly ingested OATP-B substrate drugs or increase the plasma concentration levels of concomitantly ingested CYP3A-substrate drugs. *In vivo* studies on the interaction between black mulberry and black raspberry and CYP3A substrates are needed to determine whether inhibition of CYP3A activity by fruit juices is clinically relevant.

5.10. Apple (*Malus domestica*)

Apple and its products contain high amounts of polyphenols, which show diverse biological activities and may contribute to beneficial health effects such as protecting the intestine against inflammation due to chronic inflammatory bowel diseases [108, 109]. It has been found that apple juice extract inhibits CYP1A1 at levels of CYP1A1 mRNA, protein, and enzymatic activity [110]. On the other hand, it has also been reported that apple juice and its constituents can interact with members of the OATP transporter family (OATP-1, OATP-3 and NTCP) by reducing their activities *in vitro*. The functional consequence of such an interaction was a significant reduction in the oral bioavailability of fexofenadine in human plasma levels, possibly by preferential direct inhibition of intestinal OATP activity [29]. These findings suggest that apple might interact with OATP substrates (e.g., estrone-3-sulfate, deltorphin II, fexofenadine, vasopressin, and rosuvastatin).

5.11. Papaya (*Carican papaya* L.)

Papaya is prized worldwide for its flavor and nutritional properties. An ethno-botanical survey showed that papaya is commonly used in traditional medicine for the treatment of various human diseases, including abdominal discomfort, pain, malaria, diabetes, obesity, infections, and oral drug poisoning [111,112]. Papaya leaves and seeds are known to contain proteolytic enzymes (papain, chymopapain), alkaloids (carpain, carpasemine), sulfurous compounds (benzyl iso- thiocyanate), flavonoids, tannins, triterpenes, anthocyanins, organic acids and oils. Papaya fruit is a good source of nutrients and some phytochemicals such as beta-cryptoxanthin and benzyl isothiocyanates [113]. Hidaka et al. found that *papaya* produced an inhibition of CYP3A activity in human microsomes [114]. So far, there has been no clinical report suggesting adverse food-drug interaction caused by the intake of papaya. Accordingly, the inhibition of CYP3A by papaya may not be observed in vivo. However, the results obtained by others raised the hypothesis that papaya extracts were capable of altering the pharmacokinetics of therapeutic drugs coadministered via CYP3A inhibition, as in the case of grapefruit. Thus, the possibility of adverse food-drug interaction involving papaya and medicine acting via CYP3A metabolism should be examined in vivo. The empirical evidence regarding the wide use of fermented papaya preparation (FPP), especially by elderly people, has indicated an unknown collateral effect, i.e., drops in blood sugar levels, especially in the afternoon. Those findings have been corroborated by a clinical study that shows that FPP use can induce a significant decrease in plasma sugar levels in both healthy subjects and type 2 diabetic patients [115]. Therefore, patients consuming papaya and taking antidiabetic therapy could suffer from potential drug-food interaction.

5.12. Leafy vegetables

Broccoli (*Brassica oleracea var. italica*) and cauliflower (*Brassica oleracea var. botrytis)* are unique among the common cruciferous vegetables that contain high levels of the aliphatics glucosinolate and glucoraphanin [116]. Upon hydrolysis, glucoraphanin produces several products that include the bioactive isothiocyanate sulforaphane. The percentage of isothiocyanate sulforaphane present in these vegetables may vary depending on conditions of hydrolysis, food handling, and preparation procedures [117, 118]. In animal studies, dietary freeze-dried broccoli was found to offer protection against several cancers [119]. However, broccoli, cauliflower and their glucosinolate hydrolysis products have been shown to induce phase I and phase II drug-metabolizing enzymes in intact liver cells from both rats and humans. The isothiocyanate sulforaphane decreased the enzyme activities hepatocytes associated with CYP1A1 and 2B1/2, namely ethoxyresorufin-O-deethylase and pentoxyresorufin-O-dealkylase, respectively, in a dose-dependent manner [120]. An increase in hGSTA1/2 mRNA has been observed in isothiocyanate sulforaphane-treated human hepatocytes, whereas the expression of CYP3A4, the major CYP in the human liver, markedly decreased at both mRNA and activity levels [121]. Conversely, it was recently shown that sulforaphane induces mRNA levels of MRP1 and MRP2 in primary hepatocytes and Caco-2 cells [122]. It has been additionally reported that broccoli is able to induce the activity of phenolsulfotransferases [123]. These results suggest that other vegetables with a high content of isothiocyanates, such as those of the family *Cruciferae* (e.g., cabbage, cauliflower, Brussels sprouts, watercress, broccoli, and kale) and the genus *Raphanus* (radishes and daikons) may have pharmacological and toxicological implications in humans.

Watercress is another important member of the cruciferous vegetables, an excellent source for glucosinolates and other bioactive phytochemicals [124]. Watercress (*Nasturtium officinale)* is an exceptionally rich dietary source of beta-phenylethyl isothiocyanate (PEITC) [125]. Previous studies have shown that a single ingestion of watercress inhibits the hydroxylation of chlorzoxazone, an *in vivo* probe for CYP2E1, in healthy volunteers [126]. It has also been shown that watercress is a bifunctional agent with the ability to induce both phase I (CYP450) and II enzymes. Adding watercress juice to human liver cells induced the activity of CYP4501A and ethoxyresorufin-O-deethylase and NAD(P)H-quinone reductase [127]. According to reports, PEITC also has several anti-carcinogenic effects given that it can inhibit phase I enzymes and/or activate phase II enzymes. Watercress juice can increase the enzymes *SOD* and *GPX* in blood cells *in vitro* and *in vivo* [128]. Isothiocyanates also interact with ATP-binding cassette (ABC) efflux transporters such as P-glycoprotein, MRP1, MRP2 and BCRP, and may influence the pharmacokinetics of substrates of these transporters [26]. According to current data, watercress and isothiocyanate may have clinical repercussions by inducing changes in the bioavailability of some drugs.

Spinach (*Spinacia oleracea*) is an important antioxidant vegetable usually consumed after boiling the fresh or frozen leaves [129]. Freshly cut spinach leaves contain approximately 1,000 mg of total flavonoids per kilogram, and the occurrence of at least 10 flavonoid glycosides has been reported [130]. These are glucuronides and acylated di-and triglycosides of methylated and methylene dioxide derivatives of 6-oxygenated flavonols [131]. While epidemiological and preclinical data support the nutritional benefits of spinach and the safety of its consumption there are no publications about its effects on drug metabolizing enzymes and drug transporters. Little is currently known about the *in vivo* effects these compounds have on the bioavailability of xenobiotics the clearance and/or tissue distribution of which is determined by active transport and biotransformation. Platt and others [132] reported the protective effect of spinach against the genotoxic effects of 2-amino-3-methylimidazo[4,5-f]quinoline (IQ) by interaction with CYP1A2 as a mechanism of anti-genotoxicity. Its high isothiocyanate and flavonoid content demands additional research to evaluate possible nutrient-drug interactions.

5.13. Vegetable fruits

Tomatoes (*Lycopersicon esculentum*) and tomato-based products are a source of important nutrients and contain numerous phytochemicals, such as carotenoids, that may influence health (carotenoids such as phytofluene, phytoene, neurosporene, γ-carotene, and ζ-carotene) [133,134]. Tomatoes are also a source of a vast array of flavonols (e.g., quercetin and kaempferol), phytosterols, and phenylpropanoids [135]. Lycopene is the most important carotenoid present in tomatoes and tomato products, and their dietary intake has been linked to a decreased risk of chronic illnesses such as cancer and cardiovascular disease [136,137]. Studies performed on human recombinant CYP1 showed that lycopene inhibits CYP1A1 and CYP1B1. Lycopene has also been shown to slightly reduce the induction of ethoxyresorufin-O-deethylase activity by 20% by DMBA in MCF-7 cells [138]. It appears to inhibit bioactivation enzymes and induce detoxifying enzymes. It has been suggested that lycopene might have a potential advantage over other phytochemicals by facilitating the elimination of genotoxic chemicals and their metabolites [138]. Recent *in vitro* evidence suggests that high dose lycopene supplementation increases hepatic cytochrome P4502E1 protein and inflammation in alcohol-fed rats [139].

Carrots (*Daucus carrota*) are widely consumed as food. The active components of carrots, which include beta-carotene and panaxynol have been studied by many researchers [140-142]. Carrots induce phenolsulfotransferase activity [123] and decrease CYP1A2 activity [122]. It has been reported that a carrot diet increased the activity of ethoxycoumarin O-deethylase ECD activity in a mouse model [143].

Avocado (*Persea americana*) is a good source of bioactive compounds such as monounsaturated fatty acids and sterols [144]. Growing evidence on the health benefits of avocadoes have led to increased consumption and research on potential health benefits [145, 146]. Phytochemicals extracted from avocado can selectively induce several biological functions [147,148]. Two papers published in the 1990's reported avocados interact with warfarin, stating that the fruit inhibited the effect of warfarin. They, however, did not establish the cause of such inhibition [149, 150].

Red pepper (*Capsicum annuum* L.) is used as a spice that enhances the palatability of food and drugs such as the counterirritant present in stomach medicines across many countries [151]. The pungencyof red pepper is derived from a group of compounds called capsaicinoids, which possess an array of biological properties and give it its spicy flavor. Two major capsaicinoids, dihydrocapsaicin (DHC) and capsaicin (CAP) are responsible for up to 90% of the total pungency of pepper fruits. Red pepper has several uses as a fruit stimulant and rubifacient in traditional medicine; it is also used in the treatment of some diseases such as scarlatina, putrid sore throat, hoarseness, dispepsia, yellow fever, piles and snakebite [152]. Capsaicin (8-methyl-N-vanillyl-6-nonenamide) is a fundamental component of *Capsicum* fruits. Capsaicin is known to have antioxidant properties and has therefore been associated with potent antimutagenic and anticarcinogenic activities [153]. Early studies have reported that capsaicin strongly inhibited the constitutive enzymes CYP 2A2, 3A1, 2C11, 2B1, 2B2 and 2C6 [154]. There is also a report indicating that capsaicin is a substrate of CYP1A2 [155]. Pharmacokinetic studies in animals have shown that a single dose of *Capsicum* fruit could affect the pharmacokinetic parameters of theophylline, while a repeated dose affected the metabolic pathway of xanthine oxidase [156]. Therefore, a potential interaction may occur when is taken along with some medicines that are CYP450 substrates. Recently, it has been evidenced that red pepper induces alterations in intestinal brush border fluidity and passive permeability properties associated with the induction of increased microvilli length and perimeter, resulting in an increased absorptive surface for the small intestine and an increased bioavailability not only of micronutrients but also of drugs [157]. Cruz et al. have shown that pepper ingestion reduces oral salicylate bioavailability, a likely result of the gastrointestinal effects of capsaicin [158]. On the other hand, Imaizumi et al. have reported capsaicinoid-induced changes of glucose in rats. Therefore, there is a possible interaction risk between red pepper and hypoglycemic drugs in diabetic patients [159]. Patients consuming red pepper and taking antidiabetic therapy could suffer potential drug-food interaction.

5.14. Other vegetables

Yeh and Yen have reported that asparagus, cauliflower, celery and eggplant induced significant phenol sulfotransferase –P (PST-P) activity, whereas asparagus, eggplant and potato induced PST-M activity [123]. It has been have also reported that a diet supplemented with apiaceous vegetables (dill weed, celery, parsley, parsnip) resulted in a 13-15% decrease in CYP1A2 activity [122]. The authors speculate that furanocumarins present in the apiaceous vegetables were responsible for the inhibitory effects on CYP1A2 ^115 [117,160].

Vegetables such as cabbage, celery, onion and parsley are known to have a high content of polyphenols. It has been reported that polyphenols can potentially affect phase I metabolism either by direct inhibition of phase I enzymes or by regulating the expression of enzyme levels *via* their interactions with regulatory cascades. Several studies have directly and indirectly shown that dietary polyphenols can modulate phase II metabolism [161]. In addition polyphenols have been shown to interact with ABC drug transporters involved in drug resistance and drug absorption, distribution and excretion [32].

6. Drug-food interaction in specific diets with high content of fruits and vegetables

Weight-reduction diets, vegetarian diets, hospitalization, or post-operative regimes all lead to dietary modifications. These diets are often maintained for long periods of time and are likely to result in metabolic changes due to subsequently administered drugs or exposure to environmental chemicals. Several epidemiologic, clinical, and experimental studies have established that certain types of diet may have beneficial effects on health. For example, the traditional Mediterranean diet has been shown to reduce overall mortality and coronary heart disease events [162]. This diet, however, varies across at least 16 countries bordering the Mediterranean Sea. Cultural, ethnic, religious, economic and agricultural differences in these regions account for variations in dietary patterns, which are widely characterized by the following: daily consumption of fruits, vegetables, whole grain breads, non-refined cereals, olive oil, and dairy products; moderate weekly consumption of fish, poultry, nuts, potatoes, and eggs; low monthly consumption of red meat, and daily moderate wine consumption [163]. Increasing evidence suggests that a Mediterranean-style diet rich in fruits, vegetables, nuts, fish and oils with monounsaturated fat and low in meat promotes cardiovascular health and aids cancer prevention because of its positive effects on lipid profile, endothelial function, vascular inflammation, insulin resistance, and its antioxidant properties [164,165].

Vegetarians, on the other hand, exhibit a wide diversity of dietary practices often described by what is omitted from their diet. When a vegetarian diet is appropriately planned and includes fortified foods, it can be nutritionally suitable for adults and children and can promote health and lower the risk of major chronic diseases [166]. A vegetarian diet usually provides a low intake of saturated fat and cholesterol and a high intake of dietary fiber and many health-promoting phytochemicals. This is achieved by an increased consumption of fruits, vegetables, whole-grains, legumes, nuts, and various soy products. As a result of these factors, vegetarians typically have a lower body mass index, low-density lipoprotein cholesterol levels, and lower blood pressure; a reduced ischemic heart disease death rate; and decreased incidence of hypertension, stroke, type 2 diabetes, and certain cancers that are more common among non-vegetarians [167]. The vegan dietary category may be more comparable across countries and cultures because avoiding all animal products leaves little choice but to include large quantities of vegetables, fruit, nuts, and grains for nutritional adequacy. Admittedly, vegetable and fruit variety may also vary widely according to location [168].

Due to their high content of fruits and vegetables, all these diets contain a large proportion of antioxidant vitamins, flavonoids, and polyphenols [169]. Phenolic compounds may help protect the gastrointestinal tract against damage by reactive species present in foods or generated within the stomach and intestines. However, they may be beneficial in the gut in correct amounts. The overall health benefits of polyphenols are uncertain, and consumption of large quantities of them in fortified foods or supplements should not yet be encouraged [170].

Flavonoids have been known as plant pigments for over a century and belong to a vast group of phenolic compounds that are widely distributed in all foods of plant origin. Unfortunately, the potentially toxic effects of excessive flavonoid intake are largely ignored. At higher doses, flavonoids may act as mutagens, pro-oxidants that generate free radicals, and as inhibitors of key enzymes involved in hormone metabolism [171]. It has been shown that phenol ring-containing flavonoids yield cytotoxic phenoxyl radicals upon oxidation by peroxidases; co-oxidize unsaturated lipids, GSH, NADH, ascorbate, and nucleic acids; and cause ROS formation and mitochondrial toxicity [172]. In high doses, the adverse effects of flavonoids may outweigh their beneficial ones, and caution should be exercised when ingesting them at levels above those which would be obtained from a typical vegetarian diet [173]. Moreover, it is possible that people ingesting a vegetarian or Mediterranean diet may be taking medication and thus have drug-food interaction.

Inhibition of CYP enzymes, which are necessary for carcinogen activation, is a beneficial chemopreventive property of various flavonoids but may be a potential toxic property in flavonoid-drug interactions. Inhibition of CYP activities by flavonoids has been extensively studied because of their potential use as blocking agents during the initial stage of carcinogenesis [174]. The general conclusion after an analysis of available data on CYP-flavonoid interactions is that flavonoids possessing hydroxyl groups inhibit CYP activity, whereas those lacking hydroxyl groups may induce the metabolizing enzyme [175]. Flavonoids can either inhibit or induce human CYP enzymes depending on their structure, concentration, or experimental conditions [176]. The interaction of flavonoids with CYP3A4, the predominant human hepatic and intestinal CYP responsible for metabolizing 50% of therapeutic agents as well as the activation of some carcinogens, is of particular interest [177].

The simultaneous administration of flavonoids present in fruits or vegetables and clinically used drugs may cause flavonoid-drug interactions by modulating the pharmacokinetics of certain drugs, which results in an increase in their toxicity or a decline in their therapeutic effect, depending on the flavonoid structure [178]. Additional reasons for concern regarding mega flavonoid supplements include potential flavonoid-drug interactions, since flavonoids have been shown to both induce and inhibit drug-metabolizing enzymes [38, 39]. Further research regarding the potential toxicities associated with flavonoids and other dietary phenolics is required if these plant-derived products are to be used as therapy.

It is a fact that diets based on fruits and vegetables may have a variety of phytochemicals, as was mentioned earlier, so the possibility of developing a drug-food interaction is high. While dietary polyphenols may be beneficial in the correct amount, but too much may not be good and combining them with medication should be avoided.

7. Conclusion

WHO and the Food and Agriculture Organization of the United Nations (FAO) recommend a daily intake of at least 400 grams or five servings of fruits and vegetables to aid in the prevention of chronic illnesses such as heart disease, cancer, diabetes, and obesity. As a consequence, there is an increased global consumer demand for fruits and vegetables, and some consumers purchase organic foods with the understanding that they are healthy. The use of natural products for improving human health has evolved independently in different regions of the world and production, use, attitudes, and regulatory aspects vary globally. Although modern medicine may be available in most countries for the treatment of many chronic degenerative diseases, folk medicine (phytomedicine) has remained popular for historical and cultural reasons. Although the significance of interactions between drugs is widely appreciated, little attention has been given to interactions between drugs and nutrients. Most of the documented information about the effects of fruit and vegetables on metabolizing enzymes and drug transporters comes from preclinical studies. However, the possibility that these effects could occur in humans should not be ignored. Several clinical studies on the interactions of grapefruit juice and drugs have been conducted with impressive results. Most of the fruits and vegetables examined in this review contain a similar phytochemical mix to that of grapefruit juice. *In vitro* models and animal models have shown that many of these agents influence drug metabolizing enzymes and drug transporters. It is possible that other fruits and vegetables could have the same potential for fruit and drug interactions, and this should be taken into account. This review shows evidence of the influence of fruit, vegetables or their components (phytochemicals) on the CYP3A4 enzyme, which metabolizes most drugs used by the human population. A more consistent approach to the evaluation of nutrient-drug interactions in human beings is therefore needed. Said approach must be systematic in order to a) assess the influence of nutritional status, foodstuffs, or specific nutrients on a drug's pharmacokinetics and pharmacodynamics, and b) evaluate the influence of a drug on overall nutritional status or the status of a specific nutrient. In addition to all this, we must account for the fact that we live in an era of very varied lifestyles. Some people are vegetarians, others take high doses of flavonoids or antioxidants as supplements, some ingest large amounts of bottled water from plastic bottles, or use chlorinated disinfectants. In industrialized countries, fruits and vegetables tend have been subjected to some sort of processing (e.g., refrigeration, acidification, fermentation, and thermal, high pressure, chemical, or physical processing) that might have an effect on the bioactive compound. All of these factors could have an impact on the metabolism or transport of drugs in a individual, potentially altering pharmacological responses. Our knowledge regarding the potential risk of nutrient-drug interactions is still limited. Therefore, efforts to elucidate potential risk of food-drug interactions should be intensified in order to prevent undesired and harmful clinical consequences

Author details

Lourdes Rodríguez-Fragoso* and Jorge Reyes-Esparza

*Address all correspondence to: mrodriguezf@uaem.mx

Universidad Autónoma del Estado de Morelos, Facultad de Farmacia, Cuernavaca, México

References

[1] Liu RH (2004) Potential synergy of phytochemicals in cancer prevention: mechanism of action. J. Nutr. 134:3479S-3485S.

[2] Milner JA (2004) Molecular targets for bioactive food components. J. Nutr. 134: 2492s-2498s.

[3] Liu RH (2003) Health benefits of fruit and vegetables are from additive and synergistic combinations of phytochemicals. Am. J. Clin. Nutr. 78: 517S-5120S.

[4] Custodio JM, Wu CY, Benet LZ (2008) Predicting drug disposition, absorption/elimination/transporter interplay and the role of food on drug absorption. Adv. Drug Deliv. Rev. 60:717-733.

[5] Franco OH, Bonneux L, de Laet C, Peeters A, Steyerberg EW, Mackenbach JP (2004) The Polymeal: a more natural, safer, and probably tastier (than the Polypill) strategy to reduce cardiovascular disease by more than 75%. BMJ 329:1447-1450.

[6] Ortega RM (2006) Importance of functional foods in the Mediterranean diet. Public Health Nutr. 9(8A):1136-1140.

[7] Dangour AD, Lock K, Hayter A, Aikenhead A, Allen E, Uauy R (2010) Nutrition-related health effects of organic foods: a systematic review. Am. J. Clin. Nutr. 92:203-210.

[8] Santos CA, and Boullata JI (2005) An Approach to Evaluating Drug-Nutrient Interactions. Pharmacother. 25: 1789-1800.

[9] Genser D (2008) Food and Drug Interaction: Consequences for the Nutrition/Health Status. Ann. Nutr. Metab. 52: 29-32.

[10] Singh BN, Malhotra BK (2004) Effects of food on the clinical pharmacokinetics of anticancer agents: underlying mechanisms and implications for oral chemotherapy. Clin. Pharmacokinet. 43:1127-1156.

[11] Malhotra S, Bailey DG, Paine MF, Watkins PB (2001) Seville orange juice-felodipine interaction: comparison with dilute grapefruit juice and involvement of furocoumarins. Clin. Pharmacol. Ther. 69: 14-23.

[12] Schmidt LE, Dalhoff K (2002) Food-drug interactions. Drugs 62:1481-1502.

[13] Chan LN (2006) Drug-Nutrient Interactions; in Shils ME, Shike M, Ross AC, Caballero B, Cousins RJ (eds) In: Modern Nutrition in Health and Disease. Lippincott Williams & Wilkins, 1540 p.

[14] Muntané J (2009) Regulation of drug metabolism and transporters. Curr. Drug Metab. 10: 932-995.

[15] Sai Y (2005) Biochemical and molecular pharmacological aspects of transporters as determinants of drug disposition. Drug Metab. Pharmacokinet. 20: 91-99.

[16] Zhang L, Zhang YD, Strong JM, Reynolds KS, Huang S M (2008). A regulatory viewpoint on transporter based drug interactions. Xenobiotica 38: 709-724.

[17] Ayrton A, Morgan P (2001) Role of transport proteins in drug absorption, distribution and excretion. Xenobiotica 8: 469-497.

[18] Li P, Wang GJ, Robertson TA, Roberts MS (2009) Liver transporters in hepatic drug disposition: an update. Curr. Drug Metab. 10:482-498.

[19] Kohl C (2009) Transporters--the view from industry. Chem. Biodivers. 6: 1988-1999.

[20] The International Transporter Consortium (2010) Membrane transporters in drug development. Drug Discovery. Macmillan Publishers Limited , 215 p.

[21] VanWert AL, Gionfriddo MR, Sweet DH (2010) Organic Anion transporters: Discovery, Pharmacology, Regulation and Roles in Pathophysiology. Biopharm. Drug Dispos. 31: 1-71.

[22] Hagenbuch B, Gui C (2008) Xenobiotic transporters of the human organic anion transporting polypeptides (OATP) family. Xenobiotica 38: 778–801.

[23] Schinkel A H, Jonker J W (2003) Mammalian drug efflux transporters of the ATP binding cassette (ABC) family: an overview. Adv. Drug Deliv. Rev. 55: 3-29.

[24] Huang SM, Strong JM, Zhang L, Reynolds KS, Nallani S, Temple R, Abraham S, Habet SA, Baweja RK, Burckart GJ, Chung S, Colangelo P, Frucht D, Green MD, Hepp P, Karnaukhova E, Ko HS, Lee JI, Marroum PJ, Norden JM, Qiu W, Rahman A, Sobel S, Stifano T, Thummel K, Wei XX, Yasuda S, Zheng JH, Zhao H, Lesko LJ (2008). New era in drug interaction evaluation: US Food and Drug Administration update on CYP enzymes, transporters, and the guidance process. J Clin. Pharmacol. 48: 662–670.

[25] Wink M (2008) Evolutionary Advantage and Molecular Modes of Action of Multi-Component Mixtures Used in Phytomedicine. Curr Drug Metab 9: 996-1009.

[26] Telang U, Ji Y, Morris ME (2009) ABC Transporters and Isothiocyanates: Potential for Pharmacokinetic Diet–Drug Interactions. Biopharm. Drug Dispos. 30: 335-344.

[27] Huang SM Hall SD, Watkins P, Love LA, Serabjit-Singh C, Betz JM, Hoffman FA, Honig P, Coates PM, Bull J, Chen ST, Kearms GL, Murray MD (2004). Drug interac-

tions with herbal products & grapefruit juice: a conference report. Clin. Pharmacol. Ther. 75: 1-12.

[28] Tomlinson B, Hu M, Lee VW (20089 In vivo assessment of herb-drug interactions: Possible utility of a pharmacogenetic approach? Mol. Nut. Food Res. 52: 799-809.

[29] Dresser GK, Bailey DG, Leake BF, Schwarz UI, Dawson PA, Freeman DJ, Kim RB (2002). Fruit juices inhibit organic anion transporting polypeptide-mediated drug uptake. Clin. Pharmacol. Ther. 71: 11-20.

[30] Meijerman I, Beijnen JH, Schellensa JH (2006) Herb–Drug Interactions in Oncology: Focus on Mechanisms of Induction. Oncol. 11: 742-752.

[31] Zhou S, Lim LY, Chowbay B (2004) Herbal modulation of P-glycoprotein. Drug Metab. Rev. 36: 57-104

[32] Alvarez AI, Real R, Perez M, Mendoza G, Prieto JG, Merino G (2010) Modulation of the activity of ABC transporters (P-glycoprotein, MRP2, BCRP) by flavonoids and drug response. Pharm. Sci. 99: 598-617.

[33] Rushmore TH, Kong AN (2002). Pharmacogenomics, Regulation and Signaling Pathways of Phase I and II Drug Metabolizing Enzymes. Curr. Drug Metab. 3: 481- 490.

[34] Watkins PB (1992) Drug metabolism by cytochromes P450 in liver and small bowel. Gastrointerol. Clin. North Am. 21: 511-526.

[35] Rendic S (2002) Summary of information on human CYP enzymes: human P450 metabolism data. Drug Metab. Rev. 34: 83-448.

[36] Iyanagi T (2007) Molecular mechanism of phase I and phase II drug-metabolizing enzymes: implications for detoxification. Int. Rev. Cytol. 260: 35-112.

[37] [37] Xu C, Li CYL and Kong ANT (2005) Induction of Phase I, II and III Drug Metabolism/Transport by Xenobiotics. Arch. Pharm. Res. 28: 249-268.

[38] [38] Saxena A, Tripathi KP, Roy S, Khan F, Sharma A (2008) Pharmacovigilance: Effects of herbal components on human drugs interactions involving Cytochrome P450. Bioinformation 3: 198-204.

[39] Foti RS, Wienkers LC, Wahlstrom JL (2010). Application of Cytochrome P450 Drug Interaction Screening in Drug Discovery. Comb Chem High Throughput Screen 13:145-158.

[40] Walter-Sack I, Klotz U (1996). Influence of diet and nutritional status on drug metabolism. Clin. Pharmacokinet. 31: 47-64.

[41] Mandlekar S, Hong JL, Kong AN (2006) Modulation of Metabolic Enzymes by Dietary Phytochemicals: A Review of Mechanisms Underlying Beneficial Versus Unfavorable Effects. Curr. Drug Metab. 7: 661-675.

[42] Nahrstedt A, Butterweck V (2010) Lessons learned from herbal medicinal products: the example of St. John's Wort (perpendicular). J. Nat. Prod. 28: 1015-1021.

[43] Kimura Y, Ito H, Ohnishi R, Hatano T (2010) Inhibitory effects of polyphenols on human cytochrome P450 3A4 and 2C9 activity. Food Chem. Toxicol. 48: 429-435.

[44] World Health Organization (2003) Diet, nutrition, and the prevalence of chronic diseases. Geneva, Switzerland: World Health Organization. Contract No.: WHO Technical Report Series No. 916.

[45] Flanagan D (2005) Understanding the grapefruit-drug interaction. Gen. Dent. 53: 282-285.

[46] Cuciureanu M, Vlase L, Muntean D, Varlan I, Cuciureanu R (2010) Grapefruit juice--drug interactions: importance for pharmacotherapy. Rev. Med. Chir. Soc. Med. Nat. Iasi 114:885-891.

[47] Hanley MJ, Cancalon P, Widmer WW, Greenblatt DJ (2011). The effect of grapefruit juice on drug disposition. Expert Opin. Drug Metab. Toxicol. 7: 267-286.

[48] Bressler R (2006) Grapefruit juice and drug interactions. Exploring mechanisms of this interaction and potential toxicity for certain drugs. Geriatrics 61:12-18.

[49] Kim H, Yoon YJ, Shon JH, Cha IJ, Shin JG, Liu KH (2006). Inhibitory effects of fruit juices on CYP3A activity. Drug Metab. Dispos. 34: 521-523.

[50] Honda Y, Ushigome F, Koyabu N, Morimoto S, Shoyama Y, Uchiumi T, Kuwano M, Ohtani H, Sawada Y (2004) Effects of grapefruit juice and orange juice components on P-glycoprotein- and MRP2-mediated drug efflux. Br. J. Pharmacol. 143: 856-864.

[51] Konishi T, Satsu H, Hatsugai Y, Aizawa K, Inakuma T, Nagata S, Sakuda SH, Nagasawa H, Shimizu M (2004) Inhibitory effect of a bitter melon extract on the P-glycoprotein activity in intestinal Caco-2 cells. Br. J. Pharmacol. 143: 379-387.

[52] Yoo HH, Lee M, Chung HJ, Lee SK, Kim DH (2007) Effects of diosmin, a flavonoid glycoside in citrus fruits, on P-glycoprotein-mediated drug efflux in human intestinal Caco-2 cells. J. Agric. Food Chem. 55: 7620-7625.

[53] Satoh H, Yamashita F, Tsujimoto M, Murakami H, Koyabu N, Ohtani H, Sawada Y (2005) Citrus juices inhibit the function of human organic anion-transporting polypeptide OATP-B. Drug Metab. Dispos. 33. 518-523.

[54] Greenblatt DJ (2009) Analysis of drug interactions involving fruit beverages and organic anion-transporting polypeptides. J. Clin. Pharmacol. 49: 1403-1407.

[55] Takanaga H, Ohnishi A, Yamada S, Matsuo H, Morimoto S, Shoyama Y, Ohtani H, Sawada Y (2000) Polymethoxylated flavones in orange juice are inhibitors of P-glycoprotein but not cytochrome P450 3A4. J. Pharmacol. Exp. Ther. 293: 230-236.

[56] Hidaka M, Okumura M, Fujita K, Ogikubo T, Yamasaki K, Iwakiri T, Setoguchi N, Arimori K (2005) Effects of pomegranate juice on human cytochrome p450 3A

(CYP3A) and carbamazepine pharmacokinetics in rats. Drug Metab. Dispos. 33: 644-648.

[57] Sica DA (2006) Interaction of grapefruit juice and calcium channel blockers. Am. J. Hypertens. 19: 768-773.

[58] Pawełczyk T, Kłoszewska I (2008) Grapefruit juice interactions with psychotropic drugs: advantages and potential risk. Przegl Lek. 65: 92-95.

[59] Reamy BV, Stephens MB (2007) The grapefruit-drug interaction debate: role of statins. Am. Fam. Phys. 76: 190-192.

[60] Paine MF, Widmer WW, Pusek SN, Beavers KL, Criss AB, Snyder J, Watkins PB (2008) Further characterization of a furanocoumarin-free grapefruit juice on drug disposition: studies with cyclosporine. Am. J. Clin. Nutr. 87: 863-871.

[61] Van den Bout-Van den Beukel CJ, Koopmans PP, van der Ven AJ, De Smet PA, Burger DM (2006) Possible drug-metabolism interactions of medicinal herbs with antiretroviral agents. Drug Metab. Rev. 38: 477-514.

[62] Bailey DG, Dresser GK. (2004) Interactions between grapefruit juice and cardiovascular drugs. Am. J. Cardiovasc. Drugs 4: 281-297.

[63] Dresser GK, Kim RB, Bailey DG (2005) Effect of grapefruit juice volume on the reduction of fexofenadine bioavailability: possible role of organic anion transporting polypeptides. Clin. Pharmacol. Ther. 77: 170-177.

[64] Amory JK, Amory DW (2005) Oral erythromycin and the risk of sudden death. N. Engl. J. Med. 352: 301-304.

[65] Saito M, Hirata-Koizumi M, Matsumoto M, Urano T, Hasegawa R (2005) Undesirable effects of citrus juice on the pharmacokinetics of drugs: focus on recent studies. Drug Saf. 28: 677-694.

[66] Kiani J, Imam S (2007) Medicinal importance of grapefruit juice and its interaction with various drugs. Nutr. J. 6: 33-35.

[67] Pillai U, Muzaffar J, Sen S, Yancey A (2009) Grapefruit juice and verapamil: a toxic cocktail. South Med. J. 102: 308-309.

[68] Ho PC, Saville DJ, Coville PF, Wanwimolruk S (2000) Content of CYP3A4 inhibitors, naringin, naringenin and bergapten in grapefruit and grapefruit juice products. Pharm. Acta Helv. 74:379-385.

[69] Kamath AV, Yao M, Zhang Y, Chon S (2005) Effect of fruit juices on the oral bioavailability of fexofenadine in rats. J. Pharm. Sci. 94: 233-239.

[70] Farkas D, Greenblatt DJ (2008) Influence of fruit juices on drug disposition: discrepancies between in vitro and clinical studies. Expert Opin. Drug Metab. Toxicol. 4: 381-393.

[71] Lilja JJ, Juntti-Patinen L, Neuvonen PJ (2004) Orange juice substantially reduces the bioavailability of the beta-adrenergic-blocking agent celiprolol. Clin. Pharmacol. Ther. 75: 184-190.

[72] Lilja JJ, Raaska K, Neuvonen PJ (2005) Effects of orange juice on the pharmacokinetics of atenolol. Eur. J. Clin. Pharmacol. 61: 337-340.

[73] Obermeier MT, White RE, Yang CS (1995) Effects of bioflavonoids on hepatic P450 activities. Xenobiotica 25: 575-584.

[74] Backman JT, Maenppa J, Belle DJ, Wrighton SA, Kivisto KT, Neuvonen PJ (2000) Lack of correlation between in vitro and in vivo studies on the effects of tangeretin and tangerine juice on midazolam hydroxylation. Clin. Pharmacol. Ther. 67, 382–390.

[75] Yadav M, Jain S, Bhardwaj A, Nagpal R, Puniya M, Tomar R, Singh V, Parkash O, Prasad GB, Marotta F, Yadav H (2009) Biological and medicinal properties of grapes and their bioactive constituents: an update. J. Med. Food 12: 473-484.

[76] Vislocky LM, Fernandez ML (2010) Biomedical effects of grape products. Nutr. Rev. 68:656-670.

[77] Chan WK, Delucchi BA (2000) Resveratrol, a red wine constituent, is a mechanism-based inactivator of cytochrome P450 3A4. Life Sci. 67: 3103-3112.

[78] Piver B, Berthou F, Dreano Y, Lucas D (2001) Inhibition of CYP3A, CYP1A and CYP2E1 activities by resveratrol and other non volatile red wine components. Toxicol. Let. 125: 83-91.

[79] Rossi R, Porta S, Canovi B (2010) Overview on cranberry and urinary tract infections in females. J. Clin. Gastroenterol. 44:S61-S62.

[80] Côté J, Caillet S, Doyon G, Sylvain JF, Lacroix M (2010) Bioactive compounds in cranberries and their biological properties. Crit. Rev. Food Sci. Nutr. 50:666-679.

[81] Izzo AA (2005) Herb–drug interactions: an overview of the clinical evidence. Fundam. Clin. Pharmacol. 19:1–16.

[82] Pham DQ, Pham AQ (2007) Interaction potential between cranberry juice and warfarin. Am. J. Health Syst. Pharm. 64: 490-494.

[83] Ushijima K, Tsuruoka S, Tsuda H, Hasegawa G, Obi Y, Kaneda T, Takahashi M, Maekawa T, Sasaki T, Koshimizu TA, Fujimura A (2009) Cranberry juice suppressed the diclofenac metabolism by human liver microsomes, but not in healthy human subjects. Br. J. Clin. Pharmacol. 68: 194-200.

[84] Uesawa Y, Mohri K (2006) Effects of cranberry juice on nifedipine pharmacokinetics in rats. J. Pharm. Pharmacol. 58: 1067-1072.

[85] Shabtay A, Eitam H, Tadmor Y, Orlov A, Meir A, Weinberg P, Weinberg ZG, Chen Y, Brosh A, Izhaki I, Kerem Z (2008) Nutritive and antioxidative potential of fresh and

stored pomegranate industrial byproduct as a novel beef cattle feed. J. Agric. Food Chem. 56:10063-10070

[86] Ross SM (2009) Pomegranate: its role in cardiovascular health. Holist Nurs. Pract. 23:195-197.

[87] Oliveira RA, Narciso CD, Bisinotto RS, Perdomo MC, Ballou MA, Dreher M, Santos JE (2010) Effects of feeding polyphenols from pomegranate extract on health, growth, nutrient digestion, and immunocompetence of calves. J. Dairy Sci. 93:4280-4291

[88] Nagata M, Hidaka M, Sekiya H, Kawano Y, Yamasaki K, Okumura M, Arimori K (2007) Effects of pomegranate juice on human cytochrome P450 2C9 and tolbutamide pharmacokinetics in rats. Drug Metab. Dispos. 35:302-305.

[89] Saruwatari A, Okamura S, Nakajima Y, Narukawa Y, Takeda T, Tamura H (2008) Pomegranate juice inhibits sulfoconjugation in Caco-2 human colon carcinoma cells. J. Med. Food 11: 623-628.

[90] Knodler M, Conrad J, Wenzig EM, Bauer R, Lacorn M, Beifuss U, Carle R, Schieber A (2008) Anti-inflammatory 5-(11'Z-heptadecenyl)- and 5-(8'Z,11'Z-heptadecadienyl)-resorcinols from mango (Mangifera indica L.) peels. Phytochemistry 69: 988-993.

[91] Engels C, Knodler M, Zhao YY, Carle R, Ganzle MG, Schieber A (2009) Antimicrobial activity of gallotannins isolated from mango (Mangifera indica L.) kernels. J. Agric. Food Chem 57: 7712– 7718.

[92] Schieber A, Berardini N, Carle R (2003) Identification of flavonol and xanthone glyco-sides from mango (Mangifera indica L. Cv. "Tommy Atkins") peels by high-perform-ance liquid chromatography-electrospray ionization mass spectrometry. J. Agric. Food Chem. 51: 5006-5011.

[93] Berardini N, Fezer R, Conrad J, Beifuss U, Carle R, Schieber A (2005) Screening of mango (Mangifera indica L.) cultivars for their contents of flavonol O- and xanthone C-glycosides, anthocyanins, and pectin. J. Agric. Food Chem. 53: 1563-1570

[94] Bischoff SC (2008) Quercetin: potentials in the prevention and therapy of disease. Curr. Opin. Clin. Nutr. Metab. Care 11: 733-740

[95] Rodeiro I, Donato MT, Lahoz A, Garrido G, Delgado R, Gómez-Lechón MJ (2008) In-teractions of polyphenols with the P450 system: possible implications on human therapeutics. Mini Rev. Med. Chem. 8: 97–106.

[96] Rodeiro I, Donato MT, Jimenez N, Garrido G, Molina-Torres J, Menendez R, Castell JV, Gómez-Lechón MJ (2009) Inhibition of human P450 enzymes by natural extracts used in traditional medicine. Phytother. Res. 23: 279-282.

[97] Chieli E, Romiti N, Rodeiro I, Garrido G (2009) In vitro effects of Mangifera indica and polyphenols derived on ABCB1/P-glycoprotein activity. Food Chem. Toxicol. 47: 2703-2710.

[98]   Jouad H, Haloui M, Rhiouani H, El Hilaly J, Eddouks M (2001) Ethnobotanical sur-
       vey of medicinal plants used for the treatment of diabetes, cardiac and renal diseases
       in the North centre region of Morocco (Fez-Boulemane). J. Ethnopharmacol.
       77:175-182.

[99]   De Wet H, Nkwanyana MN, van Vuuren SF (2010) Medicinal plants used for the
       treatment of diarrhoea in northern Maputaland, KwaZulu-Natal Province, South Af-
       rica. J. Ethnopharmacol. 130:284-289.

[100] Qian H, Nihorimbere V (2004) Antioxidant power of phytochemicals from Psidium
       guajava leaf. J. Zhejiang Univ. Sci. 5:676-683.

[101] Junyaprasert VB, Soonthornchareonnon N, Thongpraditchote S, Murakami T, Taka-
       no M (2006) Inhibitory effect of Thai plant extracts on P-glycoprotein mediated ef-
       flux. Phytother. Res. 20: 79-81.

[102] Patel AV, Rojas-Vera J, Dacke CG (2004) Therapeutic constituents and actions of Ru-
       bus species. Curr. Med. Chem. 11:1501-1512.

[103] Zafra-Stone S, Yasmin T, Bagchi M, Chatterjee A, Vinson JA, Bagchi D (2007) Berry
       anthocyanins as novel antioxidants in human health and disease prevention. Mol.
       Nutr. Food Res. 51:675-683.

[104] Del Rio D, Borges G, Crozier A (2010) Berry flavonoids and phenolics: bioavailability
       and evidence of protective effects. Br. J. Nutr. 104:S67-S90.

[105] Wang SY, Lin HS (2000) Antioxidant activity in fruits and leaves of blackberry, rasp-
       berry, and strawberry varies with cultivar and developmental stage. J. Agric. Food
       Chem. 48:140-146.

[106] Juranic Z, Zixack Z (2005) Biological activities of berries: from antioxidant capacity to
       anti-cancer effects. BioFactors 23: 207-211.

[107] Seeram NP, Adams LS, Zhang Y, Lee R, Sand D, Scheuller HS, Heber D (2006) Black-
       berry, black raspberry, blueberry, cranberry, red raspberry, and strawberry extracts
       inhibit growth and stimulate apoptosis of human cancer cells in vitro. J. Agric. Food
       Chem. 54:9329-9339.

[108] Lewis N, Ruud J (2004) Apples in the American diet. Nutr. Clin. Care 7:82-88.

[109] Gerhauser C (2008) Cancer chemopreventive potential of apples, apple juice, and ap-
       ple components. Planta Med. 74:1608-1624.

[110] Pohl C, Will F, Dietrich H, Schrenk D (2006) Cytochrome P450 1A1 Expression and
       Activity in Caco-2 Cells: Modulation by Apple Juice Extract and Certain Apple Poly-
       phenols. J Agric Food Chem 54: 10262-10268.

[111] Nakasone HY, Paull RE. The production of papain—an agri- cultural industry for
       tropical America. In: Tropical Fruits. CAB International, Wallingford, UK, 1998, pp.
       62–79.

[112] Adeneye AA, Olagunju IA (2009) Preliminary hypoglycemic and hypolipidemic activities of the aqueous seed extract of Carica papaya Linn. in Wistar rats. Biol Med, 1: 1–10.

[113] Chavez-Quintal P, Gonzalez-Flores T, Rodriguez-Buenfil I, Gallegos-Tintore S (2011) Antifungal Activity in Ethanolic Extracts of Carica papaya L. cv. Maradol Leaves and Seeds. Indian J Microbiol 51:54–60.

[114] Hidaka M, Fujita K, Ogikubu T, Yamasaki K, Iwakiri T, Okumura M, Arimori K. (2004) Potent inhibition by star fruit of human cytochrome p450 3a (cyp3a) activity. DMD 32:581-583.

[115] Danese C, Esposito D, D'Alfonso V, Cirene M, Ambrosino M, Colotto M (2006) Plasma glucose level decreases as collateral effect of fermented papaya preparation use. Clin Ter 157:195-198

[116] Cartea ME, Francisco M, Soengas P, Velasco P (2010) Phenolic compounds in Brassica vegetables. Molecules 16:251-280.

[117] Tian Q, Rosselot RA, Schwartz SJ (2005) Quantitative determination of intact glucosinolates in broccoli, broccoli sprouts, Brussels sprouts, and cauliflower by high-performance liquid chromatography-electrospray ionization-tandem mass spectrometry. Anal. Biochem. 343:93-99.

[118] Vasanthi HR, Mukherjee S, Das DK (2009) Potential health benefits of broccoli- a chemico-biological overview. Mini Rev. Med. Chem. 9:749-759.

[119] Velasco P, Francisco M, Moreno DA, Ferreres F, García-Viguera C, Cartea ME (2011) Phytochemical fingerprinting of vegetable Brassica oleracea and Brassica napus by simultaneous identification of glucosinolates and phenolics. Phytochem. Anal. 22: 144-152

[120] Anwar-Mohamed A, El-Kadi AO (2009) Sulforaphane induces CYP1A1 mRNA, protein, and catalytic activity levels via an AhR-dependent pathway in murine hepatoma Hepa 1c1c7 and human HepG2 cells. Cancer Lett. 275: 93-101.

[121] Fimognari C, Lenzi M, Hrelia P (2008) Interaction of the isothiocyanate sulforaphane with drug disposition and metabolism: pharmacological and toxicological implications. Curr. Drug Metab. 9: 668-678.

[122] Harris KE, Jeffery EH (2008) Sulforaphane and erucin increase MRP1 and MRP2 in human carcinoma cell lines. J. Nutr. Biochem. 19: 246-254.

[123] Yeh CT, Yen GC (2005) Effect of vegetables on human phenolsulfotransferases in relation to their antioxidant activity and total phenolics. Free Radic. Res. 39: 893-904.

[124] Getahun SM, Chung FL (1999) Conversion of glucosinolates to isothiocyanates in humans after ingestion of cooked watercress. Cancer Epidemiol. Biomarkers Prev. 8:447-451.

[125] Palaniswamy UR, McAvoy RJ, Bible BB, Stuar JD (2003) Ontogenic variations of as-corbic acid and phenethyl isothiocyanate concentrations in watercress (Nasturtium officinale R.Br.) leaves. J. Agric. Food Chem. 51: 5504-5509.

[126] Leclercq I, Desager JP, Horsmans Y (1998) Inhibition of chlorzoxazone metabolism, a clinical probe for CYP2E1, by a single ingestion of watercress. Clin. Pharmacol. Ther. 64: 144-149.

[127] Lhoste EF, Gloux K, De Waziers I, Garrido S, Lory S, Philippe C, Rabot S, Knasmüller S (2004) The activities of several detoxication enzymes are differentially induced by juices of garden cress, water cress and mustard in human HepG2 cells. Chem. Biol. Interact. 150: 211-219.

[128] Hofmann T, Kuhnert A, Schubert A, Gill C, Rowland IR, Pool-Zobel BL, Glei M (2009) Modulation of detoxification enzymes by watercress: in vitro and in vivo in-vestigations in human peripheral blood cells. Eur. J. Nutr. 48: 483-491.

[129] Schirrmacher G, Skurk T, Hauner H, Grassmann J (2010) Effect of Spinacia oleraceae L. and Perilla frutescens L. on antioxidants and lipid peroxidation in an intervention study in healthy individuals. Plant Foods Hum. Nutr .65:71-76

[130] Bergquist SA, Gertsson UE, Knuthsen P, Olsson ME (2005) Flavonoids in baby spi-nach (Spinacia oleracea L.): changes during plant growth and storage. J. Agric. Food Chem. 53:9459-9464.

[131] Lomnitski L, Bergman M, Nyska A, Ben-Shaul V, Grossman S (2003) Composition, efficacy, and safety of spinach extracts. Nutr. Cancer 46: 222-231.

[132] Platt KL, Edenharder R, Aderhold S, Muckel E, Glatt H (2010) Fruits and vegetables protect against the genotoxicity of heterocyclic aromatic amines activated by human xenobiotic-metabolizing enzymes expressed in immortal mammalian cells. Mutat. Res. 703: 90-98.

[133] Heber D (2004) Vegetables, fruits and phytoestrogens in the prevention of diseases. J. Postgrad. Med. 50:145-149

[134] Tan HL, Thomas-Ahner JM, Grainger EM, Wan L, Francis DM, Schwartz SJ, Erdman JW Jr, Clinton SK (2010) Tomato-based food products for prostate cancer prevention: what have we learned? Cancer Metastasis Rev. 29:553-568.

[135] Ellinger S, Ellinger J, Stehle P (2006) Tomatoes, tomato products and lycopene in the prevention and treatment of prostate cancer: do we have the evidence from interven-tion studies? Curr. Opin. Clin. Nutr. Metab. Care 9: 722-727.

[136] Riccioni G, Mancini B, Di Ilio E, Bucciarelli T, D'Orazio N (2008) Protective effect of lycopene in cardiovascular disease. Eur. Rev. Med. Pharmacol. Sci. 12:183-190.

[137] Waliszewski KN, Blasco G (2010) Nutraceutical properties of lycopen]. Salud Publica Mex. 52:254-265

[138] Wang H, Leung LK (2010) The carotenoid lycopene differentially regulates phase I and II enzymes in dimethylbenz[a]anthracene-induced MCF-7 cells. Nutrition 26: 1181-1187.

[139] Veeramachaneni S, Ausman LM, Choi SW, Russell RM, Wang XD (2008) High dose lycopene supplementation increases hepatic cytochrome P4502E1 protein and inflammation in alcohol-fed rats. J. Nutr. 138: 1329-1335.

[140] Surles RL, Weng N, Simon PW, Tanumihardjo SA (2004) Carotenoid profiles and consumer sensory evaluation of specialty carrots (Daucus carota, L.) of various colors. J. Agric. Food Chem .52:3417-3421

[141] Sikora M, Hallmann E, Rembiałkowska E (2009) The content of bioactive compounds in carrots from organic and conventional production in the context of health prevention. Rocz. Panstw. Zakl. Hig. 60:217-220

[142] Sun T, Simon PW, Tanumihardjo SA (2009) Antioxidant Phytochemicals and Antioxidant Capacity of Biofortified Carrots (Daucus carota L.) of Various Colors. J Agric. Food Chem. 57: 4142-4147.

[143] Bradfield CA, Chang Y, Bjeldanes LF (1985) Effects of commonly consumed vegetables on hepatic xenobiotic-metabolizing enzymes in the mouse. Food Chem. Toxicol. 23: 899-904.

[144] Duester KC (2001) Avocado fruit is a rich source of beta-sitosterol. J. Am. Diet Assoc. 101:404-405.

[145] Whiley AW, Schaffer B (2002) History, distribution and uses. In The Avocado: Botany, Production, and Uses; CABI Publishing: New York, Chapter 1, p 1-30.

[146] Ernst E (2003) Avocado–soybean unsaponifiables (ASU) for osteoarthritis—A systematic review. Clin. Rheumatol. 22: 285-288.

[147] Lu QY, Arteaga JR, Zhang Q, Huerta S, Go V L, Heber D (2005) Inhibition of prostate cancer cell growth by an avocado extract: Role of lipid-soluble bioactive substances J. Nutr. Biochem. 16: 23-30.

[148] Plaza L, Sánchez-Moreno C, de Pascual-Teresa S, de Ancos B, Cano MP (2009) Fatty acids, sterols, and antioxidant activity in minimally processed avocados during refrigerated storage. J. Agric. Food Chem. 57:3204-3209

[149] Blickstein D, Shaklai M, Inbal A (1991) Warfarin antagonism by avocado. Lancet 337: 914-915.

[150] Wells PS, Holbrook AM, Crowther NR, Hirsh J (1994) Interactions of warfarin with drugs and food. Ann. Intern. Med. 121: 676-683.

[151] Watanabe T, Sakurada N, and Kobata K (2001) Capsaici-, resiniferatoxin-, and olvanil-induced adrenaline secretion in rats via the vanilloid receptor. Biosci Biotechnol Biochem 65: 2443-2447.

[152] Ishtiaq M, Hanif W, Khan MA, Ashraf M, Butt AM (2007) An ethnomedicinal survey and documentation of important medicinal folklore food phytonims of flora of Samahni Valley (Azad Kashmir) Pakistan. Pak J Biol Sci 10: 2241-2256.

[153] Materska M, Perucka I (2005) Antioxidant activity of the main phenolic compounds isolated from hot pepper fruit (Capsicum annuum L.). J Agric Food Chem 53:1750-1756.

[154] Zhang Z, Hamilton SM, Stewart C, Strother A, Teel RW (1993) Inhibition of liver microsomal cytochrome P450 activity and metabolism of the tobacco-specific nitrosamine NNK by capsaicin and ellagic acid. Anticancer Res 13:2341-2346.

[155] Oikawa S, Nagao E, Sakano K, Kawanishi S (2006) Mechanism of oxidative DNA damage induced by capsaicin, a principal ingredient of hot chili pepper. Free Radic Res 40(9):966-973.

[156] Bouraoui A, Brazier JL, Zouaghi H, Rousseau M (1995) Theophylline pharmacokinetics and metabolism in rabbits following single and repeated administration of Capsicum fruit. Eur J Drug Metab Pharmacokinet 20:173-178.

[157] Prakash UN, Srinivasan K (2010) Beneficial influence of dietary spices on the ultrastructure and fluidity of the intestinal brush border in rats. Br J Nutr 104: 31–39.

[158] Cruz L, Castañeda-Hernández G, Navarrete A (1999) Ingestion of chilli pepper (Capsicum annuum) reduces salicylate bioavailability after oral asprin administration in the rat. Can J Physiol Pharmacol 77:441-446.

[159] Imaizumi K, Sato S, Kumazawa M, Arai N, Aritoshi S, Akimoto S, Sakakibara Y, Kawashima Y, Tachiyahiki K (2011) Capsaicinoids-induced changes of plasma glucose, fre fatty acids and glicerol concentrations in rats. J Toxicol Sci 36: 109-116.

[160] Lampe JW, King IB, Li S, Grate MT, Barale KV, Chen C, Feng Z, Potter JD (2000) Brassica vegetables increase and apiaceous vegetables decrease cytochrome P450 1A2 activity in humans: changes in caffeine metabolite ratios in response to controlled vegetable diets. Carcinogenesis 21: 1157-1162.

[161] Lambert JD, Sang S, Lu AY, Yang CS (2007) Metabolism of dietary polyphenols and possible interactions with drugs. Curr. Drug Metab. 8: 499-507.

[162] Pauwels EK (2011) The protective effect of the Mediterranean diet: focus on cancer and cardiovascular risk. Med. Princ. Pract. 20:103-111.

[163] Bach-Faig A, Berry EM, Lairon D, Reguant J, Trichopoulou A, Dernini S, Medina FX, Battino M, Belahsen R, Miranda G, Serra-Majem L; Mediterranean Diet Foundation Expert Group (2011) Mediterranean diet pyramid today. Science and cultural updates. Public Health Nutr. 14:2274-2284

[164] Trichopoulou A, Lagiou P, Kuper H, Trichopoulos D (2000) Cancer and Mediterranean Dietary Traditions. Cancer Epidemiol. Biomark. Prevent. 9: 869-873.

[165]   Nadtochiy SM, Redman EK (2011) Mediterranean diet and cardioprotection: the role of nitrite, polyunsaturated fatty acids, and polyphenols. Nutrition 27(7-8):733-744.

[166]   Craig WJ (2010) Nutrition Concerns and Health Effects of Vegetarian Diets. Nutr. Clin. Pract. 25:613-620.

[167]   Fraser GE (2009) Vegetarian diets: what do we know of their effects on common chronic diseases? Am. J. Clin. Nutr. 89:1607S-1612S

[168]   Li D (2011) Chemistry behind Vegetarianism. J. Agric. Food Chem. 59:777-784.

[169]   Halliwell B (2007) Dietary polyphenols: Good, bad, or indifferent for your health? Cardiovascular Res. 73: 341-347

[170]   Skibola CF. and Smith TS (2000) Potential health impacts of excessive flavonoid intake. Free Radical Biol. Med. 29: 375-383.

[171]   Galati G. O'Brien PJ (2004) Potential toxicity of flavonoids and other dietary phenolics: significance for their chemopreventive and anticancer properties. Free Radical Biol. Med. 37: 287-303.

[172]   Chan T. Galati G. O'Brien PJ (1999) Oxygen activation during peroxidase catalysed metabolism of flavones or flavanones. Chem. Biol . Interact. 122:15-25.

[173]   Galati, G. Sabzevari O. Wilson J X. O'Brien PJ (2002) Prooxidant activity and cellular effects of the phenoxyl radicals of dietary flavonoids and other polyphenolics. Toxicology 177:91-104.

[174]   Oostdar H. Burke MD. Mayer RT (2000) Bioflavonoids: selective substrates and inhibitors for cytochrome P450 CYP1A and CYP1B1. Toxicology 144:31-38.

[175]   Hodek P, Trefil P, Stiborova´M (2002) Flavonoids-potent and versatile biologically active compounds interacting with cytochromes P450. Chem. Biol. Interact. 139:1-21.

[176]   Doostdar H. Burke MD. Mayer RT (2000) Bioflavonoids: selective substrates and inhibitors for cytochrome P450 CYP1A and CYP1B1. Toxicology 144:31-38.

[177]   Tang W. Stearns RA (2001) Heterotropic cooperativity of cytochrome P450 3A4 and potential drug – drug interactions. Curr. Drug Metab

Chapter 6

Interactions with Drugs and Dietary Supplements Used For Weight Loss

Melanie A. Jordan

Additional information is available at the end of the chapter

1. Introduction

Obesity and overweight have increasingly become major global health issues. Data from the World Health Organization (WHO) reports a near doubling of the prevalence of obesity worldwide from 1998 to 2008 [1]. In the European Region, an average of over 50% of adults are overweight and nearly 23% obese, with the prevalence of overweight and obesity being highest in Finland (67.1%), Germany (67.2%), the United Kingdom (67.8%), Malta (73.3%), and Greece (77.5%) [2]. Similar alarming trends are seen in the United States NHANES data where 68% of adults have a body mass index (BMI) greater than 25 (overweight or obese) and nearly 37% of the population is considered obese [3-7]. A large burden of health care costs can be attributed to overweight and obesity since multiple disease states such as diabetes, cancer, heart disease can be linked overweight and obesity [8-10]. The WHO estimates that up to 6% of health care expenditures in the European Region, while estimates for the United States have been estimated at 5.7% of the National Health Expenditure [8-11]. Most major organizations, like the WHO, and governmental agencies such as the U.S. Department of Agriculture Center for Nutrition Policy and Promotion have a major focus on the treatment of the obesity epidemic through promotion of proper healthy lifestyle changes [11, 12]. Although multiple anti-obesity agents have progressed through the development process, few drug products have made it through the approval process due to safety or lack of efficacy concerns. Several products, such as amphetamine, fenfluramine and sibutramine, have had their approval removed and/or have been removed from the market following reports linking the drugs to cardiovascular side effects (e.g. hypertension and myocardial infarction), addiction, and death [13-15]. As an alternative, overweight or obese patients may turn to less regulated dietary supplements as a means to assist in weight loss. Multiple herbal products are available that are indicated, often without significant scientific basis, for the treatment of overweight and obesity. The safety and efficacy of herbal products is often unknown, especially given the presence of multiple chemical compounds, lack of known active constituents or lack of standardization of known compounds [16-19].This chapter presents a review of the chemistry and pharmacology of approved anti-obesity drug products, the proposed mechanism of action for common dietary supplements used in the management of weight loss, and potential drug-drug or herb-drug interactions.

2. Drugs used in weight LOcSS

2.1. Sympathomiometic agents

2.1.1. Diethylpropion hydrochloride (Tenuate®; Tenuate® Dospan®; Durad®)

Diethylpropion HCl (amfepramone, Figure 1a) is a sympathomimetic aminoketone agent with some similarity both chemically and pharmacologically to amphetamines and other related stimulant drugs. Similarly to amphetamine, diethylpropion stimulates release while inhibiting reuptake of dopamine, norepinephrine, and 5-hydroxytryptamine [20, 21]. The increase in norepinephrine and dopamine levels along with inhibition of their reuptake is proposed as the mechanism of diethylpropion anorectic effects [22]. Diethylpropion is indicated for short term management of obesity in patients with a body mass index (BMI) of > 30 kg/m² who have not responded to diet and exercise alone [23]. Because of its similarity to amphetamine, some patients become psychologically dependent on diethylpropion with an increased risk of self-medicating at higher dosages, increasing potential for drug interactions.

Diethylpropion is a monoamine and therefore can interact with monoamine oxidase inhibitors (MAOI), resulting in hypertension [23]. The manufacturer recommends avoiding use of diethylpropion during or within 14 days of discontinuation of MAOI administration. There is also one reported case of diethylpropion -induced psychosis in a 26 year old female patient taking phenelzine [24]. The authors hypothesized that chronic diethylpropion use led to an increased sensitivity to MAOI psychosis-inducing effects. Although the additive effects of diethylpropion in combination with other anorectic agents has not been studied, combined use of these agents is contraindicated due to the potential increased risk of cardiovascular issues [23]. In an early study of diethylpropion in 32 obese hypertensive patients, a drop in blood pressure was observed [25]. However, it was unclear if the drop in blood pressure in these subjects was due to weight loss or the additive effect of additional hypertensive agents that the patients were taking. The manufacturer also recommends potential modification of insulin dosing, although no strong evidence to support this statement can be found. In one study done in the rat, it was determined that anorectic drugs acting via the dopaminergic system antagonize hyperphagia induced by 2-deoxy-D-glucose, although the authors did not find any modifications to insulin-induced hypoglycemia [26]. There are no reported cases of drug-herb interactions with diethylpropion. However, theoretically herbal products with CNS stimulant properties (e.g. ephedra, caffeine, bitter orange), potential for interaction with sympathomimetic agents (e.g. Indian snakeroot), or MAOI activity (e.g. yohimbe) should be avoided due to an increased risk of hypertension, cardiovascular effects, and changes in blood pressure [27].

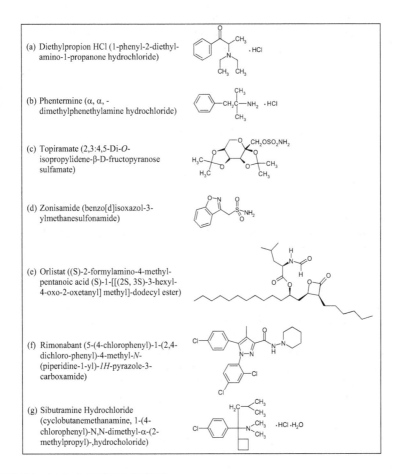

(a) Diethylpropion HCl (1-phenyl-2-diethyl-amino-1-propanone hydrochloride)

(b) Phentermine (α, α, - dimethylphenethylamine hydrochloride)

(c) Topiramate (2,3:4,5-Di-*O*-isopropylidene-β-D-fructopyranose sulfamate)

(d) Zonisamide (benzo[d]isoxazol-3-ylmethanesulfonamide)

(e) Orlistat ((S)-2-formylamino-4-methyl-pentanoic acid (S)-1-[[(2S, 3S)-3-hexyl-4-oxo-2-oxetanyl] methyl]-dodecyl ester)

(f) Rimonabant (5-(4-chlorophenyl)-1-(2,4-dichloro-phenyl)-4-methyl-*N*-(piperidine-1-yl)-*1H*-pyrazole-3-carboxamide)

(g) Sibutramine Hydrochloride (cyclobutanemethanamine, 1-(4-chlorophenyl)-N,N-dimethyl-α-(2-methylpropyl)-,hydrocholoride)

Figure 1. Molecular structures of anorectic drugs.

2.1.2. Phentermine / Phentermine hydrochloride (Fastin®, Ionamin®, Adipex-P®, Suprenza®)

Phentermine (Figure 1b), a member of the β-phenylethylamine family of compounds, exerts anorectic activity centrally through appetite suppression and is indicated in the short term treatment of obesity in patients with a BMI ≥ 30 kg/m² [28]. A meta-analysis of six randomized controlled trials of phentermine cumulatively show an added 3.6 kg weight loss over 2 to 24 weeks compared to control groups [29]. Phentermine acts by increasing the release of and inhibiting the reuptake of norepinephrine or dopamine [22]. Although one of the oldest approved anti-obesity drugs, the safety of monotherapy of phentermine is relatively scarce due to the long history of combination products, most notably phentermine/fenfluramine (Phen-Fen), which was removed from the market due to serious and potentially fatal cardio-vascular effects [30, 31]. More recently a combination product containing phentermine and topiramate has been investigated (see *Topiramate* below) and is currently under review by the US Food and Drug Administration (FDA).

Because of the similarity in activity and mechanism of action, drug interactions with phenter-mine are similar to those for diethylpropion (see *Diethylpropion* above) including avoidance of alcohol, potential changes to antidiabetic agent therapy, and avoidance of coadministration of MAOIs [28]. There is one case report of a female patient experiencing two penropative hypertensive crises, which were attributed to an interaction between phentermine and anesthetic agents [32].

2.2. Antiepileptic agents

Several antiepileptic agents are known to have an effect on weight gain [33]. However, two newer antiepileptic agents, topiramate and zonisamide, have shown an associated decrease in weight in patients taking these medications [34]. Therefore, these two drugs are being looked at as potential anorectic agents.

2.2.1. Topiramate (Topamax®)

Topiramate is a carbonic anhydrase inhibitor (Figure 1c) that is typically used in the treatment of migraines and as an anticonvulsant [35]. Topiramate is proposed to exert its antiepileptic activity via gamma-aminobutyric acid (GABA)-A-mediated inhibition via a benzodiazepine insensitive pathway, although the drug also blocks voltage dependent sodium channels [35-37]. Weight loss has been a commonly reported adverse effect of topiramate; therefore, the drug has recently come into focus as a potential anorectic agent [38-42]. Topiramate has shown promise as a combination low-dose therapy with phentermine (Qsymia(R) (originally Qnexa(R), Vivus Pharmaceuticals, Mountain View, CA, USA) for long term treatment of obesity [43-46]. Despite, safety concerns related to teratogenicity and cardiovascular effects, the product has recently been approved by the U.S. Food and Drug Administration."

Drug interactions with topiramate include coadministration with other antiepileptic agents. Although no changes in carbamazepine or phenytoin levels were seen, topiramate levels decreased by 40% or 48%, respectively [35]. However, there have been two case reports of antiepileptic drug intoxications in patients initiated on topiramate who were already taking the maximum carbamazepine dose [47]. Decrease in carbamazepine dosage resolved the interaction. Hyperammonemia, hypothermia and potentially encephalopathy can result from a synergistic interaction between topiramate, valproic acid, and phenobarbital, although the exact mechanism of this interaction is unknown [35, 48-50]. Levels of ethinyl estradiol can be significantly decreased in patients taking topiramate as an adjunctive therapy with valproic acid [35]. As a carbonic anhydrase inhibitor, topiramate can cause metabolic acidosis, and therefore is contraindicated in patients taking metformin, while patients taking other carbonic anhydrase inhibitors should be monitored due to the potential additive effects when coadministered with topiramate [51-55]. High doses of topiramate (600 mg/day) can increase systemic exposure to lithium. However, since topiramate dosage proposed to anorectic effects is low, this interaction may not be a significant concern when used as anti-obesity treatment [56]. No clinical studies or case studies are available for interactions with CNS depressants (e.g alcohol), although combined use is contraindicated by the manufacturer due to combined CNS depression [35]. No data supporting herb-drug interactions are available specifically related to use of topiramate at low doses as an anorectic agent [27].

2.2.2. Zonisamide (Zonegran®)

Zonisamide (Figure 1d), a methanesulfonamide, is an antiepileptic agent which has broad spectrum activity and has proven to be useful in patients not responding to other antiepileptic treatments [57]. The drug blocks sustained and repetitive neuronal firing by blocking voltage sensitive sodium channels and decreasing voltage sensitive T-type calcium channels [58, 59]. Additionally, it was found that zonisamide has dopaminergic and serotonergic activity, which contributes to the anorectic effects of the drug [60, 61]. In one randomized placebo-controlled trial, 30 subjects were administered zonisamide 100 mg daily along with a low calorie diet (500 kcal/day) for a period of 16 weeks. Dosage was increased to up to 600 mg/day for patients not losing >5% of their initial body weight within the first 12 weeks. The zonisamide group lost significantly more body weight at the end of the trial compared to the placebo group (approx. 6% loss vs. 1% loss) [62].

Zonisamide is metabolized by the cytochrome P450 3A4 system and therefore can potentially interact with other drugs metabolized via this route. In one study, the half-life of zonisamide ($t_{1/2}$ = 60 h) was decreased in patients receiving both zonisamide and phenytoin ($t_{1/2}$ = 27 h), carbamazepine ($t_{1/2}$ = 38 h, and sodium valproate ($t_{1/2}$ = 46 h) [57, 63]. Another study in the dog demonstrated decreased plasma levels of zonisamide during administration of phenobarbital [64]. However, any associated decrease in levels of other antiepileptic drugs was not found to be clinically significant [65, 66]. Cigarette smoking may alter the pharmacokinetics of zonisamide. Coadministration of carbonic anhydrase inhibitors may increase risk of metabolic acidosis and kidney stone formation, therefore monitoring is recommended in this patient population [66]. One study on the effects of cigarette smoke on zonisamide concentrations in rats suggests that cigarette smoke may decrease plasma levels of the drug due to decreased oral absorption [67]. Brain, but not plasma levels of zonisamide may be affected by chronic ethanol consumption. In one study inbred EL mice were administered zonisamide 75 mg/kg for 1 – 4 weeks along with 10% ethanol ad libidum. In groups with 4 week coadministration, representing chronic use of alcohol, a decrease in zonisamide brain concentrations, but not serum concentration were observed [68].

2.3. Orlistat (Xenical®, Alli®)

Orlistat (Figure 1e) is a gastrointestinal lipase inhibitor approved both as a prescription (Xenical®) and over-the-counter (Alli®) weight loss aid in the long term treatment of obesity [69]. The drug exhibits antiobesity activity by inhibiting the absorption of dietary fat from the lumen of the stomach and small intestine through covalent binding with gastric and pancreatic lipase active serine residues [70]. Multiple randomized controlled trials have reported significant weight loss in patients taking orlistat compared to placebo controlled groups. One meta-analysis cites mean weight loss compared to control of -2.59 kg [95%CI, -3.46 to -1.74] or -2.9 kg [95%CI, -3.2 to -2.5] over 6 or 12 months, respectively, with a corresponding decrease in waist circumference, blood pressure, and blood glucose and lipid profiles [71-73].

A large number of preclinical and clinical studies and case reports related to potential drug interactions with orlistat have been published. There have been several cases of orlistat interaction with cyclosporine [74-79]. In all cases, significant decreases in plasma cyclosporine levels were observed following adjunct treatment with orlistat for cyclosporine-associated weight gain. Although one proposed mechanism for the reduction in plasma cyclosporine is a decrease in drug absorption, decreased levels may be due to rapid gastrointestinal transit time resulting from contraindicated high fat diets rather than a true drug-drug interaction [80]. Because orlistat is designed to inhibit gastrointestinal lipases, theoretically absorption of lipophilic molecules would also be inhibited [81-83]. In one open-label, placebo-controlled randomized two-way crossover study, orlistat (120 mg) was administered to 12 healthy subjects three times daily for 9 days followed by administration of Vitamin A (25,000 IU) or Vitamin E (400 IU) [82]. Although no effect was seen on Vitamin A levels, a significant reduction in C_{max} (approx. 43%) and AUC (approx. 60%) were observed for Vitamin E, suggesting impaired absorption of Vitamin E by orlistat. In another study, approximately a 30% reduction in beta-carotene levels was observed after administration of orlistat (120 mg) for four days followed by administration of 0 – 120 mg of beta-carotene three times a day for six days [83]. Absorption of lipophilic drugs such as the CNS agent lamotrigene can also be affected by orlistat. In one report, increased frequency of seizures was reported in an 18 year old female taking lamotrigene following initiation of an orlistat regimen [84]. One case of hypothyroidism in thyroid carcinoma was reported, presumably due to decreased absorption of thyroxine [85]. Although orlistat was not found to alter warfarin kinetics *per se*, but the drug may alter absorption of the fat soluble vitamin K which can have an effect warfarin levels and therefore these patients should be monitored for changes in coagulation parameters [86].

2.4. Rimonabant (Acomplia®, Zumulti®)

Rimonabant (Figure 1f) is a cannabanoid receptor antagonist that suppresses appetite by preventing activation of CB_1 receptors by the endogenous cannabanoids anandamide and 2-arachidonoyl-glycerol [87]. In clinical trials the drug resulted in improvement of multiple endpoints associated with obesity and metabolic syndrome compared to control groups including significant weight loss, reduction in waist circumference, decreased triglycerides, blood glucose, fasting insulin, and leptin levels with increased HDL cholesterol and adiponectin levels [88-96]. Although rimonabant proved a potentially successful drug in the treatment of obesity, especially given lack of cardiovascular risks compared to other weight loss drugs (see *Sibutramine* below), the drug has not been approved by the U.S. Food and Drug Administration (FDA). Additionally, although the drug was initially approved in 2006 by the European Medicines Agency (EMEA), later studies indicating serious neuropsychiatric adverse events, especially related to increased risk of suicide, caused the Agency to rescind the approval in 2009. Although rimonabant is not available in most major markets, ongoing investigations surrounding the development of the drug continue, while the drug has been approved in other markets [97-100]. Additionally, the drug appears to be available readily via online pharmacy services and has been identified as an adulterant in dietary supplements marketed for weight loss (see *Adulteration of Dietary Supplements* below) [101-103].

Given the limited and short-lived approval status of rimonabant, there is little information regarding potential drug-drug and herb-drug interactions available. According to package insert data submitted to the EMEA, rimonabant is known to be eliminated hepatically and into the bile by amidohydrolase and CYP3A4, with a 104% increase in rimonabant AUC (95% CI 40 – 197%) upon coadministration of ketoconazole [92, 96, 104, 105]. Therefore, the manufacturer indicated potential interactions with strong CYP3A4 inhibitors (e.g. ketoconazole, itraconazole, ritonavir, telithromycin, clarithromycin, and nefazodone) and inducers (e.g. rifampicin, phenytoin, phenobarbital, carbamazepine, and St. John's Wort). Because rimonabant can decrease levels of fasting insulin and blood sugar, use of rimonabant in diabetic patients taking anti-diabetic agents is cautioned [92, 96, 104, 105].

2.5. Sibutramine (Meridia®, Reductil®)

Sibutramine hydrocholoride (Figure 1g), and its active primary (M_1) and secondary (M_2) metabolites, is a selective serotonin (5-hydroxytryptamine, 5-HT) and norepinephrine reuptake inhibitor [106-110]. Clinical data supported the efficacy of sibutramine as a weight loss agent, reporting significant weight loss compared to placebo for patients taking at least 10 mg/day for up to one year [107, 110-114]. The drug was approved as an anti-obesity agent in 1997 by the U.S. FDA and in 2002 by the EMEA, despite evidence of increased risk of hypertension and tachycardia, with a requirement that additional post-marketing safety data be collected relative to cardiotoxicity. As a result, the SCOUT (Sibutramine Cardiovascular OUTcomes) trial was implemented, which enrolled 10,000 overweight or obese patients aged 55 and older with coexisting diabetes and/or heart disease in a randomized controlled trial with a 6-month lead in period [115-118]. At the end of the six year study period, data showed a significant decrease in body weight compared to placebo but increased cardiovascular morbidity in the randomized sibutramine group [115-118]. Following publication of the SCOUT trial results in 2010, the EMEA and most other major markets pulled sibutramine while the United States and Australia required stricter labeling. By 2011 sibutramine was pulled from all major markets globally. However, as with the case of rimonabant (see above), sibutramine is of note since it is the primary contaminant found in dietary weight loss supplements (see *Adulteration of Dietary Supplements* below).

Sibutramine is known to be metabolized by CYP 3A4 into two active metabolites (M_1 and M_2). Data reported by the manufacturer in limited clinical trials (n = 12 – 27 patients) suggest potential pharmacokinetic changes in AUC and C_{max} for sibutramine when taken in combination with CYP 3A4 inhibitors such as cimetidine, ketoconazole, erythromycin, simvastatin, and omeprazole; while sibutramine does not generally have a significant impact on the levels of these drugs in return [106]. Because of the role of CYP 3A4 in sibutramine elimination, use o the drug with other CYP 3A4 substrates, including coadministration with grapefruit juice, is contraindicated [111]. One case report describes a possible interaction between sibutramine and citalopram in a 43 year old female patient who experienced hypomanic symptoms shortly after adding 10 mg sibutramine to her current citalopram and fluoxetine regimen [119]. Symptoms ceased within one day of discontinuing sibutramine. Although the exact mechanism of the interaction is unknown, the author hypothesized a possible amphetamine-like hypomania or serotonin syndrome due to increased brain serotonin levels via the combination of a serotonin reuptake inhibitor and serotonin-norepinephrine reuptake inhibitor. Another case report notes a possible interaction between sibutramine and cyclosporine in a 26 year old transplant patient resulting in significant increases in cyclosporine trough plasma levels, likely due to inhibition of CYP 3A4 metabolism [120]. Coadministration of α_2 adrenergic blockers, such as the herb yohimbine, with sibutramine has been recognized as potentially life threatening due to potential sympathetic side effects resulting in hypertension and tachycardia [121]. Due to the potential risk of bleeding caused by sibutramine, the drug should be used with caution in patients taking warfarin and other anticoagulants [106].

3. Herbs and dietary supplements used in weight loss

3.1. Açaí (*Euterpe oleracea*)

The açaí berry is harvested from the palm species *Euterpe oleracea* and is used mainly for dietary consumption as whole fruit, juice, or as a flavoring and coloring agent [27]. The fruit, widely used in Brazil, has gained in popularity as a food product and dietary supplement in the past several years, mainly due to its antioxidant and anti-inflammatory effects related to high polyphenol content [122-126]. Although there is little scientific evidence to support the berry for any of its purported health benefits, it can be found in several dietary supplements promoted for weight loss. In a pilot study investigating the effect of açaí supplementation on metabolic parameters in healthy overweight patients, the authors found a significant decrease in fasting glucose, insulin and cholesterol levels and a mild decrease in LDL-cholesterol and ratio of total cholesterol to HDL-cholesterol [127]. However, the authors did not assess weight loss in this study and therefore the activity of açaí as an anorectic agent cannot be determined. There have been no reported adverse drug interactions or interactions with others herbs and açaí [27].

3.2. Bitter orange (*Citrus aurantium, Citrus naringin, synephrine*)

Bitter orange is the fruit of *Citrus aurantium* or *Citrus naringin*, used as both a food product and the medicinal properties of the juice and peel [27]. There are multiple active constituents in bitter orange including several flavonoids (e.g. naringin) and the adrenergic agonists synephrine and octopamine [128-134]. Synephrine is structurally similar to ephedrine, therefore prompting the replacement of ephedra with bitter orange in weight loss supplements, although the fruit has been used dichotomously as both an appetite stimulant and for weight loss [27]. However, there is insufficient evidence to confirm the efficacy of bitter orange as an anti-obesity agent, especially given its inclusion in combination products [27].

Interactions with bitter orange are varied. Synephrine, like ephedrine, is known to cause adverse cardiovascular effects at high doses, the risk of which are heightened when combination products also including caffeine are ingested and therefore patients taking cardiac medications should be cautioned on its use [135, 136]. Some evidence demonstrates that bitter orange can inhibit cytochrome P450 3A4, although to a lesser extent than with grapefruit [137-140]. A 76% increase in AUC was observed following administration of 10 mg extended release felodipine administered with 240 mL Seville orange juice compared to control [139]; while a significant increase in indinavir t_{max} was observed with administration of 8 ounces of Seville orange juice compared to control [140]. Because synephrine and octopamine, both endogenous substances, can interact with monoamine oxidase there is a theoretical interaction of bitter orange with MAOIs [141, 142].

3.3. Caffeine-containing herbs

Caffeine is a methylxanthine that is commonly found in food, beverages, and dietary supplements. It is used as an additive in beverages and dietary supplements for its energy enhancing properties. Many dietary supplements marketed for weight loss contain high levels of caffeine, often from multiple sources, for increased thermogenesis and lipid metabolism [143, 144]. Most studies investigating the anti-obesity effects of caffeine have been done using combination products that include ephedra, or have looked at enhancement of athletic endurance [145-151]. Therefore, it is difficult to assess the effect of caffeine alone on weight loss. One study demonstrated an increase in thermogenic metabolic rate in subjects drinking coffee along with food, compared to ingestion of decaffeinated coffee [144].

Adverse effects associated with caffeine consumption include restlessness, jitteriness, anxiety, insomnia, and cardiovascular effects [152-156]. Most drug and herb interactions with caffeine are mild to moderate and are related to increased adverse effects resulting from decreased caffeine elimination or additive effects with other methylxanthine containing products [157]. For example, estrogen drugs (e.g. oral contraceptives and estrogen replacement therapy) have been shown to decrease clearance of caffeine up to 50 – 65% [158, 159]. The most significant caffeine interaction occurs with coadministration of *Ephedra* or ephedrine containing products (see *Ephedra* below). The ban on ephedra in the United States has resulted in marketing of "ephedra-free" dietary supplements using ephedra alternatives, including caffeine containing herbs and bitter orange (see *Bitter Orange* above). In one randomized controlled trial study, subjects were administered products containing *Citrus aurantium* standardized to either a high dose of synephrine (46.9 mg) or a product containing caffeine and a low synephrine dose (5.5 mg) [136]. A significant increase on blood pressure was observed in patients taking the product containing both caffeine and synephrine, but not high dose synephrine alone, suggesting an interaction between the two herbs.

3.3.1. Green tea (Camellia sinensis; EGCG)

Green tea has gained in popularity for the treatment of a wide variety of diseases and for promotion of general wellbeing. The addition of green tea to weight loss supplements is due in part to the caffeine content of *Camellia sinensis*. However, in addition to alkaloid content (caffeine, theobromine, theophylline) green tea also contains polyphenols, most notably the catechin epigallocatechin-3-gallate (EGCG) [160-164]. EGCG, in concert with caffeine, is proposed to elicit anti-obesity effects via inhibition of catechol O-methyl transferase and phosphodiesterase [164]. A meta-analysis of clinical trials involving green tea in weight loss concluded that weight loss is decreased, relative to placebo, in treatment involving both green tea ECGC and caffeine but not with decaffeinated green tea products [165].

As expected, the majority of drug interactions associated with green tea are related to caffeine content. However, a few interactions described in the literature are due to other constituents of green tea. Green tea may be contraindicated, especially at high doses, in patients taking anticoagulants such as warfarin due to the high Vitamin K content of the herb. There is one case report of a patient taking warfarin who experienced a significant reduction in INR following initiation of daily consumption of one-half to one gallon of green tea [166]. Once green tea consumption was stopped INR normalized. Green tea is also thought to cause decreased estrogen levels and combination products containing the herb have been used to improve fertility and relieve menopausal symptoms [167-170]. Therefore, use of high doses of green tea in patients taking oral contraceptives or estrogen replacement therapy may be cautioned.

3.3.2. Guarana (Paullinia cupana)

Guarana (*Paullinia cupana*) is a plant native to South America that is used traditionally and in anti-obesity supplements for its high caffeine content, although other minor constituents including theophylline, theobromine, catechin and epicatechin are found in these extracts [171-176]. There are no studies investigating the effects of Guarana alone on weight loss so it is difficult to determine the anti-obesity properties of the herb. In one double-blind, parallel, placebo controlled trial 47 subjects were administered three capsules containing yerba mate (*Ilex paraguayensis*, 112 mg), guarana (95 mg) and damiana (*Turnera diffusa*, 36 mg) daily for 45 days, resulting in significant weight loss (-5.1 ± 0.5 kg) compared to placebo (-0.3 ± 0.08 kg) [145]. One of the few interactions reported with guarana not related to caffeine content suggests possible interference with anticoagulants since platelet aggregation was observed *in vitro* and in animal studies [177].

3.4. Dandelion (*Taraxacum officinale*)

Dandelion is a perennial herb of multiple global varieties that has traditionally been used for liver, spleen, kidney, and gastrointestinal disorders, although there have been no clinical trials investigating the effects of dandelion in weight loss [27, 178]. It is commonly added to weight loss supplements, mainly for its diuretic properties, although the herb does possess some mild laxative properties [179-181]. There are no known drugs interactions between *Taraxacum* and other herbs or drugs, although one study in rats suggests a probable interaction with quinolone antibiotics due to the high mineral content of *Taraxacum* [182]. In the study, ciprofloxacin (20 mg/kg) C_{max} significantly decreased while V_d and $t_{1/2}$ significantly increased when administered with crude dandelion extract (2 g/kg) compared to control. There is one case report of hypoglycemia in a 58 year old diabetic patient following a 2-week period of dandelion consumption in salads [183].

The patient denied changes in calorie consumption, exercise, or insulin dosing. Diabetic patients taking hypoglycemic agents while consuming dandelion should be monitored.

3.5. Ephedra (*Ephedra sinica*, ma huang)

Ephedra, derived from the evergreen shrub *Ephedra sinica*, contains multiple plant alkaloids including ephedrine and pseudoephedrine that are chemically related to amphetamines. These compounds act by increasing availability and activity of endogenous neurotransmitters such as epinephrine and norepinephrine, resulting in brain and cardiovascular catecholamine receptor stimulation [184]. The herb has traditionally been used for bronchodilation in the treatment of respiratory ailments such as asthma, as an athletic performance enhancer, and for its thermogenic properties in weight loss [148, 185-189]. Ephedra as a weight loss dietary supplement is commonly found in combination products also containing caffeine or caffeine-containing herbs. In one study a product containing 90 mg and 192 mg of ephedra alkaloids and caffeine, respectively, administered daily over six months in a randomized, double-blind placebo controlled trial resulted in significant decreases in body weight, body fat and LDL-cholesterol with an increase in HDL-cholesterol [148]. The addition of aspirin to ephedrine containing products can potentiate the thermogenic properties of ephedra, improving weight loss compared to products containing ephedra alone [190-201]. Due to high risk of cardiovascular toxicities and cardiomyopathies, ephedra has been banned in the United States [202-211]. However, the herb is still available in other countries [212].

Because of the controversial nature of ephedra related to cardiac toxicity and its eventual ban via the U.S. FDA, there are a significant number of clinical studies and case reports related to toxicities and interactions with ephedra and ephedrine. Ephedra can potentially interact with anesthetics since it is known that administration of ephedrine can reverse anesthesia induced hypotension and regression of analgesia following epidural blockade [213, 214]. Ephedrine has both chrontropic and inotropic effects, and therefore interactions with cardiovascular agents may be possible [184, 211, 215, 216]. However, no effects on heart rate or blood pressure were seen in clinical trials investigating the efficacy of ephedra in weight loss [192, 217, 218]. Theoretically interactions with antiadrenergic agents and MAOIs can occur due to sympathomimetic effects of ephedrine, potentially increasing risk of hypertensive crisis. There is a case report of a patient taking a product containing caffeine, ephedrine, and theophylline who experienced multiple adverse effects including encephalopathy, hypotension, tachycardia, and hypothermia 24 hours following discontinuation of phenelzine [219]. Interactions with ephedrine and tricyclic antidepressants are also possible [220]. Some evidence from clinical trials suggests that ephedra in combination with caffeine can cause hyperglycemia, and therefore interactions with antidiabetic agents is possible [147, 148, 221]. A lowering of seizure threshold has been observed in patients taking ephedrine, and therefore use of ephedra in this patient population is cautioned [222]. A major interaction between ephedra and methylxanthines (e.g. caffeine, theophylline) is possible due to increased risk of cardiovascular, neurologic and psychiatric adverse effects due to additive sympathomimetic and CNS stimulant activity [184, 223, 224]. One case study reports a 21 year old male patient admitted to the hospital emergency room with a blood pressure of 220/110 mmHg and ventricular arrhythmia following ingestion of a caffeine/ephedra containing product ("Herbal Ecstasy") [225].

3.6. Glucomannan (*Amorphophallus konjac*)

Glucomannan is a soluble but highly viscous dietary fiber derived from the root of the *Amorphophallus konjac* (elephant yam) plant that grows native to Asia [27]. Although traditionally used as a food, the plant has gained popularity as an additive in weight loss supplements since the dietary fiber absorbs water in the gastrointestinal tract, helping to promote a sense of satiety and act as a bulk laxative [226-228]. There is also evidence that fiber content of glucomannan helps to reduce cholesterol levels [67, 229-232]. In a double blind crossover study involving 63 healthy males, 3.9 grams of glucomannan administered daily for four weeks resulted in a 10% reduction in total cholesterol, 7.2% reduction in LDL cholesterol, and a 23% decrease in triglyceride levels [67]. A meta-analysis of clinical trials involving glucomannan reported overall decreases in the above markers as well as fasting blood glucose [230].

There are relatively few reported drug interactions with glucomannan, most of which are likely due to associated decreases in cholesterol and lipid levels as well as interference with absorption of some drugs. Monitoring of patients taking antihypertensives, antilipemics, and other anti-obesity agents is warranted. Several studies note a significant decrease in fasting blood glucose levels following glucomannan administration while decreased absorption of the sulfonylurea drugs is possible [230, 231, 233-237]. Glucomannan can significantly decrease circulating levels of T3, T4, and FT3 in the treatment of thyrotoxicosis and therefore its use may be contraindicated in patients taking thyroid medications [238]. Glucomannan can potentially affect the absorption of certain drugs and supplements as demonstrated in one study in which absorption of the fat soluble Vitamin E was decreased potentially via the reduction of bile acids necessary for absorption of the vitamin [239].

3.7. *Hoodia gordonii*

Hoodia gordonii, a small succulent of the Apocynaceae family native to the Kalahari Desert, has been used traditionally by native tribes for its appetite and thirst suppressing properties [240, 241]. The active constituent of Hoodia (P57 or P57AS3) is an oxypregnane steroidal glycoside which is purported to increase ATP production in the hypothalamus, resulting in a feeling of satiety [242]. There is little known regarding potential drug or herb interactions with *Hoodia*, although *in vitro* studies suggest a potential interaction with drugs metabolized by CYP 3A4 [243].

3.8. Hydroxycitric acid (HCA, *Garcinia cambogia*)

Garcinia cambogia is a plant native to Southeast Asia which yields a small purple fruit used in weight loss products for its hydroxycitric acid (HCA) content [27, 244]. The anorectic activity of HCA is due to the inhibition of the adenosine triphosphate-citrate (pro-3S)-lyase, which catalyzes the formation of acetyl-CoA, resulting in decreased fatty acid synthesis and lipogenesis [245]. The evidence for HCA as an effective weight loss agent is contradictory. One randomized controlled trial reported a 5-6% reduction in weight and BMI following approximately a 4.5 gram daily dose of HCA, while two other studies reported no significant weight loss or effect on appetite at lower doses of 1.5 – 2.4 gram daily HCA doses [246-248]. There are a minimal number of reported interactions with *Garcinia* or HCA. Antilipemic agents such as HMG-CoA reductase inhibitors should be avoided due to an increased risk of rhabdomyolysis. In one case report a healthy 54 year old female patient reported chest pain following ingestion of an herbal product containing ephedra, guarana, chitosan, *Gymnena sylvestre*, *Garcinia cambogia* (50% HCA), and chromium. Lab results indicated elevated serum creatine kinase (1028 IU/mL), which declined following cessation of the supplement [249]. Although the exact interaction was not determined, cautionary use of HCA-containing products in patients at risk of rhabdomyolysis is warranted.

3.9. Herbal laxatives

Frequently laxatives and diuretics are used alone or in combination products to promote weight loss. However, there is little to no evidence supporting these supplements as anti-obesity agents, although subgroups of this patient population may abuse laxatives and diuretics for the purpose of weight loss [250].

3.9.1. Bulk laxatives

Bulk laxatives generally consist of soluble dietary fiber which expands in the gastrointestinal tract in the presence of water resulting in improved bowel function. Common sources of bulk laxatives include *Amorphophallus konjac* (glucomannan, *see above*), guar gum (*Cyamopsis tetragonoloba*), and psyllium husk (*Plantago psyllium*). Although the efficacy of bulk laxatives for weight loss is not proven, adsorption of dietary glucose and lipids to these agents in the gastrointestinal tract results in decreased absorption of lipids, cholesterol, and carbohydrates into the body, thereby promoting weight loss [230, 234, 251-253]. Because of changes in carbohydrate and glucose absorption, dosing of antidiabetic agents may require modification and therefore patients in this population should be monitored when taking bulk laxatives [254-261]. Bulk laxatives appear to have some effect on the absorption of orally administered medications, which can result in changes in drug plasma levels [262-272]. For example, in one study the effect of guar gum on digoxin and phenoxymethyl penicillin absorption was studied in 10 healthy volunteers, with significant reductions in both peak penicillin plasma concentrations and AUC, but little effect on overall digoxin levels [269]. In one case report of a patient with adrenal insufficiency treated with fludrocortisone and prednisolone, the patient experienced symptoms of acute adrenal crisis including fatigue, nausea, abdominal pain, and weakness approximately 3 – 4 days after initiation of psyllium [262]. The authors postulated that psyllium inhibited absorption of fludrocortisone and/or prednisolone. Other evidence related to changes in absorption of ethinyl estradiol, metformin, and lithium have also been reported [264-266, 270, 272].

3.9.2. Stimulant laxatives

Stimulant laxatives act by irritating the lining of the gastrointestinal tract, resulting in increased propulsive muscle contractions that aid elimination of intestinal contents. Because of the quick and efficacious activity, stimulant laxatives are most frequently abused to promote weight loss by increasing gastrointestinal transit time [273, 274]. The most common stimulant laxative herbs are senna (*Cassia senna*), aloe latex (*Aloe vera*), and Cascara sagrada (*Frangula purshiana*). The leaves and pods from *Cassia senna* contain anthroquinone stimulant laxative compounds effective in the treatment of constipation and for bowel evacuation prior to medical procedures [27, 275-295]. The herb has been approved by the U.S. FDA as a non-prescription medication. Similarly, aloe latex, derived from the peripheral bundle sheath cells of the aloe leaf, contains anthracene compounds that are cleaved in the colon by bacterial enzymes into active anthrone compounds with stimulant laxative properties [296-299]. However, concerns over possible carcinogenic properties of certain anthraquinones in aloe latex, along with lack of safety evidence, prompted the U.S. FDA to ban aloe latex in 2002, although the herb is still used in other countries [178, 300, 301]. The bark of the deciduous buckthorn shrub Cascara sagrada is effective for the treatment of constipation due to the stimulant laxative properties of its anthraglycoside constituents [27, 302]. Like aloe latex, Cascara had previously been approved by the U.S. FDA as a non-prescription medication, but the designation was withdrawn into 2002 based on lack of safety and efficacy evidence, although the herb is still available as a supplement [300].

Stimulant laxatives share multiple common adverse effects and potential drug interactions. Because of decreased gastrointestinal transit time, absorption of some drugs, especially those with poor permeability, may be decreased [303, 304]. Experimental evidence in rats suggests absorption of carbohydrates may result in decreased blood glucose levels and therefore monitoring of patients receiving hypoglycemic agents or insulin is warranted [305-307]. Concomitant use of stimulant laxatives with diuretics, cardiac glycosides and licorice is contraindicated due to hypokalemic effects, especially with long term use of these laxatives [27, 178, 304, 308, 309]. Senna can potentially interfere with antiplatelet and anticoagulant activity by causing excessive bleeding [310]. There is one case report of a possible interaction of aloe and sevoflurane, in which a 35 year old female patient undergoing surgery for hemangioma experienced perioperative bleeding [311]. Although the size and vascularization of the hemangioma were noted as partial root causes of the bleeding episodes, the authors felt that the combination of anesthetic and aloe administration (4 tablets daily for 2 weeks prior to surgery) may have contributed to the adverse event.

3.10. Licorice (*Glycyrrhiza glabra*)

Licorice has historically been used both medicinally and as a food product and its relative safety at low doses has placed it on the U.S. FDA GRAS (generally recognized as safe) list, although at high doses licorice can cause severe adverse effects [27]. The main active components of licorice are glycyrrhizin and glycyrrhizic acid, although several other active constituents have been identified [312, 313]. One of the main adverse effects of high licorice consumption includes mineralocorticoid excess syndrome and resulting hypokalemia with associated increases in blood pressure, as well as secondary pseudohyperaldosteronism [314-338]. Licorice consumption may also alter blood glucose levels, potentially via binding to PPAR-γ [339, 340]. Although licorice is used in dietary supplements for weight loss, contradictory evidence reports weight gain with licorice consumption [341-343]. However, one study in which 3.5 grams daily licorice consumption was administered to 15 normal weight subjects for two months reports a significant decrease in body fat mass but not body mass index [344, 345].

Acquisition of mineralocorticoid excess syndrome following high dose consumption of licorice results in the potential for licorice-drug interactions with multiple drug classes, including aldosterone receptor antagonists, antiarrhythmics, antihypertensives, cardiac glycosides, corticosteroids, diuretics, and potassium lowering agents [321-324, 326]. In one study, 10 healthy subjects were given 32 grams of licorice daily for two weeks along with 25 mg of hydrochlorothiazide (HCTZ); a significant reduction in potassium levels was observed, while two patients experience hypokalemia, compared to HCTZ alone [346]. Glycyrrhizin and β-glycyrrhetinic acid may also affect complement activity and decrease neutrophil generated oxides and peroxides, resulting in anti-inflammatory activity [347-350]. Therefore, licorice should be used with caution in patients taking other anti-inflammatory medications. Licorice constituents may also have an effect on hormonal agents via anti-estrogenic activity, inhibition of 17β-hydroxysteroid dehydrogenase, or associated decreases in prolactin levels [351-358]. In *in vitro* and animal studies it has been shown that constituents in licorice can promote the intestinal absorption of some drugs and therefore it is recommended that oral drugs be taken at least an hour before or two hours after licorice consumption [359]. Theoretically licorice may interact with antidepressant agents, since increases in norepinephrine and dopamine have been observed in mice while *in vitro* cell culture studies suggest potential serotonin reuptake inhibition [360, 361].

3.11. St. John's Wort (*Hypericum perforatum*)

St. John's Wort (SJW) is a perennial herb native to Europe that is commonly used to treat depression, anxiety, post-menopausal symptoms, attention deficit hyperactivity disorder (ADHD), and other mood disorders [362-367]. The active constituents of SJW are hypericin and hyperforin, which are thought to act by inhibiting the synaptic uptake of serotonin (5-HT), GABA, noradrenaline, dopamine, and L-glutamate via a novel mechanism compared to synthetic antidepressants [362, 368-373]. Although there are no official studies regarding the use of SJW for weight loss, anecdotal reports suggest a positive effect on satiety, which may be attributable to the serotonergic uptake inhibition (see *Sibutramine* above). Following the removal of fenfluramine, an anorectic agent commonly used in the combination product "Phen-Fen" (phentermine – fenfluramine), from the market in 1997, SJW was combined with *Ephedra* or *Citrus aurantium* (see above) and marketed for weight loss as "Herbal Phen-Fen". Because of the expanding popularity of SJW in the 1990s – 2000s, a great deal of research on the mechanism of action and herb-drug interactions has been reported.

Drug interactions with SJW are primarily related to binding of active constituents to the pregnane X receptor leading to induction of cytochrome P450 metabolizing or induction of p-glycoprotein efflux mechanisms via the MDR-1 drug transporter [374-388]. As a result, pharmacokinetics of many cytochrome P450 drug substrates is altered, often leading to decreased plasma concentrations and reduced efficacy [27]. There have been numerous studies that have demonstrated potential metabolism-related drug interactions with CYP 3A4, 1A2, 2C9 and 2C19 [389]. Kinetics of antiplatelet and anticoagulant agents may be altered in the presence of SJW [390, 391]. In one open-label, three-way crossover randomized study, 12 healthy male subjects were given 1 gram of SJW (standardized to hypericin 0.825 mg/g and hyperforin 12.5 mg/g) for 21 days, with administration of a single 25 mg dose of warfarin on day 14 [390]. A significant increase in warfarin (Cl/F) was observed compared to warfarin alone, with a corresponding decrease in AUC and half-life. However, there was no significant impact on INR or platelet aggregation. The interaction is likely caused not only by alteration of drug metabolism via CYP 450 induction, but also binding of warfarin to the SJW constituents hypericin and pseudohypericin, leading to decreased absorption of the drug [392]. In another study, patients not responding to clopidogrel therapy alone experienced an increase in therapeutic activity when clopidogrel and SJW were coadministered; therefore it is possible that patients responding to stand alone clopidogrel treatment may be at increased risk of bleeding [391]. There has been one case report of a possible interaction between theophylline and SJW in which theophylline levels significantly increased following discontinuation of SJW in a smoker also taking 11 other drugs [393]. However, another study in healthy subjects showed no impact of SJW on theophylline kinetics [394]. Plasma concentrations of protease inhibitors such as indinavir may be reduced in the presence of SJW due to induction of p-glycoprotein efflux in the gastrointestinal tract [395-398]. Decreased plasma levels of the "statins" simvastatin and atorvastatin have been reported in controlled, randomized, cross-over studies [399, 400]. Reports of pharmacokinetic interactions have also been reported for digoxin, gliclazide, imatinib, irinotecan, methadone, omeprazole, verapamil, and voriconazole have also been published [401-412]. In general, coadministration of SJW with drugs signifi-cantly eliminated via these enzymes should be avoided.

Several studies and case reports describe interactions between SJW and oral contraceptives, resulting in breakthrough or irregular bleeding and unplanned pregnancy [413-416]. In one case report, an unwanted pregnancy occurred in a 36-year old patient while taking an ethinyl estradiol/dinogesterol oral contraceptive (Valette®). The patient had previously been taking fluvastatin (20 mg/day) for 2 years, but had discontinued the drug and started 1700 mg SJW extract daily for 3 months prior to conception [414]. One randomized controlled trial in 18 female subjects taking low dose oral contraceptives (0.02 mg ethinyl estradiol / 0.150 mg desogestrel) in combination with 300 mg SJW twice daily reported a significant increase in breakthrough bleeding compared to subjects taking oral contraceptive alone [417]. Progestins and estrogens contained in oral contraceptives are known to be metabolized by various CYP enzymes and therefore induction of these enzymes by SJW results in decreased plasma concentrations and therapeutic failure [417-420].

Interactions between SJW and with drugs used in the prevention of organ transplant rejection such as tacrolimus and cyclosporine have been reported [421-431]. Several transplant patients have experienced transplant rejection potentially related to coadministration of SJW. In one case report a patient treated with 75 mg cyclosporine daily for several years following kidney transplant experienced a drop in cyclosporin plasma levels attributed to SJW administration [427]. Levels returned to normal when SJW was discontinued and dropped upon rechallenge with SJW extract. Similarly, tacrolimus plasma levels markedly decreased in a study involving 10 stabilized renal transplant patients administered 600 mg SJW extract for two weeks, requiring dosage adjustments during and for up to two weeks following discontinuation of SJW [431].

SJW may interact with selective serotonin reuptake inhibitors (SSRIs), monoamines, and other antidepressant and psychiatric medications due to the serotonin uptake inhibitory properties of hypericin and hyperforin, although metabolic induction plays a role for some drugs [368, 370-373, 432-446]. In one case report, a patient who had been taking paroxetine 40 mg daily for treatment of depression discontinued her medication and began taking SJW 600 mg daily [434]. No adverse events were reported with the switch, but upon coadministration of a 20 mg dose of paroxetine to aid in sleep the patient experience extreme grogginess, weakness, fatigue, and incoherency. The author cited the potential for additive serotonin uptake inhibition resulting in "serotonin syndrome". One case of a male adult patient stabilized on methylphenidate for attention deficit hyperactivity disorder (ADHD) is reported in which the patient experienced increased ADHD symptoms after taking SJW 600 mg daily for four months [438]. The mechanism of the interaction is unknown. Interactions have also been reported for amitriptyline, clozapine, fexofenadine, and sertraline; therefore administration of SJW in patients taking these and similar drugs should be avoided [440, 443, 444, 446, 447].

An interaction between SJW and drugs known to cause phototoxic adverse reactions is also possible, due to the photosensitizing nature of hypericin [448-450]. In one study, 11 subjects were exposed to UVA1 radiation at baseline and following 10 days treatment with 1020 mg (3000 mcg hypericin) extract [449]. Minimum erythemal dose (MED) as measured 8, 24 and 48 hours after exposure to radiation and was found to be significantly lower at 8 and 48, but not 24 hours, after exposure compared to control. There is one case report of a patient experiencing severe phototoxicity upon exposure to laser light (532 nm) and pulsed dye laser light (585 nm), presumably due to ingestion of SJW [451]. SJW may also increase the sensitivity and skin toxicity of radiation treatment in patients undergoing radiation therapy, possibly through photosensitizing effects although the exact underlying mechanism is not known [452].

3.12. Willow bark (*Salix alba*)

Willow bark from the *Salix alba* tree is often contained in weight loss supplements, presumably due to earlier studies that noted enhanced thermogenic properties of ephedra in combination products also including aspirin (see *Ephedra* above). The active constituents of white willow are predominantly the salicylates (acetylsalicylic acid) and, therefore, the bark has traditionally been used in the treatment of pain [27, 453, 454]. The analgesic and anti-inflammatory activity of willow bark is due to inhibition of cyclooxygenase-2 (COX-2) mediated prostaglandin E2 release [455, 456]. Although there are few case reports dealing with willow bark extract specifically, drug and herb interactions seen with other salicylates are possible [455, 457]. Generally, caution should be used in concomitant administration of drugs contraindicated for aspirin, such as beta-blockers, NSAIDs, carbonic anhydrase inhibitors (e.g. acetazolamide), probenecid, alcohol, and salicylates, while the kinetics of protein bound drugs can also be modified [27]. Salicin may also have an effect on platelet aggregation, and therefore interactions with anticoagulants and antiplatelet drugs are possible [458, 459]. In one randomized double-blind study involving 16 patients administered standardized extracts of *Salicis cortex* (240 mg salicin/day), mean arachidonic induced platelet aggregation was reduced (61% compared to 78% in placebo group), but not as significantly as in the acetylsalicylic acid group (13% reduction) [458]. One randomized placebo-controlled trial investigating the efficacy of willow bark extract in osteoarthritis reported an increase in triglyceride levels, suggesting a potential interaction between willow bark and antihyperlipidemics [460]. Some patients in another randomized controlled trial, who were given 240 mg salicin daily for four weeks, suffered blood pressure instability and edema; use of willow bark in patients taking antihypertensives should be cautioned [461].

4. Adulteration of dietary supplements

A final note is necessary regarding the adulteration of weight loss supplements with drug products and other chemical substances. This adulteration is often the underlying cause for the purported activity of a dietary supplement and can result in serious toxicity. The most commonly cited contaminant in weight loss supplements is sibutramine (Meridia®; see above), a weight loss supplement removed from the market in October 2010 for significant cardiac toxicities [462-466]. One U.S. FDA report cites 72 different herbal products containing adulterants, 94.4% of which contained sibutramine as an additive [102]. Multiple products listed in the report were contaminated with phenolphthalein (11.1%) or the anti-seizure drug phenytoin (2.8%). Other reported contaminants (1.4%) included the experimental anti-obesity agent cetilistat, the recalled anti-obesity agent rimonabant (see above), the anti-obesity amphetamine stimulant drug fenproporex, the antidepressant fluoxetine, or the diuretics furosemide and bumetanide[103]. Phenophthalein was previously used as a laxative in over-the-counter products but was removed from the U.S. market in 1999 due to concerns of carcinogenicity and genotoxicity [467]. Another study investigating contamination of 20 different dietary supplements using 1H-NMR methods found contamination of 14 of the products (70%), with eight products containing sibutramine, five containing both sibutramine and phenolphthalein, and one formulation containing undeclared synephrine [468]. There have been other reports of contamination of weight loss supplements with the diuretic hydrochlorothiazide [462, 469]. Given that tainting of weight loss supplements is common, patients and health care professionals should be made aware of the risks associated with ingestion of herbal products, especially those with minimal evidence backing their claims of efficacy.

Author details

Melanie A. Jordan

Midwestern University, College of Pharmacy – Glendale, Glendale, AZ, USA

References

[1] World Health Organization, *Obesity: Facts and Figures*, 2012; Available from: http://www.euro.who.int/en/what-we-do/health-topics/noncommunicable-diseases/obesity/facts-and-figures [accessed 06/20/12].

[2] World Health Organization, *WHO Global Infobase*, 2012; Available from: https://apps.who.int/infobase/Comparisons.aspx [accessed 06/20/12]

[3] Ogden, C.L., et al., *Prevalence of overweight and obesity in the United States, 1999-2004.* JAMA, 2006. 295(13): p. 1549-55.

[4] Flegal, K.M., et al., *Prevalence of obesity and trends in the distribution of body mass index among US adults, 1999-2010.* JAMA, 2012. 307(5): p. 491-7.

[5] James, W.P., *WHO recognition of the global obesity epidemic.* Int J Obes (Lond), 2008. 32 Suppl 7: p. S120-6.

[6] Ogden, C.L., et al., *Prevalence of obesity in the United States, 2009-2010.* NCHS Data Brief, 2012(82): p. 1-8.

[7] Samaranayake, N.R., et al., *Management of obesity in the National Health and Nutrition Examination Survey (NHANES), 2007-2008.* Ann Epidemiol, 2012. 22(5): p. 349-53.

[8] Manton, K.G., *The global impact of noncommunicable diseases: estimates and projections.* World Health Stat Q, 1988. 41(3-4): p. 255-66.

[9] Wang, Y., et al., *Will all Americans become overweight or obese? estimating the progression and cost of the US obesity epidemic.* Obesity (Silver Spring), 2008. 16(10): p. 2323-30.

[10] Wolf, A.M. and G.A. Colditz, *Current estimates of the economic cost of obesity in the United States.* Obes Res, 1998. 6(2): p. 97-106.

[11] *European Charter on Counteracting Obesity*, in *WHO European Ministerial Conference on Counteracting Obesity.* 2006, World Health Organization: Istanbul, Turkey.

[12] U.S. Department of Agriculture, Cente rfor Nutrition Policy and Promotion, 2012. *ChooseMyPlate.gov*; Available from: http://www/ChooseMyPlate.gov [accessed 06/20/12].

[13] J. Steenhuysen, S.H., J. Lentz, L. Richwine, *Factbox: A troubled history for weight-loss drugs*, in *Reuters.* 2011, Thomson Reuters.

[14] Sam, A.H., V. Salem, and M.A. Ghatei, *Rimonabant: From RIO to Ban.* J Obes, 2011. 2011: p. 432607.

[15] U.S. Food and Drug Adminsitration, *FDA Drug Safety Communication: FDA Recommends Against the Continued Use of Meridia (sibutramine)*, 2010: Silver Spring, MD.

[16] Basch, E.M., J.C. Servoss, and U.B. Tedrow, *Safety assurances for dietary supplements policy issues and new research paradigms.* J Herb Pharmacother, 2005. 5(1): p. 3-15.

[17] Harris, I.M., *Regulatory and ethical issues with dietary supplements.* Pharmacotherapy, 2000. 20(11): p. 1295-302.

[18] Jordan, S.A., D.G. Cunningham, and R.J. Marles, *Assessment of herbal medicinal products: challenges, and opportunities to increase the knowledge base for safety assessment.* Toxicol Appl Pharmacol, 2010. 243(2): p. 198-216.

[19] Tsutani, K. and H. Takuma, *[Regulatory sciences in herbal medicines and dietary supplements].* Yakugaku Zasshi, 2008. 128(6): p. 867-80.

[20] Garcia-Mijares, M., A.M. Bernardes, and M.T. Silva, *Diethylpropion produces psychostimulant and reward effects.* Pharmacol Biochem Behav, 2009. 91(4): p. 621-8.

[21] Ollo, C., et al., *Lack of neurotoxic effect of diethylpropion in crack-cocaine abusers.* Clin Neuropharmacol, 1996. 19(1): p. 52-8.

[22] Samanin, R. and S. Garattini, *Neurochemical mechanism of action of anorectic drugs.* Pharmacol Toxicol, 1993. 73(2): p. 63-8.

[23] *Prescribing Information. Tenuate (diethylpropion hydrochloride).* November 2003, Aventis Pharmaceuticals, Inc.: Bridgewater, NJ.

[24] Martin, C.A. and E.T. Iwamoto, *Diethylpropion-induced psychosis reprecipitated by an MAO inhibitor: case report.* J Clin Psychiatry, 1984. 45(3): p. 130-1.

[25] Seedat, Y.K. and J. Reddy, *Diethylpropion hydrochloride (Tenuate Dospan) in combination with hypotensive agents in the treatment of obesity associated with hypertension.* Curr Ther Res Clin Exp, 1974. 16(5): p. 398-413.

[26] Carruba, M.O., et al., *Dopaminergic and serotoninergic anorectics differentially antagonize insulin- and 2-DG-induced hyperphagia.* Life Sci, 1985. 36(18): p. 1739-49.

[27] Jellin, J. et al. (Eds), *Natural Medicines Comprehensive Database.* 1995 - 2012, Therapeutic Research Faculty.

[28] *Suprenza (phentermine hydrochloride) Prescribing Information.* 2011, Akrimax Pharmaceuticals, LLC: Cranford, NJ.

[29] Haddock, C.K., et al., *Pharmacotherapy for obesity: a quantitative analysis of four decades of published randomized clinical trials.* Int J Obes Relat Metab Disord, 2002. 26(2): p. 262-73.

[30] Fleming, R.M. and L.B. Boyd, *The longitudinal effects of fenfluramine-phentermine use.* Angiology, 2007. 58(3): p. 353-9.

[31] Barasch, A. and M.M. Safford, *Diet medications and valvular heart disease: the current evidence.* Spec Care Dentist, 2002. 22(3): p. 108-14.

[32] Stephens, L.C. and S.G. Katz, *Phentermine and anaesthesia*. Anaesth Intensive Care, 2005. 33(4): p. 525-7.

[33] Biton, V., *Clinical pharmacology and mechanism of action of zonisamide*. Clin Neurophar-macol, 2007. 30(4): p. 230-40.

[34] Antel, J. and J. Hebebrand, *Weight-reducing side effects of the antiepileptic agents topira-mate and zonisamide*. Handb Exp Pharmacol, 2012(209): p. 433-66.

[35] *Topamax (topiramate) Prescribing Information*. 2009, Janssen Pharmaceuticals, Inc.: Ti-tusville, NJ.

[36] Czuczwar, S.J., *[GABA-ergic system and antiepileptic drugs]*. Neurol Neurochir Pol, 2000. 34 Suppl 1: p. 13-20.

[37] White, H.S., et al., *Topiramate modulates GABA-evoked currents in murine cortical neu-rons by a nonbenzodiazepine mechanism*. Epilepsia, 2000. 41 Suppl 1: p. S17-20.

[38] Eliasson, B., et al., *Weight loss and metabolic effects of topiramate in overweight and obese type 2 diabetic patients: randomized double-blind placebo-controlled trial*. Int J Obes (Lond), 2007. 31(7): p. 1140-7.

[39] Gordon, A. and L.H. Price, *Mood stabilization and weight loss with topiramate*. Am J Psy-chiatry, 1999. 156(6): p. 968-9.

[40] Littrell, K.H., et al., *Weight loss with topiramate*. Ann Pharmacother, 2001. 35(9): p. 1141-2.

[41] Roy Chengappa, K.N., et al., *Long-term effects of topiramate on bipolar mood instability, weight change and glycemic control: a case-series*. Eur Psychiatry, 2001. 16(3): p. 186-90.

[42] Shapira, N.A., T.D. Goldsmith, and S.L. McElroy, *Treatment of binge-eating disorder with topiramate: a clinical case series*. J Clin Psychiatry, 2000. 61(5): p. 368-72.

[43] Allison, D.B., et al., *Controlled-release phentermine/topiramate in severely obese adults: a randomized controlled trial (EQUIP)*. Obesity (Silver Spring), 2012. 20(2): p. 330-42.

[44] Bays, H.E. and K.M. Gadde, *Phentermine/topiramate for weight reduction and treatment of adverse metabolic consequences in obesity*. Drugs Today (Barc), 2011. 47(12): p. 903-14.

[45] Powell, A.G., C.M. Apovian, and L.J. Aronne, *The combination of phentermine and topir-amate is an effective adjunct to diet and lifestyle modification for weight loss and measures of comorbidity in overweight or obese adults with additional metabolic risk factors*. Evid Based Med, 2012. 17(1): p. 14-5.

[46] Shah, K. and D.T. Villareal, *Combination treatment to CONQUER obesity?* Lancet, 2011. 377(9774): p. 1295-7.

[47] Mack, C.J., et al., *Interaction of topiramate with carbamazepine: two case reports and a re-view of clinical experience*. Seizure, 2002. 11(7): p. 464-7.

[48] Cano-Zuleta, A., et al., *Report of three cases of hyperammonaemic encephalopathy associated with valproic acid due to possible synergism with phenobarbital and topiramate.* Farm Hosp, 2012.

[49] Deutsch, S.I., J.A. Burket, and R.B. Rosse, *Valproate-induced hyperammonemic encephalopathy and normal liver functions: possible synergism with topiramate.* Clin Neuropharmacol, 2009. 32(6): p. 350-2.

[50] Gomez-Ibanez, A., E. Urrestarazu-Bolumburu, and C. Viteri-Torres, *Hyperammonemic encephalopathy related to valproate, phenobarbital, and topiramate synergism.* Epilepsy Behav, 2011. 21(4): p. 480-2.

[51] *Metabolic acidosis due to topiramate.* Prescrire Int, 2004. 13(73): p. 186.

[52] Burmeister, J.E., et al., *Topiramate and severe metabolic acidosis: case report.* Arq Neuropsiquiatr, 2005. 63(2B): p. 532-4.

[53] Fernandez-de Orueta, L., et al., *Topiramate-induced metabolic acidosis: a case study.* Nefrologia, 2012. 32(3): p. 403-404.

[54] Ko, C.H. and C.K. Kong, *Topiramate-induced metabolic acidosis: report of two cases.* Dev Med Child Neurol, 2001. 43(10): p. 701-4.

[55] Ozer, Y. and H. Altunkaya, *Topiramate induced metabolic acidosis.* Anaesthesia, 2004. 59(8): p. 830.

[56] Vivius, I., *VI-0521 (Qnexa) Advisory Committee Briefing Document*, E.a.M.D.A. Committee, Editor. 2012, Vivius, Inc.: Mountain View, CA. p. 1 - 166.

[57] Leppik, I.E., *Zonisamide: chemistry, mechanism of action, and pharmacokinetics.* Seizure, 2004. 13 Suppl 1: p. S5-9; discussion S10.

[58] Czapinski, P., B. Blaszczyk, and S.J. Czuczwar, *Mechanisms of action of antiepileptic drugs.* Curr Top Med Chem, 2005. 5(1): p. 3-14.

[59] Suzuki, S., et al., *Zonisamide blocks T-type calcium channel in cultured neurons of rat cerebral cortex.* Epilepsy Res, 1992. 12(1): p. 21-7.

[60] Okada, M., et al., *Effects of zonisamide on dopaminergic system.* Epilepsy Res, 1995. 22(3): p. 193-205.

[61] Okada, M., et al., *Biphasic effects of zonisamide on serotonergic system in rat hippocampus.* Epilepsy Res, 1999. 34(2-3): p. 187-97.

[62] Gadde, K.M., et al., *Zonisamide for weight loss in obese adults: a randomized controlled trial.* JAMA, 2003. 289(14): p. 1820-5.

[63] Ojemann, L.M., et al., *Comparative pharmacokinetics of zonisamide (CI-912) in epileptic patients on carbamazepine or phenytoin monotherapy.* Ther Drug Monit, 1986. 8(3): p. 293-6.

[64] Orito, K., et al., *Pharmacokinetics of zonisamide and drug interaction with phenobarbital in dogs.* J Vet Pharmacol Ther, 2008. 31(3): p. 259-64.

[65] Shinoda, M., et al., *The necessity of adjusting the dosage of zonisamide when coadministered with other anti-epileptic drugs.* Biol Pharm Bull, 1996. 19(8): p. 1090-2.

[66] *Zonegran (zonisamide) Package Insert.* 2006, Eisai Inc.: Teaneck, NJ.

[67] Arvill, A. and L. Bodin, *Effect of short-term ingestion of konjac glucomannan on serum cholesterol in healthy men.* Am J Clin Nutr, 1995. 61(3): p. 585-9.

[68] Nagatomo, I., et al., *Alcohol intake decreases brain Zonisamide concentration in inbred EL mice.* Neuroreport, 1997. 8(2): p. 391-4.

[69] *Xenical Prescribing Information.* 2012, Genentech USA, Inc.: South San Francisco, CA.

[70] Drent, M.L. and E.A. van der Veen, *Lipase inhibition: a novel concept in the treatment of obesity.* Int J Obes Relat Metab Disord, 1993. 17(4): p. 241-4.

[71] Li, Z., et al., *Meta-analysis: pharmacologic treatment of obesity.* Ann Intern Med, 2005. 142(7): p. 532-46.

[72] Davidson, M.H., et al., *Weight control and risk factor reduction in obese subjects treated for 2 years with orlistat: a randomized controlled trial.* JAMA, 1999. 281(3): p. 235-42.

[73] Torgerson, J.S., et al., *XENical in the prevention of diabetes in obese subjects (XENDOS) study: a randomized study of orlistat as an adjunct to lifestyle changes for the prevention of type 2 diabetes in obese patients.* Diabetes Care, 2004. 27(1): p. 155-61.

[74] Colman, E. and M. Fossler, *Reduction in blood cyclosporine concentrations by orlistat.* N Engl J Med, 2000. 342(15): p. 1141-2.

[75] Errasti, P., et al., *Reduction in blood cyclosporine concentration by orlistat in two renal transplant patients.* Transplant Proc, 2002. 34(1): p. 137-9.

[76] Evans, S., et al., *Drug interaction in a renal transplant patient: cyclosporin-Neoral and orlistat.* Am J Kidney Dis, 2003. 41(2): p. 493-6.

[77] Le Beller, C., et al., *Co-administration of orlistat and cyclosporine in a heart transplant recipient.* Transplantation, 2000. 70(10): p. 1541-2.

[78] Nagele, H., et al., *Effect of orlistat on blood cyclosporin concentration in an obese heart transplant patient.* Eur J Clin Pharmacol, 1999. 55(9): p. 667-9.

[79] Schnetzler, B., et al., *Orlistat decreases the plasma level of cyclosporine and may be responsible for the development of acute rejection episodes.* Transplantation, 2000. 70(10): p. 1540-1.

[80] Barbaro, D., et al., *Obesity in transplant patients: case report showing interference of orlistat with absorption of cyclosporine and review of literature.* Endocr Pract, 2002. 8(2): p. 124-6.

[81] McDuffie, J.R., et al., *Effects of orlistat on fat-soluble vitamins in obese adolescents.* Pharmacotherapy, 2002. 22(7): p. 814-22.

[82] Melia, A.T., S.G. Koss-Twardy, and J. Zhi, *The effect of orlistat, an inhibitor of dietary fat absorption, on the absorption of vitamins A and E in healthy volunteers.* J Clin Pharmacol, 1996. 36(7): p. 647-53.

[83] Zhi, J., et al., *The effect of orlistat, an inhibitor of dietary fat absorption, on the pharmacokinetics of beta-carotene in healthy volunteers.* J Clin Pharmacol, 1996. 36(2): p. 152-9.

[84] Bigham, S., C. McGuigan, and B.K. MacDonald, *Reduced absorption of lipophilic anti-epileptic medications when used concomitantly with the anti-obesity drug orlistat.* Epilepsia, 2006. 47(12): p. 2207.

[85] Madhava, K. and A. Hartley, *Hypothyroidism in thyroid carcinoma follow-up: orlistat may inhibit the absorption of thyroxine.* Clin Oncol (R Coll Radiol), 2005. 17(6): p. 492.

[86] Zhi, J., et al., *The effect of orlistat on the pharmacokinetics and pharmacodynamics of warfarin in healthy volunteers.* J Clin Pharmacol, 1996. 36(7): p. 659-66.

[87] Xie, S., et al., *The endocannabinoid system and rimonabant: a new drug with a novel mechanism of action involving cannabinoid CB1 receptor antagonism--or inverse agonism--as potential obesity treatment and other therapeutic use.* J Clin Pharm Ther, 2007. 32(3): p. 209-31.

[88] Banerji, M.A. and M. Tiewala, *Rimonabant--the RIO North America trial: a new strategy to sustaining weight loss and related morbidity.* Curr Diab Rep, 2006. 6(3): p. 228-9.

[89] Kintscher, U., *The cardiometabolic drug rimonabant: after 2 years of RIO-Europe and STRADIVARIUS.* Eur Heart J, 2008. 29(14): p. 1709-10.

[90] Nissen, S.E., et al., *Effect of rimonabant on progression of atherosclerosis in patients with abdominal obesity and coronary artery disease: the STRADIVARIUS randomized controlled trial.* JAMA, 2008. 299(13): p. 1547-60.

[91] Pan, C., H.J. Yoo, and L.T. Ho, *Perspectives of CB1 Antagonist in Treatment of Obesity: Experience of RIO-Asia.* J Obes, 2011. 2011: p. 957268.

[92] Pi-Sunyer, F.X., et al., *Effect of rimonabant, a cannabinoid-1 receptor blocker, on weight and cardiometabolic risk factors in overweight or obese patients: RIO-North America: a randomized controlled trial.* JAMA, 2006. 295(7): p. 761-75.

[93] Scheen, A.J., *CB1 receptor blockade and its impact on cardiometabolic risk factors: overview of the RIO programme with rimonabant.* J Neuroendocrinol, 2008. 20 Suppl 1: p. 139-46.

[94] Topol, E.J., et al., *Rimonabant for prevention of cardiovascular events (CRESCENDO): a randomised, multicentre, placebo-controlled trial.* Lancet, 2010. 376(9740): p. 517-23.

[95]   Van Gaal, L.F., et al., *Long-term effect of CB1 blockade with rimonabant on cardiometabolic risk factors: two year results from the RIO-Europe Study.* Eur Heart J, 2008. 29(14): p. 1761-71.

[96]   Despres, J.P., A. Golay, and L. Sjostrom, *Effects of rimonabant on metabolic risk factors in overweight patients with dyslipidemia.* N Engl J Med, 2005. 353(20): p. 2121-34.

[97]   Rasmussen, E.B., et al., *Rimonabant reduces the essential value of food in the genetically obese Zucker rat: an exponential demand analysis.* Physiol Behav, 2012. 105(3): p. 734-41.

[98]   Verty, A.N., et al., *Anti-obesity effects of the combined administration of CB1 receptor antagonist rimonabant and melanin-concentrating hormone antagonist SNAP-94847 in dietinudced obese mice.* Int J Obes (Lond), 2012.

[99]   Zaitone, S.A. and S. Essawy, *Addition of a low dose of rimonabant to orlistat therapy decreases weight gain and reduces adiposity in dietary obese rats.* Clin Exp Pharmacol Physiol, 2012. 39(6): p. 551-9.

[100] Taj Pharmaceuticals Limited, *Indian Pharmaceuticals Company Taj Pharmaceuticals receives FDA Approval for Generic Rimonabant.* 2010; Available from: http://www.tajpharma.com/media/media_r/Indian%20Pharmaceuticals%20Company%20Taj%20Pharmaceuticals%20receives%20FDA%20approval%20for%20Generic%20Rimonabant.pdf [accessed 06/20/12].

[101] Venhuis, B.J., et al., *The identification of rimonabant polymorphs, sibutramine and analogues of both in counterfeit Acomplia bought on the internet.* J Pharm Biomed Anal, 2011. 54(1): p. 21-6.

[102] U.S. Food and Drug Adminsitration, Department of Health and Human Services, *Questions and Answers about FDA's Initiative Against Contaminated Weight Loss Products,* 2008: Silver Spring, MD.

[103] U.S. Food and Drug Adminsitration, Department of Health and Human Services, *FDA Uncovers Additional Tainted Weight Loss Products: Agency Alerts Consumers to the Finding of New Undeclared Drug Ingredients.,* 2009: Rockville, MD.

[104] European Medicines Agency (EMEA), *Acomplia: EPAR - Product Information,* 2009.

[105] Mandhane, S., et al., *Induction of Glucose Intolerance by Acute Administration of Rimonabant.* Pharmacology, 2012. 89(5-6): p. 339-347.

[106] *Meridia (sibutramine hydrocholoride) Package Insert.* 2010, Abbott Laboratories: North Chicago, IL.

[107] Heal, D.J., et al., *Sibutramine: a novel anti-obesity drug. A review of the pharmacological evidence to differentiate it from d-amphetamine and d-fenfluramine.* Int J Obes Relat Metab Disord, 1998. 22 Suppl 1: p. S18-28; discussion S29.

[108] Liu, Y.L., D.J. Heal, and M.J. Stock, *Mechanism of the thermogenic effect of Metabolite 2 (BTS 54 505), a major pharmacologically active metabolite of the novel anti-obesity drug, sibutramine.* Int J Obes Relat Metab Disord, 2002. 26(9): p. 1245-53.

[109] McNeely, W. and K.L. Goa, *Sibutramine. A review of its contribution to the management of obesity.* Drugs, 1998. 56(6): p. 1093-124.

[110] Nisoli, E. and M.O. Carruba, *An assessment of the safety and efficacy of sibutramine, an anti-obesity drug with a novel mechanism of action.* Obes Rev, 2000. 1(2): p. 127-39.

[111] Bailey, D.G. and G.K. Dresser, *Interactions between grapefruit juice and cardiovascular drugs.* Am J Cardiovasc Drugs, 2004. 4(5): p. 281-97.

[112] Greenway, F.L. and M.K. Caruso, *Safety of obesity drugs.* Expert Opin Drug Saf, 2005. 4(6): p. 1083-95.

[113] Wellman, P.J., S.L. Jones, and D.K. Miller, *Effects of preexposure to dexfenfluramine, phentermine, dexfenfluramine-phentermine, or fluoxetine on sibutramine-induced hypophagia in the adult rat.* Pharmacol Biochem Behav, 2003. 75(1): p. 103-14.

[114] Yalcin, A.A., et al., *Elevation of QT dispersion after obesity drug sibutramine.* J Cardiovasc Med (Hagerstown), 2010. 11(11): p. 832-5.

[115] Caterson, I.D., et al., *Maintained intentional weight loss reduces cardiovascular outcomes: results from the Sibutramine Cardiovascular OUTcomes (SCOUT) trial.* Diabetes Obes Metab, 2012. 14(6): p. 523-30.

[116] Coutinho, W.F., *The obese older female patient: CV risk and the SCOUT study.* Int J Obes (Lond), 2007. 31 Suppl 2: p. S26-30; discussion S31-2.

[117] Maggioni, A.P., *SCOUT trial reports on the safety profile of sibutramine in patients with cardiovascular diseases.* Phys Sportsmed, 2009. 37(3): p. 95-7.

[118] Torp-Pedersen, C., et al., *Cardiovascular responses to weight management and sibutramine in high-risk subjects: an analysis from the SCOUT trial.* Eur Heart J, 2007. 28(23): p. 2915-23.

[119] Benazzi, F., *Organic hypomania secondary to sibutramine-citalopram interaction.* J Clin Psychiatry, 2002. 63(2): p. 165.

[120] Clerbaux, G., E. Goffin, and Y. Pirson, *Interaction between sibutramine and cyclosporine.* Am J Transplant, 2003. 3(7): p. 906.

[121] Jordan, J. and A.M. Sharma, *Potential for sibutramine-yohimbine interaction?* Lancet, 2003. 361(9371): p. 1826.

[122] Chin, Y.W., et al., *Lignans and other constituents of the fruits of Euterpe oleracea (Acai) with antioxidant and cytoprotective activities.* J Agric Food Chem, 2008. 56(17): p. 7759-64.

[123] Jensen, G.S., et al., *In vitro and in vivo antioxidant and anti-inflammatory capacities of an antioxidant-rich fruit and berry juice blend. Results of a pilot and randomized, double-blinded, placebo-controlled, crossover study.* J Agric Food Chem, 2008. 56(18): p. 8326-33.

[124] Lichtenthaler, R., et al., *Total oxidant scavenging capacities of Euterpe oleracea Mart. (Acai) fruits.* Int J Food Sci Nutr, 2005. 56(1): p. 53-64.

[125] Mertens-Talcott, S.U., et al., *Pharmacokinetics of anthocyanins and antioxidant effects after the consumption of anthocyanin-rich acai juice and pulp (Euterpe oleracea Mart.) in human healthy volunteers.* J Agric Food Chem, 2008. 56(17): p. 7796-802.

[126] Xie, C., et al., *Acai juice attenuates atherosclerosis in ApoE deficient mice through antioxidant and anti-inflammatory activities.* Atherosclerosis, 2011. 216(2): p. 327-33.

[127] Udani, J.K., et al., *Effects of Acai (Euterpe oleracea Mart.) berry preparation on metabolic parameters in a healthy overweight population: a pilot study.* Nutr J, 2011. 10: p. 45.

[128] Allison, D.B., et al., *Exactly which synephrine alkaloids does Citrus aurantium (bitter orange) contain?* Int J Obes (Lond), 2005. 29(4): p. 443-6.

[129] Dandekar, D.V., G.K. Jayaprakasha, and B.S. Patil, *Simultaneous extraction of bioactive limonoid aglycones and glucoside from Citrus aurantium L. using hydrotropy.* Z Naturforsch C, 2008. 63(3-4): p. 176-80.

[130] Haaz, S., et al., *Citrus aurantium and synephrine alkaloids in the treatment of overweight and obesity: an update.* Obes Rev, 2006. 7(1): p. 79-88.

[131] Liu, L., et al., *Naringenin and hesperetin, two flavonoids derived from Citrus aurantium up-regulate transcription of adiponectin.* Phytother Res, 2008. 22(10): p. 1400-3.

[132] Nelson, B.C., et al., *Mass spectrometric determination of the predominant adrenergic proto-alkaloids in bitter orange (Citrus aurantium).* J Agric Food Chem, 2007. 55(24): p. 9769-75.

[133] Pellati, F., et al., *Determination of adrenergic agonists from extracts and herbal products of Citrus aurantium L. var. amara by LC.* J Pharm Biomed Anal, 2002. 29(6): p. 1113-9.

[134] Penzak, S.R., et al., *Seville (sour) orange juice: synephrine content and cardiovascular effects in normotensive adults.* J Clin Pharmacol, 2001. 41(10): p. 1059-63.

[135] Bui, L.T., D.T. Nguyen, and P.J. Ambrose, *Blood pressure and heart rate effects following a single dose of bitter orange.* Ann Pharmacother, 2006. 40(1): p. 53-7.

[136] Haller, C.A., N.L. Benowitz, and P. Jacob, 3rd, *Hemodynamic effects of ephedra-free weight-loss supplements in humans.* Am J Med, 2005. 118(9): p. 998-1003.

[137] Di Marco, M.P., et al., *The effect of grapefruit juice and seville orange juice on the pharmacokinetics of dextromethorphan: the role of gut CYP3A and P-glycoprotein.* Life Sci, 2002. 71(10): p. 1149-60.

[138] Edwards, D.J., et al., *6',7'-Dihydroxybergamottin in grapefruit juice and Seville orange juice: effects on cyclosporine disposition, enterocyte CYP3A4, and P-glycoprotein.* Clin Pharmacol Ther, 1999. 65(3): p. 237-44.

[139] Malhotra, S., et al., *Seville orange juice-felodipine interaction: comparison with dilute grapefruit juice and involvement of furocoumarins.* Clin Pharmacol Ther, 2001. 69(1): p. 14-23.

[140] Penzak, S.R., et al., *Effect of Seville orange juice and grapefruit juice on indinavir pharmacokinetics.* J Clin Pharmacol, 2002. 42(10): p. 1165-70.

[141] Suzuki, O., et al., *Oxidation of synephrine by type A and type B monoamine oxidase.* Experientia, 1979. 35(10): p. 1283-4.

[142] Visentin, V., et al., *Dual action of octopamine on glucose transport into adipocytes: inhibition via beta3-adrenoceptor activation and stimulation via oxidation by amine oxidases.* J Pharmacol Exp Ther, 2001. 299(1): p. 96-104.

[143] Acheson, K.J., et al., *Metabolic effects of caffeine in humans: lipid oxidation or futile cycling?* Am J Clin Nutr, 2004. 79(1): p. 40-6.

[144] Acheson, K.J., et al., *Caffeine and coffee: their influence on metabolic rate and substrate utilization in normal weight and obese individuals.* Am J Clin Nutr, 1980. 33(5): p. 989-97.

[145] Andersen, T. and J. Fogh, *Weight loss and delayed gastric emptying following a South American herbal preparation in overweight patients.* J Hum Nutr Diet, 2001. 14(3): p. 243-50.

[146] Astrup, A., et al., *The effect of ephedrine/caffeine mixture on energy expenditure and body composition in obese women.* Metabolism, 1992. 41(7): p. 686-8.

[147] Astrup, A., et al., *Thermogenic synergism between ephedrine and caffeine in healthy volunteers: a double-blind, placebo-controlled study.* Metabolism, 1991. 40(3): p. 323-9.

[148] Boozer, C.N., et al., *Herbal ephedra/caffeine for weight loss: a 6-month randomized safety and efficacy trial.* Int J Obes Relat Metab Disord, 2002. 26(5): p. 593-604.

[149] Coffey, C.S., et al., *A randomized double-blind placebo-controlled clinical trial of a product containing ephedrine, caffeine, and other ingredients from herbal sources for treatment of overweight and obesity in the absence of lifestyle treatment.* Int J Obes Relat Metab Disord, 2004. 28(11): p. 1411-9.

[150] Dulloo, A.G., *Herbal simulation of ephedrine and caffeine in treatment of obesity.* Int J Obes Relat Metab Disord, 2002. 26(5): p. 590-2.

[151] Dulloo, A.G., J. Seydoux, and L. Girardier, *Peripheral mechanisms of thermogenesis induced by ephedrine and caffeine in brown adipose tissue.* Int J Obes, 1991. 15(5): p. 317-26.

[152] Cannon, M.E., C.T. Cooke, and J.S. McCarthy, *Caffeine-induced cardiac arrhythmia: an unrecognised danger of healthfood products.* Med J Aust, 2001. 174(10): p. 520-1.

[153] Heseltine, D., et al., *The effect of caffeine on postprandial hypotension in the elderly*. J Am Geriatr Soc, 1991. 39(2): p. 160-4.

[154] Heseltine, D., et al., *The effect of caffeine on postprandial blood pressure in the frail elderly*. Postgrad Med J, 1991. 67(788): p. 543-7.

[155] Katan, M.B. and E. Schouten, *Caffeine and arrhythmia*. Am J Clin Nutr, 2005. 81(3): p. 539-40.

[156] Nurminen, M.L., et al., *Coffee, caffeine and blood pressure: a critical review*. Eur J Clin Nutr, 1999. 53(11): p. 831-9.

[157] Upton, R.A., *Pharmacokinetic interactions between theophylline and other medication (Part I)*. Clin Pharmacokinet, 1991. 20(1): p. 66-80.

[158] Del Rio, G., et al., *Increased cardiovascular response to caffeine in perimenopausal women before and during estrogen therapy*. Eur J Endocrinol, 1996. 135(5): p. 598-603.

[159] Pollock, B.G., et al., *Inhibition of caffeine metabolism by estrogen replacement therapy in postmenopausal women*. J Clin Pharmacol, 1999. 39(9): p. 936-40.

[160] Dulloo, A.G., et al., *Efficacy of a green tea extract rich in catechin polyphenols and caffeine in increasing 24-h energy expenditure and fat oxidation in humans*. Am J Clin Nutr, 1999. 70(6): p. 1040-5.

[161] Dulloo, A.G., et al., *Green tea and thermogenesis: interactions between catechin-polyphenols, caffeine and sympathetic activity*. Int J Obes Relat Metab Disord, 2000. 24(2): p. 252-8.

[162] Jagdeo, J. and N. Brody, *Complementary antioxidant function of caffeine and green tea polyphenols in normal human skin fibroblasts*. J Drugs Dermatol, 2011. 10(7): p. 753-61.

[163] Samanidou, V., A. Tsagiannidis, and I. Sarakatsianos, *Simultaneous determination of polyphenols and major purine alkaloids in Greek Sideritis species, herbal extracts, green tea, black tea, and coffee by high-performance liquid chromatography-diode array detection*. J Sep Sci, 2012. 35(4): p. 608-15.

[164] Westerterp-Plantenga, M.S., *Green tea catechins, caffeine and body-weight regulation*. Physiol Behav, 2010. 100(1): p. 42-6.

[165] Phung, O.J., et al., *Effect of green tea catechins with or without caffeine on anthropometric measures: a systematic review and meta-analysis*. Am J Clin Nutr, 2010. 91(1): p. 73-81.

[166] Taylor, J.R. and V.M. Wilt, *Probable antagonism of warfarin by green tea*. Ann Pharmacother, 1999. 33(4): p. 426-8.

[167] Sun, J., *Morning/evening menopausal formula relieves menopausal symptoms: a pilot study*. J Altern Complement Med, 2003. 9(3): p. 403-9.

[168] Westphal, L.M., M.L. Polan, and A.S. Trant, *Double-blind, placebo-controlled study of Fertilityblend: a nutritional supplement for improving fertility in women.* Clin Exp Obstet Gynecol, 2006. 33(4): p. 205-8.

[169] Westphal, L.M., et al., *A nutritional supplement for improving fertility in women: a pilot study.* J Reprod Med, 2004. 49(4): p. 289-93.

[170] Wu, A.H., et al., *Tea and circulating estrogen levels in postmenopausal Chinese women in Singapore.* Carcinogenesis, 2005. 26(5): p. 976-80.

[171] Abourashed, E.A., et al., *Two new flavone glycosides from paullinia pinnata.* J Nat Prod, 1999. 62(8): p. 1179-81.

[172] Avato, P., et al., *Seed oil composition of Paullinia cupana var. sorbilis (Mart.) Ducke.* Lipids, 2003. 38(7): p. 773-80.

[173] Belliardo, F., A. Martelli, and M.G. Valle, *HPLC determination of caffeine and theophylline in Paullinia cupana Kunth (guarana) and Cola spp. samples.* Z Lebensm Unters Forsch, 1985. 180(5): p. 398-401.

[174] Saldana, M.D., et al., *Extraction of methylxanthines from guarana seeds, mate leaves, and cocoa beans using supercritical carbon dioxide and ethanol.* J Agric Food Chem, 2002. 50(17): p. 4820-6.

[175] Weckerle, C.S., M.A. Stutz, and T.W. Baumann, *Purine alkaloids in Paullinia.* Phytochemistry, 2003. 64(3): p. 735-42.

[176] Zamble, A., et al., *Paullinia pinnata extracts rich in polyphenols promote vascular relaxation via endothelium-dependent mechanisms.* J Cardiovasc Pharmacol, 2006. 47(4): p. 599-608.

[177] Bydlowski, S.P., R.L. Yunker, and M.T. Subbiah, *A novel property of an aqueous guarana extract (Paullinia cupana): inhibition of platelet aggregation in vitro and in vivo.* Braz J Med Biol Res, 1988. 21(3): p. 535-8.

[178] Blumenthal, M., W.R. Busse, and Bundesinstitut für Arzneimittel und Medizinprodukte (Germany), *The complete German Commission E monographs, Therapeutic guide to herbal medicines.* 1998, Austin, Texas; Boston: American Botanical Council ;Integrative Medicine Communications. xxii, 685 p.

[179] Escudero, N.L., DeArellano, M.L., Fernandez, S., Albarracin, G., and Mucciarelli, S., *Taraxacum officinale as a food source.* Plant Foods for Human Nutrition, 2003. 58(3): p. 1 - 10.

[180] Tabassum, N., Qazi, M.A., and Shah, A., *Curative Activity of Ethanol Extract of Taraxacum officinale Weber. Against CCl4 Induced Hepatocellular Damage in Albino Rats.* J. Pharmacy Res., 2011. 4(3): p. 687 - 689.

[181] Clare, B.A., R.S. Conroy, and K. Spelman, *The diuretic effect in human subjects of an extract of Taraxacum officinale folium over a single day.* J Altern Complement Med, 2009. 15(8): p. 929-34.

[182] Zhu, M., P.Y. Wong, and R.C. Li, *Effects of taraxacum mongolicum on the bioavailability and disposition of ciprofloxacin in rats.* J Pharm Sci, 1999. 88(6): p. 632-4.

[183] Goksu, E., et al., *First report of hypoglycemia secondary to dandelion (Taraxacum officinale) ingestion.* Am J Emerg Med, 2010. 28(1): p. 111 e1-2.

[184] Kalix, P., *The pharmacology of psychoactive alkaloids from ephedra and catha.* J Ethnopharmacol, 1991. 32(1-3): p. 201-8.

[185] Greenway, F.L., et al., *Effect of a dietary herbal supplement containing caffeine and ephedra on weight, metabolic rate, and body composition.* Obes Res, 2004. 12(7): p. 1152-7.

[186] Hackman, R.M., et al., *Multinutrient supplement containing ephedra and caffeine causes weight loss and improves metabolic risk factors in obese women: a randomized controlled trial.* Int J Obes (Lond), 2006. 30(10): p. 1545-56.

[187] Magkos, F. and S.A. Kavouras, *Caffeine and ephedrine: physiological, metabolic and performance-enhancing effects.* Sports Med, 2004. 34(13): p. 871-89.

[188] Williams, A.D., et al., *The effect of ephedra and caffeine on maximal strength and power in resistance-trained athletes.* J Strength Cond Res, 2008. 22(2): p. 464-70.

[189] Willis, S.L., et al., *Hypertensive retinopathy associated with use of the ephedra-free weight-loss herbal supplement Hydroxycut.* MedGenMed, 2006. 8(3): p. 82.

[190] *Ephedrine, Xanthines, Aspirin and Other Thermogenic Drugs to Assist the Dietary Management of Obesity. Proceedings of an international symposium. Geneva, 24-26 September 1992.* Int J Obes Relat Metab Disord, 1993. 17 Suppl 1: p. S1-83.

[191] Battig, K., *Acute and chronic cardiovascular and behavioural effects of caffeine, aspirin and ephedrine.* Int J Obes Relat Metab Disord, 1993. 17 Suppl 1: p. S61-4.

[192] Daly, P.A., et al., *Ephedrine, caffeine and aspirin: safety and efficacy for treatment of human obesity.* Int J Obes Relat Metab Disord, 1993. 17 Suppl 1: p. S73-8.

[193] Dulloo, A.G., *Ephedrine, xanthines and prostaglandin-inhibitors: actions and interactions in the stimulation of thermogenesis.* Int J Obes Relat Metab Disord, 1993. 17 Suppl 1: p. S35-40.

[194] Dulloo, A.G. and D.S. Miller, *Aspirin as a promoter of ephedrine-induced thermogenesis: potential use in the treatment of obesity.* Am J Clin Nutr, 1987. 45(3): p. 564-9.

[195] Dulloo, A.G. and D.S. Miller, *Ephedrine, caffeine and aspirin: "over-the-counter" drugs that interact to stimulate thermogenesis in the obese.* Nutrition, 1989. 5(1): p. 7-9.

[196] Geissler, C.A., *Effects of weight loss, ephedrine and aspirin on energy expenditure in obese women.* Int J Obes Relat Metab Disord, 1993. 17 Suppl 1: p. S45-8.

[197] Horton, T.J. and C.A. Geissler, *Aspirin potentiates the effect of ephedrine on the thermogenic response to a meal in obese but not lean women.* Int J Obes, 1991. 15(5): p. 359-66.

[198] Horton, T.J. and C.A. Geissler, *Post-prandial thermogenesis with ephedrine, caffeine and aspirin in lean, pre-disposed obese and obese women.* Int J Obes Relat Metab Disord, 1996. 20(2): p. 91-7.

[199] Krieger, D.R., et al., *Ephedrine, caffeine and aspirin promote weight loss in obese subjects.* Trans Assoc Am Physicians, 1990. 103: p. 307-12.

[200] Loose, I. and M. Winkel, *Clinical, double-blind, placebo-controlled study investigating the combination of acetylsalicylic acid and pseudoephedrine for the symptomatic treatment of nasal congestion associated with common cold.* Arzneimittelforschung, 2004. 54(9): p. 513-21.

[201] Lucker, P.W., et al., *Pharmacokinetic interaction study of a fixed combination of 500 mg acetylsalicylic acid/30 mg pseudoephedrine versus each of the single active ingredients in healthy male volunteers.* Arzneimittelforschung, 2003. 53(4): p. 260-5.

[202] Chen, C., et al., *Ischemic stroke after using over the counter products containing ephedra.* J Neurol Sci, 2004. 217(1): p. 55-60.

[203] Clark, B.M. and R.S. Schofield, *Dilated cardiomyopathy and acute liver injury associated with combined use of ephedra, gamma-hydroxybutyrate, and anabolic steroids.* Pharmacotherapy, 2005. 25(5): p. 756-61.

[204] Dhar, R., et al., *Cardiovascular toxicities of performance-enhancing substances in sports.* Mayo Clin Proc, 2005. 80(10): p. 1307-15.

[205] Figueredo, V.M., *Chemical cardiomyopathies: the negative effects of medications and non-prescribed drugs on the heart.* Am J Med, 2011. 124(6): p. 480-8.

[206] Flanagan, C.M., et al., *Coronary artery aneurysm and thrombosis following chronic ephedra use.* Int J Cardiol, 2010. 139(1): p. e11-3.

[207] Miller, S.C., *Safety concerns regarding ephedrine-type alkaloid-containing dietary supplements.* Mil Med, 2004. 169(2): p. 87-93.

[208] Peters, C.M., et al., *Is there an association between ephedra and heart failure? a case series.* J Card Fail, 2005. 11(1): p. 9-11.

[209] Shekelle, P.G., et al., *Efficacy and safety of ephedra and ephedrine for weight loss and athletic performance: a meta-analysis.* JAMA, 2003. 289(12): p. 1537-45.

[210] Thomas, J.E., et al., *STEMI in a 24-year-old man after use of a synephrine-containing dietary supplement: a case report and review of the literature.* Tex Heart Inst J, 2009. 36(6): p. 586-90.

[211] White, L.M., et al., *Pharmacokinetics and cardiovascular effects of ma-huang (Ephedra sinica) in normotensive adults.* J Clin Pharmacol, 1997. 37(2): p. 116-22.

[212] Siegrid Keline, C.R., Robert Rister, *The Complete German Commissions E Monographs: Therapeutic Guide to Herbal Medicines.* 1998, Boston, MA: Integrative Medicine Communications. 685.

[213] Kanaya, N., et al., *Propofol anesthesia enhances the pressor response to intravenous ephedrine.* Anesth Analg, 2002. 94(5): p. 1207-11, table of contents.

[214] Ueda, W., et al., *Ephedrine-induced increases in arterial blood pressure accelerate regression of epidural block.* Anesth Analg, 1995. 81(4): p. 703-5.

[215] Lee, A., W.D. Ngan Kee, and T. Gin, *Prophylactic ephedrine prevents hypotension during spinal anesthesia for Cesarean delivery but does not improve neonatal outcome: a quantitative systematic review.* Can J Anaesth, 2002. 49(6): p. 588-99.

[216] Lee, A., W.D. Ngan Kee, and T. Gin, *A dose-response meta-analysis of prophylactic intravenous ephedrine for the prevention of hypotension during spinal anesthesia for elective cesarean delivery.* Anesth Analg, 2004. 98(2): p. 483-90, table of contents.

[217] Astrup, A., et al., *The effect and safety of an ephedrine/caffeine compound compared to ephedrine, caffeine and placebo in obese subjects on an energy restricted diet. A double blind trial.* Int J Obes Relat Metab Disord, 1992. 16(4): p. 269-77.

[218] Martinet, A., K. Hostettmann, and Y. Schutz, *Thermogenic effects of commercially available plant preparations aimed at treating human obesity.* Phytomedicine, 1999. 6(4): p. 231-8.

[219] Dawson, J.K., S.M. Earnshaw, and C.S. Graham, *Dangerous monoamine oxidase inhibitor interactions are still occurring in the 1990s.* J Accid Emerg Med, 1995. 12(1): p. 49-51.

[220] Boada, S., et al., *[Hypotension refractory to ephedrine after sympathetic blockade in a patient on long-term therapy with tricyclic antidepressants].* Rev Esp Anestesiol Reanim, 1999. 46(8): p. 364-6.

[221] Astrup, A. and S. Toubro, *Thermogenic, metabolic, and cardiovascular responses to ephedrine and caffeine in man.* Int J Obes Relat Metab Disord, 1993. 17 Suppl 1: p. S41-3.

[222] Samenuk, D., et al., *Adverse cardiovascular events temporally associated with ma huang, an herbal source of ephedrine.* Mayo Clin Proc, 2002. 77(1): p. 12-6.

[223] Tormey, W.P. and A. Bruzzi, *Acute psychosis due to the interaction of legal compounds--ephedra alkaloids in 'vigueur fit' tablets, caffeine in 'red bull' and alcohol.* Med Sci Law, 2001. 41(4): p. 331-6.

[224] Theoharides, T.C., *Sudden death of a healthy college student related to ephedrine toxicity from a ma huang-containing drink.* J Clin Psychopharmacol, 1997. 17(5): p. 437-9.

[225] Zahn, K.A., R.L. Li, and R.A. Purssell, *Cardiovascular toxicity after ingestion of "herbal ecstasy".* J Emerg Med, 1999. 17(2): p. 289-91.

[226] Cairella, M. and G. Marchini, *[Evaluation of the action of glucomannan on metabolic parameters and on the sensation of satiation in overweight and obese patients]*. Clin Ter, 1995. 146(4): p. 269-74.

[227] Chen, H.L., et al., *Konjac acts as a natural laxative by increasing stool bulk and improving colonic ecology in healthy adults*. Nutrition, 2006. 22(11-12): p. 1112-9.

[228] Chen, H.L., et al., *Supplementation of konjac glucomannan into a low-fiber Chinese diet promoted bowel movement and improved colonic ecology in constipated adults: a placebo-controlled, diet-controlled trial*. J Am Coll Nutr, 2008. 27(1): p. 102-8.

[229] Chen, H.L., et al., *Konjac supplement alleviated hypercholesterolemia and hyperglycemia in type 2 diabetic subjects--a randomized double-blind trial*. J Am Coll Nutr, 2003. 22(1): p. 36-42.

[230] Sood, N., W.L. Baker, and C.I. Coleman, *Effect of glucomannan on plasma lipid and glucose concentrations, body weight, and blood pressure: systematic review and meta-analysis*. Am J Clin Nutr, 2008. 88(4): p. 1167-75.

[231] Vuksan, V., et al., *Beneficial effects of viscous dietary fiber from Konjac-mannan in subjects with the insulin resistance syndrome: results of a controlled metabolic trial*. Diabetes Care, 2000. 23(1): p. 9-14.

[232] Yoshida, M., et al., *Effect of plant sterols and glucomannan on lipids in individuals with and without type II diabetes*. Eur J Clin Nutr, 2006. 60(4): p. 529-37.

[233] Shima, K., et al., *Effect of dietary fiber, glucomannan, on absorption of sulfonylurea in man*. Horm Metab Res, 1983. 15(1): p. 1-3.

[234] Doi, K., *Effect of konjac fibre (glucomannan) on glucose and lipids*. Eur J Clin Nutr, 1995. 49 Suppl 3: p. S190-7.

[235] Doi, K., et al., *Treatment of diabetes with glucomannan (konjac mannan)*. Lancet, 1979. 1(8123): p. 987-8.

[236] Huang, C.Y., et al., *Effect of Konjac food on blood glucose level in patients with diabetes*. Biomed Environ Sci, 1990. 3(2): p. 123-31.

[237] Vuksan, V., et al., *Konjac-Mannan and American ginsing: emerging alternative therapies for type 2 diabetes mellitus*. J Am Coll Nutr, 2001. 20(5 Suppl): p. 370S-380S; discussion 381S-383S.

[238] Azezli, A.D., T. Bayraktaroglu, and Y. Orhan, *The use of konjac glucomannan to lower serum thyroid hormones in hyperthyroidism*. J Am Coll Nutr, 2007. 26(6): p. 663-8.

[239] Doi, K., et al., *Influence of dietary fiber (konjac mannan) on absorption of vitamin B12 and vitamin E*. Tohoku J Exp Med, 1983. 141 Suppl: p. 677-81.

[240] van Heerden, F.R., *Hoodia gordonii: a natural appetite suppressant*. J Ethnopharmacol, 2008. 119(3): p. 434-7.

[241] Vermaak, I., J.H. Hamman, and A.M. Viljoen, *Hoodia gordonii: an up-to-date review of a commercially important anti-obesity plant*. Planta Med, 2011. 77(11): p. 1149-60.

[242] MacLean, D.B. and L.G. Luo, *Increased ATP content/production in the hypothalamus may be a signal for energy-sensing of satiety: studies of the anorectic mechanism of a plant steroidal glycoside*. Brain Res, 2004. 1020(1-2): p. 1-11.

[243] Madgula, V.L., et al., *In vitro metabolic stability and intestinal transport of P57AS3 (P57) from Hoodia gordonii and its interaction with drug metabolizing enzymes*. Planta Med, 2008. 74(10): p. 1269-75.

[244] Jena, B.S., et al., *Chemistry and biochemistry of (-)-hydroxycitric acid from Garcinia*. J Agric Food Chem, 2002. 50(1): p. 10-22.

[245] Soni, M.G., et al., *Safety assessment of (-)-hydroxycitric acid and Super CitriMax, a novel calcium/potassium salt*. Food Chem Toxicol, 2004. 42(9): p. 1513-29.

[246] Heymsfield, S.B., et al., *Garcinia cambogia (hydroxycitric acid) as a potential antiobesity agent: a randomized controlled trial*. JAMA, 1998. 280(18): p. 1596-600.

[247] Preuss, H.G., et al., *Effects of a natural extract of (-)-hydroxycitric acid (HCA-SX) and a combination of HCA-SX plus niacin-bound chromium and Gymnema sylvestre extract on weight loss*. Diabetes Obes Metab, 2004. 6(3): p. 171-80.

[248] Mattes, R.D. and L. Bormann, *Effects of (-)-hydroxycitric acid on appetitive variables*. Physiol Behav, 2000. 71(1-2): p. 87-94.

[249] Mansi, I.A. and J. Huang, *Rhabdomyolysis in response to weight-loss herbal medicine*. Am J Med Sci, 2004. 327(6): p. 356-7.

[250] Levy, A.S. and A.W. Heaton, *Weight control practices of U.S. adults trying to lose weight*. Ann Intern Med, 1993. 119(7 Pt 2): p. 661-6.

[251] Boban, P.T., B. Nambisan, and P.R. Sudhakaran, *Hypolipidaemic effect of chemically different mucilages in rats: a comparative study*. Br J Nutr, 2006. 96(6): p. 1021-9.

[252] Pittler, M.H. and E. Ernst, *Guar gum for body weight reduction: meta-analysis of randomized trials*. Am J Med, 2001. 110(9): p. 724-30.

[253] Salas-Salvadó, J., et al., *Effect of two doses of a mixture of soluble fibres on body weight and metabolic variables in overweight or obese patients: a randomised trial*. Br J Nutr, 2008. 99(6): p. 1380-7.

[254] Blackburn, N.A., et al., *The mechanism of action of guar gum in improving glucose tolerance in man*. Clin Sci (Lond), 1984. 66(3): p. 329-36.

[255] Frati-Munari, A.C., et al., *Effect of Plantago psyllium mucilage on the glucose tolerance test*. Arch Invest Med (Mex), 1985. 16(2): p. 191-7.

[256] Jenkins, D.J. and A.L. Jenkins, *Dietary fiber and the glycemic response*. Proc Soc Exp Biol Med, 1985. 180(3): p. 422-31.

[257] Leclere, C.J., et al., *Role of viscous guar gums in lowering the glycemic response after a solid meal.* Am J Clin Nutr, 1994. 59(4): p. 914-21.

[258] McCarty, M.F., *Glucomannan minimizes the postprandial insulin surge: a potential adjuvant for hepatothermic therapy.* Med Hypotheses, 2002. 58(6): p. 487-90.

[259] Ou, S., et al., *In vitro study of possible role of dietary fiber in lowering postprandial serum glucose.* J Agric Food Chem, 2001. 49(2): p. 1026-9.

[260] Russo, A., et al., *Guar attenuates fall in postprandial blood pressure and slows gastric emptying of oral glucose in type 2 diabetes.* Dig Dis Sci, 2003. 48(7): p. 1221-9.

[261] Torsdottir, I., et al., *Dietary guar gum effects on postprandial blood glucose, insulin and hydroxyproline in humans.* J Nutr, 1989. 119(12): p. 1925-31.

[262] Ahi, S., et al., *A bulking agent may lead to adrenal insufficiency crisis: a case report.* Acta Med Iran, 2011. 49(10): p. 688-9.

[263] Chiu, A.C. and S.I. Sherman, *Effects of pharmacological fiber supplements on levothyroxine absorption.* Thyroid, 1998. 8(8): p. 667-71.

[264] Garcia, J.J., et al., *Influence of two dietary fibers in the oral bioavailability and other pharmacokinetic parameters of ethinyloestradiol.* Contraception, 2000. 62(5): p. 253-7.

[265] Gin, H., M.B. Orgerie, and J. Aubertin, *The influence of Guar gum on absorption of metformin from the gut in healthy volunteers.* Horm Metab Res, 1989. 21(2): p. 81-3.

[266] González, A., et al., *Effect of glucomannan and the dosage form on ethinylestradiol oral absorption in rabbits.* Contraception, 2004. 70(5): p. 423-7.

[267] Heaney, R.P. and C.M. Weaver, *Effect of psyllium on absorption of co-ingested calcium.* J Am Geriatr Soc, 1995. 43(3): p. 261-3.

[268] Holt, S., et al., *Effect of gel fibre on gastric emptying and absorption of glucose and paracetamol.* Lancet, 1979. 1(8117): p. 636-9.

[269] Huupponen, R., P. Seppala, and E. Iisalo, *Effect of guar gum, a fibre preparation, on digoxin and penicillin absorption in man.* Eur J Clin Pharmacol, 1984. 26(2): p. 279-81.

[270] Perlman, B.B., *Interaction between lithium salts and ispaghula husk.* Lancet, 1990. 335(8686): p. 416.

[271] Reissell, P. and V. Manninen, *Effect of administration of activated charcoal and fibre on absorption, excretion and steady state blood levels of digoxin and digitoxin. Evidence for intestinal secretion of the glycosides.* Acta Med Scand Suppl, 1982. 668: p. 88-90.

[272] Toutoungi, M., et al., *[Probable interaction of psyllium and lithium].* Therapie, 1990. 45(4): p. 358-60.

[273] Roerig, J.L., et al., *Laxative abuse: epidemiology, diagnosis and management.* Drugs, 2010. 70(12): p. 1487-503.

[274]   Tozzi, F., et al., *Features associated with laxative abuse in individuals with eating disorders.* Psychosom Med, 2006. 68(3): p. 470-7.

[275]   Amato, A., et al., *Half doses of PEG-ES and senna vs. high-dose senna for bowel cleansing before colonoscopy: a randomized, investigator-blinded trial.* Am J Gastroenterol, 2010. 105(3): p. 675-81.

[276]   Branco, A., et al., *Anthraquinones from the bark of Senna macranthera.* An Acad Bras Cienc, 2011. 83(4): p. 1159-64.

[277]   Brouwers, J.R., et al., *A controlled trial of senna preparations and other laxatives used for bowel cleansing prior to radiological examination.* Pharmacology, 1980. 20 Suppl 1: p. 58-64.

[278]   El-Gengaihi, S., A.H. Agiza, and A. El-Hamidi, *Distribution of anthraquinones in Senna plants.* Planta Med, 1975. 27(4): p. 349-53.

[279]   Franz, G., *The senna drug and its chemistry.* Pharmacology, 1993. 47 Suppl 1: p. 2-6.

[280]   Godding, E.W., *Laxatives and the special role of senna.* Pharmacology, 1988. 36 Suppl 1: p. 230-6.

[281]   Gould, S.R. and C.B. Williams, *Castor oil or senna preparation before colonoscopy for inactive chronic ulcerative colitis.* Gastrointest Endosc, 1982. 28(1): p. 6-8.

[282]   Hietala, P., et al., *Laxative potency and acute toxicity of some anthraquinone derivatives, senna extracts and fractions of senna extracts.* Pharmacol Toxicol, 1987. 61(2): p. 153-6.

[283]   Izard, M.W. and F.S. Ellison, *Treatment of drug-induced constipation with a purified senna derivative.* Conn Med, 1962. 26: p. 589-92.

[284]   Khafagy, S.M., et al., *Estimation of sennosides A, B, C and D in Senna leaves, pods and formulations.* Planta Med, 1972. 21(3): p. 304-9.

[285]   Kinnunen, O., et al., *Safety and efficacy of a bulk laxative containing senna versus lactulose in the treatment of chronic constipation in geriatric patients.* Pharmacology, 1993. 47 Suppl 1: p. 253-5.

[286]   Kositchaiwat, S., et al., *Comparative study of two bowel preparation regimens for colonoscopy: senna tablets vs sodium phosphate solution.* World J Gastroenterol, 2006. 12(34): p. 5536-9.

[287]   Krumbiegel, G. and H.U. Schulz, *Rhein and aloe-emodin kinetics from senna laxatives in man.* Pharmacology, 1993. 47 Suppl 1: p. 120-4.

[288]   Lamphier, T.A. and R. Ehrlich, *Evaluation of standardized senna in the management of constipation.* Am J Gastroenterol, 1957. 27(4): p. 381-4.

[289]   Lemli, J., *The Estimation of Anthracene Derivatives in Senna and Rhubarb.* J Pharm Pharmacol, 1965. 17: p. 227-32

[290] Marlett, J.A., et al., *Comparative laxation of psyllium with and without senna in an ambulatory constipated population.* Am J Gastroenterol, 1987. 82(4): p. 333-7.

[291] Mc, N.G., *The effect of a standardised senna preparation on the human bowel.* J Pharm Pharmacol, 1958. 10(8): p. 499-506.

[292] Monias, M.B., *Standardized senna concentrate in postpartum bowel rehabilitation.* Md State Med J, 1966. 15(2): p. 32-3.

[293] Putalun, W., et al., *Sennosides A and B production by hairy roots of Senna alata (L.) Roxb.* Z Naturforsch C, 2006. 61(5-6): p. 367-71.

[294] Radaelli, F., et al., *High-dose senna compared with conventional PEG-ES lavage as bowel preparation for elective colonoscopy: a prospective, randomized, investigator-blinded trial.* Am J Gastroenterol, 2005. 100(12): p. 2674-80.

[295] Valverde, A., et al., *Senna vs polyethylene glycol for mechanical preparation the evening before elective colonic or rectal resection: a multicenter controlled trial. French Association for Surgical Research.* Arch Surg, 1999. 134(5): p. 514-9.

[296] Ishii, Y., H. Tanizawa, and Y. Takino, *[Studies of aloe. II. Mechanism of cathartic effect].* Yakugaku Zasshi, 1988. 108(9): p. 904-10.

[297] Ishii, Y., H. Tanizawa, and Y. Takino, *Studies of aloe. III. Mechanism of cathartic effect. (2).* Chem Pharm Bull (Tokyo), 1990. 38(1): p. 197-200.

[298] Ishii, Y., H. Tanizawa, and Y. Takino, *Studies of aloe. V. Mechanism of cathartic effect. (4).* Biol Pharm Bull, 1994. 17(5): p. 651-3.

[299] Ishii, Y., H. Tanizawa, and Y. Takino, *Studies of aloe. IV. Mechanism of cathartic effect. (3).* Biol Pharm Bull, 1994. 17(4): p. 495-7.

[300] *Status of certain additional over-the-counter drug category II and III active ingredients. Final rule.* Fed Regist, 2002. 67(90): p. 31125-7.

[301] *Final report on the safety assessment of AloeAndongensis Extract, Aloe Andongensis Leaf Juice,aloe Arborescens Leaf Extract, Aloe Arborescens Leaf Juice, Aloe Arborescens Leaf Protoplasts, Aloe Barbadensis Flower Extract, Aloe Barbadensis Leaf, Aloe Barbadensis Leaf Extract, Aloe Barbadensis Leaf Juice,aloe Barbadensis Leaf Polysaccharides, Aloe Barbadensis Leaf Water, Aloe Ferox Leaf Extract, Aloe Ferox Leaf Juice, and Aloe Ferox Leaf Juice Extract.* Int J Toxicol, 2007. 26 Suppl 2: p. 1-50.

[302] Quercia, V., *[Separation of anthraquinone compounds of Cascara sagrada by means of high-pressure liquid chromatography].* Boll Chim Farm, 1976. 115(4): p. 309-16.

[303] Fugh-Berman, A., *Herb-drug interactions.* Lancet, 2000. 355(9198): p. 134-8.

[304] Laitinen, L., et al., *Anthranoid laxatives influence the absorption of poorly permeable drugs in human intestinal cell culture model (Caco-2).* Eur J Pharm Biopharm, 2007. 66(1): p. 135-45.

[305] Huseini, H.F., et al., *Anti-hyperglycemic and anti-hypercholesterolemic effects of Aloe vera leaf gel in hyperlipidemic type 2 diabetic patients: a randomized double-blind placebo-controlled clinical trial.* Planta Med, 2012. 78(4): p. 311-6.

[306] Musabayane, C.T., P.T. Bwititi, and J.A. Ojewole, *Effects of oral administration of some herbal extracts on food consumption and blood glucose levels in normal and streptozotocin-treated diabetic rats.* Methods Find Exp Clin Pharmacol, 2006. 28(4): p. 223-8.

[307] Rajasekaran, S., et al., *Hypoglycemic effect of Aloe vera gel on streptozotocin-induced diabetes in experimental rats.* J Med Food, 2004. 7(1): p. 61-6.

[308] Lewis, S.J., et al., *Lower serum oestrogen concentrations associated with faster intestinal transit.* Br J Cancer, 1997. 76(3): p. 395-400.

[309] Lewis, S.J., R.E. Oakey, and K.W. Heaton, *Intestinal absorption of oestrogen: the effect of altering transit-time.* Eur J Gastroenterol Hepatol, 1998. 10(1): p. 33-9.

[310] Kittisupamongkol, W., V. Nilaratanakul, and W. Kulwichit, *Near-fatal bleeding, senna, and the opposite of lettuce.* Lancet, 2008. 371(9614): p. 784.

[311] Lee, A., et al., *Possible interaction between sevoflurane and Aloe vera.* Ann Pharmacother, 2004. 38(10): p. 1651-4.

[312] Kitagawa, I., et al., *Chemical studies of Chinese licorice-roots. I. Elucidation of five new flavonoid constituents from the roots of Glycyrrhiza glabra L. collected in Xinjiang.* Chem Pharm Bull (Tokyo), 1994. 42(5): p. 1056-62.

[313] Mitscher, L.A., et al., *Antimicrobial agents from higher plants. Antimicrobial isoflavanoids and related substances from Glycyrrhiza glabra L. var. typica.* J Nat Prod, 1980. 43(2): p. 259-69.

[314] Grossman, E. and F.H. Messerli, *Drug-induced hypertension: an unappreciated cause of secondary hypertension.* Am J Med, 2012. 125(1): p. 14-22.

[315] Kaleel, M., et al., *Licorice: a patient's shocking presentation.* Del Med J, 2011. 83(7): p. 211-5.

[316] Knobel, U., et al., *Gitelman's syndrome with persistent hypokalemia - don't forget licorice, alcohol, lemon juice, iced tea and salt depletion: a case report.* J Med Case Rep, 2011. 5: p. 312.

[317] Brayley, J. and J. Jones, *Life-threatening hypokalemia associated with excessive licorice ingestion.* Am J Psychiatry, 1994. 151(4): p. 617-8.

[318] Famularo, G., F.M. Corsi, and M. Giacanelli, *Iatrogenic worsening of hypokalemia and neuromuscular paralysis associated with the use of glucose solutions for potassium replacement in a young woman with licorice intoxication and furosemide abuse.* Acad Emerg Med, 1999. 6(9): p. 960-4.

[319] Joseph, R. and J. Kelemen, *Paraparesis due to licorice-induced hypokalemia*. N Y State J Med, 1984. 84(6): p. 296.

[320] Mumoli, N. and M. Cei, *Licorice-induced hypokalemia*. Int J Cardiol, 2008. 124(3): p. e42-4.

[321] Pelner, L., *Licorice induced hypokalemia*. N Y State J Med, 1984. 84(12): p. 591.

[322] Yasue, H., et al., *Severe hypokalemia, rhabdomyolysis, muscle paralysis, and respiratory impairment in a hypertensive patient taking herbal medicines containing licorice*. Intern Med, 2007. 46(9): p. 575-8.

[323] Yoshida, S. and Y. Takayama, *Licorice-induced hypokalemia as a treatable cause of dropped head syndrome*. Clin Neurol Neurosurg, 2003. 105(4): p. 286-7.

[324] Armanini, D., et al., *Further studies on the mechanism of the mineralocorticoid action of licorice in humans*. J Endocrinol Invest, 1996. 19(9): p. 624-9.

[325] Stoving, R.K., et al., *Is glycyrrhizin sensitivity increased in anorexia nervosa and should licorice be avoided? Case report and review of the literature*. Nutrition, 2011. 27(7-8): p. 855-8.

[326] Wynn, G.J., G.K. Davis, and B. Maher, *Trick or treat? Pseudohyperaldosteronism due to episodic licorice consumption*. J Clin Hypertens (Greenwich), 2011. 13(3): p. E3-4.

[327] Armanini, D., M. Wehling, and P.C. Weber, *Mineralocorticoid effector mechanism of liquorice derivatives in human mononuclear leukocytes*. J Endocrinol Invest, 1989. 12(5): p. 303-6.

[328] Berlango Jimenez, A., et al., *[Acute rhabdomyolysis and tetraparesis secondary to hypokalemia due to ingested licorice]*. An Med Interna, 1995. 12(1): p. 33-5.

[329] Brasseur, A. and J. Ducobu, *[Severe hypokalemia after holidays return]*. Rev Med Brux, 2008. 29(5): p. 490-3.

[330] Carretta, R. and S. Muiesan, *[Pseudohyperaldosteronism caused by the abuse of licorice]*. G Clin Med, 1986. 67(1): p. 55-6.

[331] Cataldo, F., et al., *[Pseudohyperaldosteronism secondary to licorice poisoning associated with hemorrhagic gastritis]*. Pediatr Med Chir, 1997. 19(3): p. 219-21.

[332] Ferrari, P. and B.N. Trost, *[A case from practice (169). Liquorice-induced pseudohyperaldosteronism in a previously alcoholic woman caused by the drinking of an alcohol-free Pastis substitute beverage]*. Schweiz Rundsch Med Prax, 1990. 79(12): p. 377-8.

[333] Ghielmini, C. and A. Hoffmann, *[A case from practice (171). Pseudohyperaldosteronism in licorice abuse]*. Schweiz Rundsch Med Prax, 1990. 79(15): p. 472-3.

[334] Gomez Fernandez, P., et al., *[Primary pseudohyperaldosteronism produced by chronic licorice consumption]*. Rev Clin Esp, 1981. 163(4): p. 277-8.

[335] Holmes, A.M., et al., *Pseudohyperaldosteronism induced by habitual ingestion of liquorice.* Postgrad Med J, 1970. 46(540): p. 625-9.

[336] Russo, S., et al., *Low doses of liquorice can induce hypertension encephalopathy.* Am J Nephrol, 2000. 20(2): p. 145-8.

[337] Scali, M., et al., *Pseudohyperaldosteronism from liquorice-containing laxatives.* J Endocrinol Invest, 1990. 13(10): p. 847-8.

[338] Sontia, B., et al., *Pseudohyperaldosteronism, liquorice, and hypertension.* J Clin Hypertens (Greenwich), 2008. 10(2): p. 153-7.

[339] Kimura, I., et al., *The antihyperglycaemic blend effect of traditional chinese medicine byak-ko-ka-ninjin-to on alloxan and diabetic KK-CA(y) mice.* Phytother Res, 1999. 13(6): p. 484-8.

[340] Kuroda, M., et al., *Phenolics with PPAR-gamma ligand-binding activity obtained from licorice (Glycyrrhiza uralensis roots) and ameliorative effects of glycyrin on genetically diabetic KK-A(y) mice.* Bioorg Med Chem Lett, 2003. 13(24): p. 4267-72.

[341] Bardhan, K.D., et al., *Clinical trial of deglycyrrhizinised liquorice in gastric ulcer.* Gut, 1978. 19(9): p. 779-82.

[342] Engqvist, A., et al., *Double-blind trial of deglycyrrhizinated liquorice in gastric ulcer.* Gut, 1973. 14(9): p. 711-5.

[343] MacKenzie, M.A., et al., *The influence of glycyrrhetinic acid on plasma cortisol and cortisone in healthy young volunteers.* J Clin Endocrinol Metab, 1990. 70(6): p. 1637-43.

[344] Armanini, D., et al., *Effect of licorice on the reduction of body fat mass in healthy subjects.* J Endocrinol Invest, 2003. 26(7): p. 646-50.

[345] Armanini, D., et al., *Glycyrrhetinic acid, the active principle of licorice, can reduce the thickness of subcutaneous thigh fat through topical application.* Steroids, 2005. 70(8): p. 538-42.

[346] Hukkanen, J., O. Ukkola, and M.J. Savolainen, *Effects of low-dose liquorice alone or in combination with hydrochlorothiazide on the plasma potassium in healthy volunteers.* Blood Press, 2009. 18(4): p. 192-5.

[347] Kawakami, F., Y. Shimoyama, and K. Ohtsuki, *Characterization of complement C3 as a glycyrrhizin (GL)-binding protein and the phosphorylation of C3alpha by CK-2, which is potently inhibited by GL and glycyrrhetinic acid in vitro.* J Biochem, 2003. 133(2): p. 231-7.

[348] Kroes, B.H., et al., *Inhibition of human complement by beta-glycyrrhetinic acid.* Immunology, 1997. 90(1): p. 115-20.

[349] Akamatsu, H., et al., *Mechanism of anti-inflammatory action of glycyrrhizin: effect on neutrophil functions including reactive oxygen species generation.* Planta Med, 1991. 57(2): p. 119-21.

[350] Rackova, L., et al., *Mechanism of anti-inflammatory action of liquorice extract and glycyrrhizin.* Nat Prod Res, 2007. 21(14): p. 1234-41.

[351] Armanini, D., et al., *Licorice consumption and serum testosterone in healthy man.* Exp Clin Endocrinol Diabetes, 2003. 111(6): p. 341-3.

[352] Armanini, D., G. Bonanni, and M. Palermo, *Reduction of serum testosterone in men by licorice.* N Engl J Med, 1999. 341(15): p. 1158.

[353] Armanini, D., et al., *History of the endocrine effects of licorice.* Exp Clin Endocrinol Diabetes, 2002. 110(6): p. 257-61.

[354] Armanini, D., et al., *Licorice reduces serum testosterone in healthy women.* Steroids, 2004. 69(11-12): p. 763-6.

[355] Kraus, S.D., *Glycyrrhetinic acid--a triterpene with antioestrogenic and anti-inflammatory activity.* J Pharm Pharmacol, 1960. 12: p. 300-6.

[356] Kraus, S.D. and A. Kaminskis, *The anti-estrogenic action of beta-glycyrrhetinic acid.* Exp Med Surg, 1969. 27(4): p. 411-20.

[357] Yamada, K., et al., *Effectiveness of shakuyaku-kanzo-to in neuroleptic-induced hyperprolactinemia: a preliminary report.* Psychiatry Clin Neurosci, 1996. 50(6): p. 341-2.

[358] Yamada, K., et al., *Effectiveness of herbal medicine (shakuyaku-kanzo-to) for neuroleptic-induced hyperprolactinemia.* J Clin Psychopharmacol, 1997. 17(3): p. 234-5.

[359] Imai, T., et al., *In vitro and in vivo evaluation of the enhancing activity of glycyrrhizin on the intestinal absorption of drugs.* Pharm Res, 1999. 16(1): p. 80-6.

[360] Ofir, R., et al., *Inhibition of serotonin re-uptake by licorice constituents.* J Mol Neurosci, 2003. 20(2): p. 135-40.

[361] Dhingra, D. and A. Sharma, *Antidepressant-like activity of Glycyrrhiza glabra L. in mouse models of immobility tests.* Prog Neuropsychopharmacol Biol Psychiatry, 2006. 30(3): p. 449-54.

[362] Tadros, M.G., et al., *Involvement of serotoninergic 5-HT1A/2A, alpha-adrenergic and dopaminergic D1 receptors in St. John's wort-induced prepulse inhibition deficit: a possible role of hyperforin.* Behav Brain Res, 2009. 199(2): p. 334-9.

[363] Shelton, R.C., et al., *Effectiveness of St John's wort in major depression: a randomized controlled trial.* JAMA, 2001. 285(15): p. 1978-86.

[364] Kasper, S., et al., *Better tolerability of St. John's wort extract WS 5570 compared to treatment with SSRIs: a reanalysis of data from controlled clinical trials in acute major depression.* Int Clin Psychopharmacol, 2010. 25(4): p. 204-13.

[365] Niederhofer, H., *St. John's wort may improve some symptoms of attention-deficit hyperactivity disorder.* Nat Prod Res, 2010. 24(3): p. 203-5.

[366] Canning, S., et al., *The efficacy of Hypericum perforatum (St John's wort) for the treatment of premenstrual syndrome: a randomized, double-blind, placebo-controlled trial.* CNS Drugs, 2010. 24(3): p. 207-25.

[367] Balk, J., *The effects of St. John's wort on hot flashes.* Menopause, 2010. 17(5): p. 1089-90.

[368] Chatterjee, S.S., A. Biber, and C. Weibezahn, *Stimulation of glutamate, aspartate and gamma-aminobutyric acid release from synaptosomes by hyperforin.* Pharmacopsychiatry, 2001. 34 Suppl 1: p. S11-9.

[369] Gobbi, M., et al., *In vitro binding studies with two hypericum perforatum extracts--hyperforin, hypericin and biapigenin--on 5-HT6, 5-HT7, GABA(A)/benzodiazepine, sigma, NPY-Y1/Y2 receptors and dopamine transporters.* Pharmacopsychiatry, 2001. 34 Suppl 1: p. S45-8.

[370] Muller, W.E., A. Singer, and M. Wonnemann, *Hyperforin--antidepressant activity by a novel mechanism of action.* Pharmacopsychiatry, 2001. 34 Suppl 1: p. S98-102.

[371] Muller, W.E., et al., *Hyperforin represents the neurotransmitter reuptake inhibiting constituent of hypericum extract.* Pharmacopsychiatry, 1998. 31 Suppl 1: p. 16-21.

[372] Roz, N., et al., *Inhibition of vesicular uptake of monoamines by hyperforin.* Life Sci, 2002. 71(19): p. 2227-37.

[373] Singer, A., M. Wonnemann, and W.E. Muller, *Hyperforin, a major antidepressant constituent of St. John's Wort, inhibits serotonin uptake by elevating free intracellular Na+1.* J Pharmacol Exp Ther, 1999. 290(3): p. 1363-8.

[374] Wentworth, J.M., et al., *St John's wort, a herbal antidepressant, activates the steroid X receptor.* J Endocrinol, 2000. 166(3): p. R11-6.

[375] Weber, C.C., et al., *Modulation of P-glycoprotein function by St John's wort extract and its major constituents.* Pharmacopsychiatry, 2004. 37(6): p. 292-8.

[376] Wang, Z., et al., *The effects of St John's wort (Hypericum perforatum) on human cytochrome P450 activity.* Clin Pharmacol Ther, 2001. 70(4): p. 317-26.

[377] Wang, L.S., et al., *St John's wort induces both cytochrome P450 3A4-catalyzed sulfoxidation and 2C19-dependent hydroxylation of omeprazole.* Clin Pharmacol Ther, 2004. 75(3): p. 191-7.

[378] Wang, E.J., M. Barecki-Roach, and W.W. Johnson, *Quantitative characterization of direct P-glycoprotein inhibition by St John's wort constituents hypericin and hyperforin.* J Pharm Pharmacol, 2004. 56(1): p. 123-8.

[379] Ott, M., et al., *St. John's Wort constituents modulate P-glycoprotein transport activity at the blood-brain barrier.* Pharm Res, 2010. 27(5): p. 811-22.

[380] Obach, R.S., *Inhibition of human cytochrome P450 enzymes by constituents of St. John's Wort, an herbal preparation used in the treatment of depression.* J Pharmacol Exp Ther, 2000. 294(1): p. 88-95.

[381] Noldner, M. and S. Chatterjee, *Effects of two different extracts of St. John's wort and some of their constituents on cytochrome P450 activities in rat liver microsomes.* Pharmacopsychiatry, 2001. 34 Suppl 1: p. S108-10.

[382] Markowitz, J.S., et al., *Effect of St John's wort on drug metabolism by induction of cytochrome P450 3A4 enzyme.* JAMA, 2003. 290(11): p. 1500-4.

[383] Markowitz, J.S., et al., *Effect of St. John's wort (Hypericum perforatum) on cytochrome P-450 2D6 and 3A4 activity in healthy volunteers.* Life Sci, 2000. 66(9): p. PL133-9.

[384] Karyekar, C.S., N.D. Eddington, and T.C. Dowling, *Effect of St. John's Wort extract on intestinal expression of cytochrome P4501A2: studies in LS180 cells.* J Postgrad Med, 2002. 48(2): p. 97-100.

[385] Dresser, G.K., et al., *Coordinate induction of both cytochrome P4503A and MDR1 by St John's wort in healthy subjects.* Clin Pharmacol Ther, 2003. 73(1): p. 41-50.

[386] Dostalek, M., et al., *Effect of St John's wort (Hypericum perforatum) on cytochrome P-450 activity in perfused rat liver.* Life Sci, 2005. 78(3): p. 239-44.

[387] Chaudhary, A. and K.L. Willett, *Inhibition of human cytochrome CYP 1 enzymes by flavonoids of St. John's wort.* Toxicology, 2006. 217(2-3): p. 194-205.

[388] Durr, D., et al., *St John's Wort induces intestinal P-glycoprotein/MDR1 and intestinal and hepatic CYP3A4.* Clin Pharmacol Ther, 2000. 68(6): p. 598-604.

[389] Zhou, S.F. and X. Lai, *An update on clinical drug interactions with the herbal antidepressant St. John's wort.* Curr Drug Metab, 2008. 9(5): p. 394-409.

[390] Jiang, X., et al., *Effect of St John's wort and ginseng on the pharmacokinetics and pharmacodynamics of warfarin in healthy subjects.* Br J Clin Pharmacol, 2004. 57(5): p. 592-9.

[391] Lau, W.C., et al., *The effect of St John's Wort on the pharmacodynamic response of clopidogrel in hyporesponsive volunteers and patients: increased platelet inhibition by enhancement of CYP3A4 metabolic activity.* J Cardiovasc Pharmacol, 2011. 57(1): p. 86-93.

[392] Groning, R., J. Breitkreutz, and R.S. Muller, *Physico-chemical interactions between extracts of Hypericum perforatum L. and drugs.* Eur J Pharm Biopharm, 2003. 56(2): p. 231-6.

[393] Nebel, A., et al., *Potential metabolic interaction between St. John's wort and theophylline.* Ann Pharmacother, 1999. 33(4): p. 502.

[394] Morimoto, T., et al., *Effect of St. John's wort on the pharmacokinetics of theophylline in healthy volunteers.* J Clin Pharmacol, 2004. 44(1): p. 95-101.

[395]	*Toxicity. St. John's wort--interactions with indinavir and other drugs.* TreatmentUpdate, 2000. 12(2): p. 9-11.

[396]	Ho, Y.F., et al., *Effects of St. John's wort extract on indinavir pharmacokinetics in rats: differentiation of intestinal and hepatic impacts.* Life Sci, 2009. 85(7-8): p. 296-302.

[397]	Miller, J.L., *Interaction between indinavir and St. John's wort reported.* Am J Health Syst Pharm, 2000. 57(7): p. 625-6.

[398]	Piscitelli, S.C., et al., *Indinavir concentrations and St John's wort.* Lancet, 2000. 355(9203): p. 547-8.

[399]	Andren, L., A. Andreasson, and R. Eggertsen, *Interaction between a commercially available St. John's wort product (Movina) and atorvastatin in patients with hypercholesterolemia.* Eur J Clin Pharmacol, 2007. 63(10): p. 913-6.

[400]	Eggertsen, R., A. Andreasson, and L. Andren, *Effects of treatment with a commercially available St John's Wort product (Movina) on cholesterol levels in patients with hypercholesterolemia treated with simvastatin.* Scand J Prim Health Care, 2007. 25(3): p. 154-9.

[401]	Andelic, S., *[Bigeminy--the result of interaction between digoxin and St. John's wort].* Vojnosanit Pregl, 2003. 60(3): p. 361-4.

[402]	Birdsall, T.C., *St. John's wort and irinotecan-induced diarrhea.* Toxicol Appl Pharmacol, 2007. 220(1): p. 108; author reply 109-10.

[403]	Dasgupta, A., *Herbal supplements and therapeutic drug monitoring: focus on digoxin immunoassays and interactions with St. John's wort.* Ther Drug Monit, 2008. 30(2): p. 212-7.

[404]	Frye, R.F., et al., *Effect of St John's wort on imatinib mesylate pharmacokinetics.* Clin Pharmacol Ther, 2004. 76(4): p. 323-9.

[405]	Hu, Z., et al., *St. John's Wort modulates the toxicities and pharmacokinetics of CPT-11 (irinotecan) in rats.* Pharm Res, 2005. 22(6): p. 902-14.

[406]	Hu, Z.P., et al., *A mechanistic study on altered pharmacokinetics of irinotecan by St. John's wort.* Curr Drug Metab, 2007. 8(2): p. 157-71.

[407]	Mathijssen, R.H., et al., *Effects of St. John's wort on irinotecan metabolism.* J Natl Cancer Inst, 2002. 94(16): p. 1247-9.

[408]	Mueller, S.C., et al., *Effect of St John's wort dose and preparations on the pharmacokinetics of digoxin.* Clin Pharmacol Ther, 2004. 75(6): p. 546-57.

[409]	Rengelshausen, J., et al., *Opposite effects of short-term and long-term St John's wort intake on voriconazole pharmacokinetics.* Clin Pharmacol Ther, 2005. 78(1): p. 25-33.

[410]	Tannergren, C., et al., *St John's wort decreases the bioavailability of R- and S-verapamil through induction of the first-pass metabolism.* Clin Pharmacol Ther, 2004. 75(4): p. 298-309.

[411] Xie, H.G., *Additional discussions regarding the altered metabolism and transport of omeprazole after long-term use of St John's wort.* Clin Pharmacol Ther, 2005. 78(4): p. 440-1.

[412] Eich-Hochli, D., et al., *Methadone maintenance treatment and St. John's Wort - a case report.* Pharmacopsychiatry, 2003. 36(1): p. 35-7.

[413] Sarino, L.V., et al., *Drug interaction between oral contraceptives and St. John's Wort: appropriateness of advice received from community pharmacists and health food store clerks.* J Am Pharm Assoc (2003), 2007. 47(1): p. 42-7.

[414] Schwarz, U.I., B. Buschel, and W. Kirch, *Unwanted pregnancy on self-medication with St John's wort despite hormonal contraception.* Br J Clin Pharmacol, 2003. 55(1): p. 112-3.

[415] Will-Shahab, L., et al., *St John's wort extract (Ze 117) does not alter the pharmacokinetics of a low-dose oral contraceptive.* Eur J Clin Pharmacol, 2009. 65(3): p. 287-94.

[416] Hall, S.D., et al., *The interaction between St John's wort and an oral contraceptive.* Clin Pharmacol Ther, 2003. 74(6): p. 525-35.

[417] Pfrunder, A., et al., *Interaction of St John's wort with low-dose oral contraceptive therapy: a randomized controlled trial.* Br J Clin Pharmacol, 2003. 56(6): p. 683-90.

[418] Bhavnani, B.R., *Pharmacokinetics and pharmacodynamics of conjugated equine estrogens: chemistry and metabolism.* Proc Soc Exp Biol Med, 1998. 217(1): p. 6-16.

[419] Tsuchiya, Y., M. Nakajima, and T. Yokoi, *Cytochrome P450-mediated metabolism of estrogens and its regulation in human.* Cancer Lett, 2005. 227(2): p. 115-24.

[420] Ranney, R.E., *Comparative Metabolism of 17alpha-Ethynyl Steroids Used in Oral-Contraceptives.* Journal of Toxicology and Environmental Health, 1977. 3(1-2): p. 139-166.

[421] Alscher, D.M. and U. Klotz, *Drug interaction of herbal tea containing St. John's wort with cyclosporine.* Transpl Int, 2003. 16(7): p. 543-4.

[422] Barone, G.W., et al., *Drug interaction between St. John's wort and cyclosporine.* Ann Pharmacother, 2000. 34(9): p. 1013-6.

[423] Bauer, S., et al., *Alterations in cyclosporin A pharmacokinetics and metabolism during treatment with St John's wort in renal transplant patients.* Br J Clin Pharmacol, 2003. 55(2): p. 203-11.

[424] Breidenbach, T., et al., *Profound drop of cyclosporin A whole blood trough levels caused by St. John's wort (Hypericum perforatum).* Transplantation, 2000. 69(10): p. 2229-30.

[425] Karliova, M., et al., *Interaction of Hypericum perforatum (St. John's wort) with cyclosporin A metabolism in a patient after liver transplantation.* J Hepatol, 2000. 33(5): p. 853-5.

[426] Mai, I., et al., *Hyperforin content determines the magnitude of the St John's wort-cyclosporine drug interaction.* Clin Pharmacol Ther, 2004. 76(4): p. 330-40.

[427] Mai, I., et al., *Hazardous pharmacokinetic interaction of Saint John's wort (Hypericum perforatum) with the immunosuppressant cyclosporin.* Int J Clin Pharmacol Ther, 2000. 38(10): p. 500-2.

[428] Moschella, C. and B.L. Jaber, *Interaction between cyclosporine and Hypericum perforatum (St. John's wort) after organ transplantation.* Am J Kidney Dis, 2001. 38(5): p. 1105-7.

[429] Bolley, R., et al., *Tacrolimus-induced nephrotoxicity unmasked by induction of the CYP3A4 system with St John's wort.* Transplantation, 2002. 73(6): p. 1009.

[430] Hebert, M.F., et al., *Effects of St. John's wort (Hypericum perforatum) on tacrolimus pharmacokinetics in healthy volunteers.* J Clin Pharmacol, 2004. 44(1): p. 89-94.

[431] Mai, I., et al., *Impact of St John's wort treatment on the pharmacokinetics of tacrolimus and mycophenolic acid in renal transplant patients.* Nephrol Dial Transplant, 2003. 18(4): p. 819-22.

[432] Buchholzer, M.L., et al., *Dual modulation of striatal acetylcholine release by hyperforin, a constituent of St. John's wort.* J Pharmacol Exp Ther, 2002. 301(2): p. 714-9.

[433] Chatterjee, S.S., et al., *Hyperforin as a possible antidepressant component of hypericum extracts.* Life Sci, 1998. 63(6): p. 499-510.

[434] Gordon, J.B., *SSRIs and St.John's Wort: possible toxicity?* Am Fam Physician, 1998. 57(5): p. 950,953.

[435] Hirano, K., et al., *Effects of oral administration of extracts of Hypericum perforatum (St John's wort) on brain serotonin transporter, serotonin uptake and behaviour in mice.* J Pharm Pharmacol, 2004. 56(12): p. 1589-95.

[436] Kiewert, C., et al., *Stimulation of hippocampal acetylcholine release by hyperforin, a constituent of St. John's Wort.* Neurosci Lett, 2004. 364(3): p. 195-8.

[437] Kobak, K.A., et al., *St. John's wort in generalized anxiety disorder: three more case reports.* J Clin Psychopharmacol, 2003. 23(5): p. 531-2.

[438] Niederhofer, H., *St. John's wort may diminish methylphenidate's efficacy in treating patients suffering from attention deficit hyperactivity disorder.* Med Hypotheses, 2007. 68(5): p. 1189.

[439] Saraga, M. and D.F. Zullino, *[St. John's Wort, corticosteroids, cocaine, alcohol... and a first manic episode].* Praxis (Bern 1994), 2005. 94(23): p. 987-9.

[440] Schneck, C., *St. John's wort and hypomania.* J Clin Psychiatry, 1998. 59(12): p. 689.

[441] Turkanovic, J., S.N. Ngo, and R.W. Milne, *Effect of St John's wort on the disposition of fexofenadine in the isolated perfused rat liver.* J Pharm Pharmacol, 2009. 61(8): p. 1037-42.

[442] Uebelhack, R. and L. Franke, *In vitro effects of St. John's wort extract and hyperforin on 5 HT uptake and efflux in human blood platelets.* Pharmacopsychiatry, 2001. 34 Suppl 1: p. S146-7.

[443] Van Strater, A.C. and J.P. Bogers, *Interaction of St John's wort (Hypericum perforatum) with clozapine.* Int Clin Psychopharmacol, 2012. 27(2): p. 121-4.

[444] Wang, Z., et al., *Effect of St John's wort on the pharmacokinetics of fexofenadine.* Clin Pharmacol Ther, 2002. 71(6): p. 414-20.

[445] Wonnemann, M., A. Singer, and W.E. Muller, *Inhibition of synaptosomal uptake of 3H-L-glutamate and 3H-GABA by hyperforin, a major constituent of St. John's Wort: the role of amiloride sensitive sodium conductive pathways.* Neuropsychopharmacology, 2000. 23(2): p. 188-97.

[446] Johne, A., et al., *Decreased plasma levels of amitriptyline and its metabolites on comedication with an extract from St. John's wort (Hypericum perforatum).* J Clin Psychopharmacol, 2002. 22(1): p. 46-54.

[447] Barbenel, D.M., et al., *Mania in a patient receiving testosterone replacement postorchidectomy taking St John's wort and sertraline.* J Psychopharmacol, 2000. 14(1): p. 84-6.

[448] *Final report on the safety assessment of Hypericum perforatum extract and Hypericum perforatum oil.* Int J Toxicol, 2001. 20 Suppl 2: p. 31-9.

[449] Beattie, P.E., et al., *Can St John's wort (hypericin) ingestion enhance the erythemal response during high-dose ultraviolet A1 therapy?* Br J Dermatol, 2005. 153(6): p. 1187-91.

[450] Traynor, N.J., et al., *Photogenotoxicity of hypericin in HaCaT keratinocytes: implications for St. John's Wort supplements and high dose UVA-1 therapy.* Toxicol Lett, 2005. 158(3): p. 220-4.

[451] Cotterill, J.A., *Severe phototoxic reaction to laser treatment in a patient taking St John's Wort.* J Cosmet Laser Ther, 2001. 3(3): p. 159-60.

[452] Putnik, K., et al., *Enhanced radiation sensitivity and radiation recall dermatitis (RRD) after hypericin therapy -- case report and review of literature.* Radiat Oncol, 2006. 1: p. 32.

[453] Kammerer, B., et al., *HPLC-MS/MS analysis of willow bark extracts contained in pharmaceutical preparations.* Phytochem Anal, 2005. 16(6): p. 470-8.

[454] Li, L.S., et al., *[Determination of salicin in extract of willow bark by high performance liquid chromatography].* Se Pu, 2001. 19(5): p. 446-8.

[455] Fiebich, B.L. and K. Appel, *Anti-inflammatory effects of willow bark extract.* Clin Pharmacol Ther, 2003. 74(1): p. 96; author reply 96-7.

[456] Wagner, I., et al., *Influence of willow bark extract on cyclooxygenase activity and on tumor necrosis factor alpha or interleukin 1 beta release in vitro and ex vivo.* Clin Pharmacol Ther, 2003. 73(3): p. 272-4.

[457] Khayyal, M.T., et al., *Mechanisms involved in the anti-inflammatory effect of a standardized willow bark extract.* Arzneimittelforschung, 2005. 55(11): p. 677-87.

[458] Krivoy, N., Pavltzky, F., Eisenberg, E., et al., *Salix coretex (willow bark dry extract) effect on platelet aggregation.*. Drug Monitor, 1999. 21: p. 202.

[459] Krivoy, N., Pavlotzky, E., Chrubasik, S., Eisenberg, E., and Brook, G., *Effect of salicis cortex extract on human platelet aggregation.* Planta Med., 2001. 67(3): p. 209-212.

[460] Schmid, B., et al., *Efficacy and tolerability of a standardized willow bark extract in patients with osteoarthritis: randomized placebo-controlled, double blind clinical trial.* Phytother Res, 2001. 15(4): p. 344-50.

[461] Chrubasik, S., et al., *Treatment of low back pain exacerbations with willow bark extract: a randomized double-blind study.* Am J Med, 2000. 109(1): p. 9-14.

[462] U.S. Food and Drug Adminsitration, *Tainted Products Marketed as Dietary Supplements Potnetially Dangerous.* Available from: http://www.fda.gov/NewsEvents/Newsroom/PressAnnouncements/2010/ucm236967.htm [accessed 06/20/12].

[463] Deitel, M., *Sibutramine warning: hypertension and cardiac arrhythmias reported.* Obes Surg, 2002. 12(3): p. 422.

[464] Ernest, D., et al., *Sibutramine-associated QT interval prolongation and cardiac arrest.* Ann Pharmacother, 2008. 42(10): p. 1514-7.

[465] Geyer, H., et al., *Nutritional supplements cross-contaminated and faked with doping substances.* J Mass Spectrom, 2008. 43(7): p. 892-902.

[466] Wooltorton, E., *Obesity drug sibutramine (Meridia): hypertension and cardiac arrhythmias.* CMAJ, 2002. 166(10): p. 1307-8.

[467] Coogan, P.F., et al., *Phenolphthalein laxatives and risk of cancer.* J Natl Cancer Inst, 2000. 92(23): p. 1943-4.

[468] Vaysse, J., et al., *Analysis of adulterated herbal medicines and dietary supplements marketed for weight loss by DOSY 1H-NMR.* Food Addit Contam Part A Chem Anal Control Expo Risk Assess, 2010. 27(7): p. 903-16.

[469] Halbsguth, U., et al., *Necrotising vasculitis of the skin associated with an herbal medicine containing amfepramone.* Eur J Clin Pharmacol, 2009. 65(6): p. 647-8.

Chapter 7

Oxidative Stress in Human Infectious Diseases – Present and Current Knowledge About Its Druggability

Carsten Wrenger, Isolmar Schettert and Eva Liebau

Additional information is available at the end of the chapter

1. Introduction

Infectious diseases caused by parasites are a major threat for entire mankind, especially in the tropics. These infections are not only restricted to humans, they are also predominant in animal health. Just a few years ago infectious diseases caused by parasites were classified as an issue of the past. Due to the elevating level of drug resistance of these pathogens against the current chemotherapeutics, the need for new drugs became even more important. In particular parasitic diseases such as malaria, leishmaniasis, trypanosomiasis, amoebiasis, trichomoniasis, soil-transmitted helminthiasis, filariasis and schistosomiasis are major health problems, especially in "developing" areas (Renslo and McKerrow, 2006; Pal and Bandyopadhyay, 2012). A variety of these parasitic diseases, which comprises the so called neglected diseases Chagas disease, leishmaniasis, sleeping sickness, schistosomiasis, lymphatic filariasis, onchocerciasis and of course malaria (Chatelain and Ioset, 2011), are transmitted by vectors and therefore attempts to combat transmission became prominent. In contrast to the treatment of bacterial infections with antibiotics there are no "general" antiparasitic drugs. The use of a specific drug is dependent on the parasitic organism and therefore has to be individually chosen (Khaw et al., 1995).

Reactive oxygen species (ROS) and oxidative stress are the inevitable consequences of aerobic metabolism, with partially reduced and highly reactive metabolites of O_2 being formed in the mitochondria (Andreyev et al., 2005) or as by-products of other cellular sources such as the cytoplasm, the endoplasmatic reticulum, the plasma membrane and peroxisomes. Furthermore, environmental agents such as ionizing and UV radiation or xenobiotic exposure can generate intracellular ROS. O_2 metabolites include superoxide anion (O_2^-) and hydrogen peroxide (H_2O_2), formed by one- and two electron reductions of O_2 or the highly reactive hydroxyl radical ($^{\cdot}OH$) which is formed in the presence of metal ions via Fenton and/or Haber-Weiss reactions (Massimine et al., 2006). At physiologically low levels, ROS can function as second messenger in redox signaling, with H_2O_2 best providing the specificity in its interaction with effectors in signaling processes (Forman et al., 2010). Balancing the generation and elimination of ROS maintains the proper function of redox-sensitive signalling proteins. However, severe increases of ROS induce oxidative modifications in the cellular macromolecules DNA, proteins and lipids, this leading to a disruption of redox homeostasis and irreversible oxidative damage (Trachootham et al., 2008). Depending on the cellular context, the levels of ROS and the redox state of the cells, alterations of the delicate redox balance can promote cell proliferation and survival or induce cell death.

To maintain redox homeostasis and eliminate ROS, aerobes are equipped with enzymatic/nonenzymatic antioxidants and metal sequestering proteins to either prevent or intercept the formation of pro-oxidants. Furthermore, protective mechanisms are put in place to repair and replace damaged macromolecules. Two central thiol/disulfide couples are involved in controlling the redox state of the cell: glutathione/glutathione disulfide (GSH/GSSG) is the major redox couple that determines the antioxidative capacity of cells, other redox couples include the active site dithiol/disulfide of thioredoxins (Trx_{red}/Trx_{ox}) interacting with a different subset of proteins and thus forming a distinct but complementary redox system (Jones and Go, 2010).

Enzymatic antioxidants can be categorized into primary or secondary antioxidants, the first reacting directly with pro-oxidants (e.g. catalase, superoxide dismutase), the latter are involved in the regeneration of low molecular weight antioxidant species (Halliwell, 1999). Here, the reduced state of GSSG and Trx-enzymes is restored by the glutathione reductase (GSR) and the Trx reductase using electrons obtained from NADPH. Additionally glutaredoxins (Glrx) utilize GSH for the reduction of intracellular disulfides (Fernandes and Holmgren, 2004). While Trx, Trx reductase and Trx peroxidase (peroxiredoxin, Prx) constitute the Trx-system, the versatile GSH-system includes enzymes required for GSH synthesis and recycling, for its use in metabolism, in defense against ROS-induced damage and in a multitude of detoxification processes. Furthermore, for normal GSH turnover and disposition of GSH-conjugated metabolites and xenobiotics, export from the cell is required that is carried out by GSH efflux transporters and pumps (Sies, 1999) (Fig. 1).

In spite of the diversity of parasites, all are faced with similar biological problems that are related to their lifestyle. Besides coping with ROS levels generated from intrinsic sources, all have to deal with the oxidative stress imposed by the host's immune response. Furthermore, parasites are faced with ROS that are produced during the epithelial innate immune response of their vector, by vector-resident gut bacteria (Cirimotich et al., 2011) or during melanotic encapsulation processes (Kumar et al., 2003).

Since the redox system plays such a fundamental and indispensable role for parasite survival within their host (Massimine et al., 2006), drugs that either promote ROS generation or inhibit cellular antioxidant systems will lead to redox imbalance by pushing ROS levels above a certain threshold level that will ultimately lead to parasite death (Müller et al., 2003). In general, drugs that target vital redox reactions or promote oxidative stress are named redox-active antiparasitic drugs (Seeber et al., 2005) on which we will mainly focus within this chapter.

2. The role of the antioxidant system in *Leishmania*

Leishmaniasis is caused by the protozoan flagellate *Leishmania* which is transmitted by sandflies of the genus *Phlebotomus* (Sharma and Singh, 2008). There are several species of the genus *Leishmania* which are known to cause this infectious disease. Leishmaniasis shows a broad spectrum of clinical manifestations and includes visceral, cutaneous and mucocutaneous leishmaniasis. Whereas the two latter ones are not considered to be lethal (Herwaldt, 1999), infection with *Leishmania donovani/infantum* – resulting in kala azar or visceral leishmaniasis - can be lethal without treatment. Although treatment of leishmaniasis with chemotherapeutics is the only current option, drug resistance to first-line drugs is increasing which is accompanied by frequently occurring toxic side effects and by the high cost of treatment (Van Assche et al., 2011). Additionally, the small number of novel drugs combined with the low number of identified and subsequently validated number of *Leishmania* drug targets in clinical use, reveals an alarming situation for the current status in chemotherapy. The predominant target for the application of chemotherapy is the amastigote stage which proliferates intracellularly in tissue macrophages (Dedet et al., 2009), thereby hindering the accessibility of antileishmanial drugs to the pathogen.

3. Antimonials

Despite the fact that antimonials were already identified in 1921, they still remain the first-line treatment, although the precise mode of action is not known. But it is generally accepted that pentavalent antimonials (Sb^V) represent a pro-drug which is converted to trivalent antimonials (Sb^{III}) for antileishmanial activity. Recently it has been indicated that thiols act as reducing agents in this conversion. Furthermore, the participation of a unique parasite-specific trimeric glutathione transferase TDR1 in the activation of antimonial prodrugs has been suggested (Fyfe et al., 2012).

Treatment with antimonials requires parenteral administration and is accompanied by toxic side effects such as cardiac arrhythmia and acute pancreatitis (Sundar and Rai, 2002). Some studies have been carried out to investigate the activity mechanism of antimonials which correlates with an interference with the antioxidant defence system of the parasite: Trivalent antimonials decrease the thiol-reducing capacity of *Leishmania* by inducing an efflux of trypanothione. In contrast to *Leishmania*, mammalian cells depend on GSH to control their intracellular thiol-redox status. Here, ROS and oxidized cell components are efficiently reduced by GSH, thereby generating GSSG. The glutathione disulfide form can then be regenerated by the GSR (Monostori et al., 2009). In contrast, the redox metabolism of *Leishmania* relies on a modified GSH-system, $N1,N8$-bis(l-γ-glutamyl-l-hemicystinylglycyl) spermidine, also known as trypanothione (Fairlamb et al., 1985). The oxidised form, trypanothione disulfide, is generated when trypanothione reduces ROS and its reconversion is catalysed by the trypanothione reductase. Antimonials inhibit this enzyme, leading to an accumulation of trypanothione disulfide, which subsequently is not accessible for the reduction of ROS (Krauth-Siegel and Comini, 2008). The influence of antimonials on the parasite's redox biology has been verified on cellular level by the fact that trivalent antimonials-resistant parasites display an increased IC_{50}-value for nitric oxide donors such as $NaNO_2$, SNAP, and DETA NONOate compared to antimonial-sensitive strains (Souza et al., 2010; Holzmüller et al., 2005; Vanaerschot et al., 2010). Whether nitric oxide resistance is due to elevated trypanothione levels or due to another antioxidant mode of action is not yet clear.

4. Amphotericin B

Amphotericin B (Fig. 2), a polyene macrolide, has been employed in the treatment of *Leishmania* since 1960, but just as a second-line drug. This drug exhibits an excellent antileishmania activity with more than 90% cure rates. Because the pure compound creates severe side effects and requires long-term treatment and extensive monitoring, liposomal application of amphotericin B is used at the moment which results in cure rates of 3–5 days (up to 100%), is convenient for the patient and is less expensive (Gradoni et al., 2008; Manandhar et al., 2008; Sundar et al., 2002; Thakur et al., 1996). The mode of action can be explained based on its chemical structure, polyene macrolide has been shown to bind to ergosterol, one of the main sterols within *Leishmania* membranes. Interference with this molecule results in an increasing permeability of the cell membrane which leads to the parasite's death (Balana-Fouce et al., 1998; Amato et al., 2008). Additionally there is some evidence that amphotericin B has an effect on the oxidative response of macrophages (Mukherjee et al., 2010), however further experiments are required to verify this effect.

5. Miltefosine

Miltefosine (hexadecylphosphocholine) is the first and currently the only, orally administered antileishmanial drug (Fig. 2). However, despite cure rates of up to 98% (Roberts, 2006), the drug reveals serious side effects such as vomiting, diarrhea and can cause abnormal physiological development of the foetus. Furthermore, the drug has a relatively long half-life of about 150 hours (Seifert et al., 2007; Maltezou, 2010) which could lead to the development of rapid resistance. Related to its structure, the drug possibly interferes with membranes and membrane-linked enzymes. Currently no verified implications of the drug within the redox biology of the parasite have been found (Rakotomanga et al., 2004; Saint-Pierre-Chazalet et al., 2009).

6. Oxidative chemotherapeutic intervention
of Trypanosoma infections

Trypanosoma infections, caused by the flagellate protozoan *Trypanosoma* are responsible for a high degree of health problems in endemic countries. They can be divided into two types of pathogens: *Trypanosoma cruzi*, the causative agent of Chagas disease, also known as American trypanosomiasis, since it occurs in Latin America and *Trypanosoma brucei ssp.*, the causative agent of sleeping sickness, or human African trypanosomiasis, since it is endemic to sub-Saharan Africa. The current medication is known for its toxicity, poor activity in immune-suppressed patients and long-term treatment combined with high costs. Moreover, vaccines are not foreseeable in the near future. The *T. cruzi* life cycle includes three fundamental forms characterized by the relative positions of the flagellum, kinetoplast and nucleus: Trypomastigotes, epimastigotes and amastigotes, the latter one characterized by their proliferation in any nucleated cell (Prata, 2001). On the one hand Chagas' disease is controlled through elimination of its vectors by using insecticides and on the other side by chemotherapy. Currently, the drugs used are nifurtimox (4[(5-nitrofurfurylidene)amino]-3-methylthiomorpholine-1,1-dioxide), derived from nitrofuran, and benznidazole (*N*-benzyl-2-nitroimidazole-1-acetamide), a nitroimidazole derivative. Nifurtimox and benznidazole (Fig. 2) are trypanocidal to all forms of the parasite (Rodriques Coura and de Castro, 2002). However, severe side effects and toxicity have been observed (Kirchhoff, 2000). In addition, there are also reports of mutagenesis resulting in DNA damage (Zahoor et al., 1987). An additional aspect that complicates treatment is the different susceptibility of different parasite strains to the applied chemotherapeutics (Filardi and Brener, 1987). The mode of action of nifurtimox and benznidazole (Fig. 2) is via the formation of free radicals and/or charged metabolites. The nitro group of both drugs is reduced to an amino group by the catalysis of nitro-reductases, leading to the formation of various free radical intermediates. Cytochrome P450-related nitro-reductases initiate this process by producing a nitro anion radical (Moreno et al., 1982). Subsequently, the radical reacts with oxygen, which regenerates the drug (Mason and Holtzman, 1975). For example, nifurtimox-derived free radicals may undergo redox cycling with O_2, thereby producing H_2O_2 in a reaction catalysed by the SOD (Temperton et al., 1998). Furthermore, in the presence of Fe^{3+} the highly reactive ·OH is also being formed according to the Haber-Weiss reaction. These free radicals can subsequently bind to cellular macromolecules such as lipids, proteins and DNA, resulting in severe damage of parasitic cells (Díaz de Toranzo et al., 1988). In contrast, the trypanocidal effect of benznidazole does not depend on ROS but it is likely that reduced metabolites of benznidazole are covalently binding to cellular macromolecules, thereby revealing their trypanocidal effect (Díaz de Toranzo et al., 1988; Maya et al., 2004). Additionally, it has been demonstrated that benznidazole inhibits the *T. cruzi* NADH-fumarate reductase (Turrens et al., 1996).

7. Approaches to increase oxidative stress within the malaria parasite

Malaria is a devastating and quite often a deadly parasitic disease, which causes important public health problems in the tropics. The population in more than 90 countries, with more than 2000 million citizens, is exposed to the infection. Malaria infection is responsible for an estimated 500 million clinical cases per annum, causing more than one million deaths; most of these are children in Africa. The malaria parasite *Plasmodium falciparum*, the causative agent of Malaria tropica, is proliferating within human red blood cells, thereby exploiting host's nutrient sources and hiding from the human immune response. A vaccine is not available and the control of the disease depends solely on the administration of a small number of drugs. Due to mutational modification of the genome of the malaria parasite, an ongoing rapid adaptation to environmental changes and drug resistance is occurring (Greenwood et al., 2008). At the moment – which is just a question of time - solely artemesinin is still effective against the malaria parasite. However, first reports already demonstrated drug resistance against artemisinin (Wangroongsarb et al., 2011). Therefore, continuous discovery and development of new drugs are urgently needed. A variety of the current anti-malaria drugs are targeting the redox balance of the parasite. As outlined above, redox systems are essential for the intracellular proliferation of the plasmodial pathogen.

In general, *P. falciparum* uses the two interacting systems, GSH- and TRX-system, to protect against reactive ROS (Kanzok et al., 2002; Kanzok et at., 2000; Kawazu et al., 2001; Kehr et al., 2011; Krnajski et al., 2001; Krnajski et al., 2002; Kumar et al., 2008; Liebau et al., 2002). Both systems can be link by the redox protein plasmoredoxin (Becker et al., 2003). Active interference by employing redox-active antiparasitic drugs, however, harms the parasite and results in its death. Compounds which disturb the redox balance can be categorised into three different groups: (i) molecules that are responsible for the *de novo* synthesis of ROS and thus lead to parasite death, (ii) molecules which inhibit the activities of redox balancing enzymes and (iii) molecules that interfere in the scavenging of pro-oxidant metabolic products like hemozoin.

8. Molecules which inhibit the activities of redox balancing enzymes

The GSH-system plays an important role in the maintenance of the redox status in *Plasmodium* (Kehr et al., 2011). It is involved in detoxifying free heme (ferriprotoporphyrin IX) (Atamna et al., 1995; Müller, 2003) and in the termination of radical-based chain reactions (Frey, 1997). Therefore, enzymatic reactions within this system are highly druggable. The GSR is one of the key enzymes of the GSH-system and consequently several compounds have been synthesized to successfully interfere with its catalysis *in vitro* and *in vivo* (Biot et al., 2004; Gallo et al., 2009; Grellier et al., 2010; Muller et al., 2011). Inhibitory compounds comprise for example isoalloxazines, quinacrines, tertiary amides that reveal antimalarial activity at low doses against the chloroquine sensitive *P. falciparum* strain 3D7 (Sarma et al., 2003; Friebolin et al., 2008; Chibale et al., 2001). Methylene blue (Fig. 2), a noncompetitive inhibitor of the *P. falciparum* GR, shows antiplasmodial activity against all blood stage forms, whereas only a marginal cytotoxic effect against mammalian cells has been reported (Biot et al., 2004; Buchholz et al., 2008; Atamna et al., 1996; Akoachere et al., 2005; Badyopadhyay et al., 2004; Krauth-Siegel et al., 2005; Garavito et al., 2007).

The GST is one of the most abundant proteins expressed in *P. falciparum*. Additionally to its detoxifying role, it efficiently binds parasitotoxic heme not only in the presence of GSH, but also when GSSG is present, thereby protecting the parasite from hemin even under severe oxidative stress conditions. Here, a peculiar loop region, that is both crucial for the gluta-thione-dependent tetramerization/inactivation process and for hemin-binding, represents an ideal drug target (Liebau et al., 2005; 2009). Recently chemical synthesis to design effective compounds to target GST has been performed which show some promising antiplasmodial activity (Ahmad et al., 2007; Sturm et al., 2009). Furthermore, the development of drugs that overcome resistance to available antimalarial drugs also are of great interest. The action of multidrug resistance protein (MRP)-like transporters is associated with the efflux of xenobi-otics in both unaltered and GSH-conjugated form and it is conceivable that they are in-volved in the development of drug resistance in malarial parasites (Koenderink et al., 2010). Since coordinated expression and synergistic interactions between GST and efflux pumps have been observed (Sau et al., 2010), a promising new intervening strategy might be the in-hibition of GST and/or the development of GST-activated pro-drugs that overcome drug re-sistance by blocking the drug binding sites of the transporters.

Another promising antimalarial drug target is the *P. falciparum* TrxR (Banerjee et al., 2009). Chalcone derivatives and Eosin B exhibit antiplasmodial activity by inhibiting the plasmo-dial TrxR (Li et al., 1995; Massimine et al., 2006).

For many years it was thought that the malaria parasite had no need for an endogenous SOD and simply adopted the host's enzyme for its purpose. However, in 2002, an iron-de-pendent SOD was described in *P. falciparum* (Boucher et al., 2006). Being quite distinct from the human tetrameric Mn and Cu/Zn SOD, it is exploited as anti-malaria drug target (Sou-lere et al., 2003).

9. Drugs inhibiting hemozoin formation and thereby inducing oxidative stress

Besides the attacks of the immune systems of the respective host, where ROS are deployed to kill invading pathogens, the parasite faces another even bigger challenge: *Plasmodium* relies al-so on the digestion of human haemoglobin to obtain amino acids for its metabolism (Sherman, 1977). Haemoglobin is the major protein inside the erythrocyte and the parasite has evolved a unique pathway to utilise this molecule (Muller et al., 2011). Heme is the degradation product of haemoglobin, which has to be detoxified and stored as hemozoin within the food vacuole of the parasite – the place where the haemoglobin degradation occurs. Non-detoxified heme is extremely toxic (Papalexis et al., 2001) and leads not only to the generation of H_2O_2, $\cdot OH$ and O_2^{2-} (Francis et al., 1997), but also to the highly reactive, non-radical molecule, singlet oxygen ($^1O_2$)

(Freinbicherler et al., 2011). Moreover, one $^1O_2$ molecule can be either synthesised by the reaction of $^.OH$ and O^{2-} or two O^{2-} with two hydrogen ions (Khan and Kasha, 1994). In order to detoxify these ROS, *Plasmodium* has developed – as outlined above - multiple antioxidant defence systems. However - excluding the membrane located lipophilic tocopherol (vitamin E) (Wang and Quinn, 1999) - none of the above mentioned defense systems are capable to detoxify $^1O_2$. The fact that vitamin B6 is linked to the defense against $^1O_2$ in plants and fungi (Tambasco-Studart et al., 2005; Ehrenshaft et al., 1999), suggests that the vitamin B6 biosynthesis might also play a yet unrecognized role in combating $^1O_2$ in the malaria parasite *P. falciparum*. Very recently this role of $^1O_2$ detoxification has been verified in the malaria parasite (Wrenger et al., 2005; Knöckel et al., 2012; Butzloff et al., 2012).

extracellular space

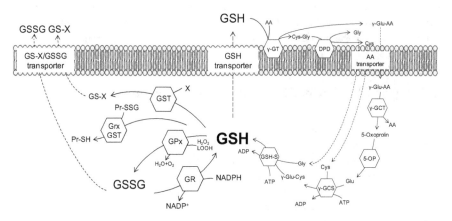

cytosolic compartment

Figure 1. Schematic illustration of the glutathione (GSH) system. GSH homeostasis involves intra- and extracellular mechanisms. GSH is synthesized from amino acids (AA) by the action of γ-glutamylcysteine synthetase (γ-GCS) and glutathione synthase (GSH-S), both requiring ATP. As antioxidant, GSH participates in the reduction of peroxides, catalysed by glutathione peroxidase (GPx), in the reduction of protein-disulfides, catalysed by glutaredoxins (Grx) and in conjugation reactions with electrophils (eg. xenobiotics, X), catalysed by glutathione transferases (GSTs). The glutathione conjugates (GS-X) and GSSG are transported out of the cell via GS-X/GSSG pumps. The NADPH-dependent GSH reductase (GR) is responsible for the intracellular recycling of GSH, while extracellular GSH gets sequentially hydrolysed by γ-glutamyl transpeptidase (γ-GT) and dipeptidase (DPD), with glutamate, cysteine and glycine being recycled for GSH synthesis (γ-glutamyl cycle).

A number of drugs have been identified that act as inhibitors of the hemozoin formation by binding to heme. This leads to an accumulation of free heme, causes high levels of oxidative stress and ends in the death of the parasite (Meunier et al., 2010). Quinoline-containing derivatives such as amopyroquine, amodiaquine, tebuquine, halofantrine, py-ronaridine, quinine, mepacrine, epiquinine, quinidine, bisquinoline chloroquine (see figure 2) are highly potent antimalarials that inhibit hemozoin formation at EC_{50}-values in the low nano-molar range (Egan et al., 2000; Kotecka et al., 1997; O'Neill et al., 2003; Vennerstrom et al., 1992). Azole derivatives are also inhibitors of the hemozoin formation and reveal efficacy against chloroquine sensitive as well as resistant plasmodial strains (Banerjee et al., 2009; Rodrigues et al., 2011). Another novel class, which has been identified to interact with heme and thereby prevent the hemozoin formation, are xanthones (Docampo et al., 1990; Ignatushchenko et al., 1997; Xu Kelly et al., 2001). Moreover, a variety of isonitrile derivatives gain their antimalarial activity from inhibition of the hemozoin synthesis (Kumar et al., 2007; Wright et al., 2001) resulting in EC_{50}-values in the low nano-molar range (Badyopadhyay et al., 2001; Singh et al., 2002; Kumar et al., 2007). Benzylmenadione derivatives do not show any cytotoxicity against two human cell lines while they are effective against the chloroquine resistant *P. falciparum* strain Dd2 (Muller et al., 2011). The precise mode of action of benzylmenadione remains for elucidation, but it has been suggested that the molecule is initially oxidized to a naphthoquinone derivative within the food vacuole of the parasite which leads subsequently to the inhibition of the hemozoin formation (Davioud-Charvet et al., 2003).

10. Druggability of oxidative stress systems in helminths

Helminths are parasitic worms that encompass nematodes (roundworms), cestodes and trematodes (flatworms) and affect humans in all areas of the world, with more than one-third of humans harbouring these parasites that cause chronic, debilitating morbidity. Furthermore, co-endemicity and polyparasitism increase the burden of millions (Hotez et al., 2008). In the absence of vaccines, control relies on pharmacotherapy and pharmacoprophylaxis to easy symptoms and reduce transmission. Helminthosis are treated with a limited number of anthelmintics by chemotherapy of symptomatic individuals or, more general, by control programmes that rely on mass drug administration (MDA) and require annual or bi-annual treatment of at-risk populations over prolonged period of time (Prichard et al., 2012). A major problem, however, is the development of resistance or tolerance by the parasites to these common antiparasitic drugs (Vercruysse et al., 2011). It is therefore essential to understand the underlying mechanisms of drug resistance and find new drugs to circumvent it.

Praziquantel has been used for over 20 years to treat a variety of human trematode infections. Its precise mechanism of action has not been fully elucidated, however, there is experimental evidence that praziquantel acts by increasing the permeability of cell membranes towards calcium ions and/or by interfering with adenosine uptake (Jeziorski and Greenberg, 2006; Angelucci et al., 2007). Furthermore, it has been suggested that praziquantel reduces GSH concentrations, making the parasite more susceptible to the host immune response (Ribeiro et al., 1998). Interestingly, exposure to sub-lethal concentrations of praziquantel shows that schistosomes undergo a transcriptomic response similar to that observed during oxidative stress (Aragon et al., 2009).

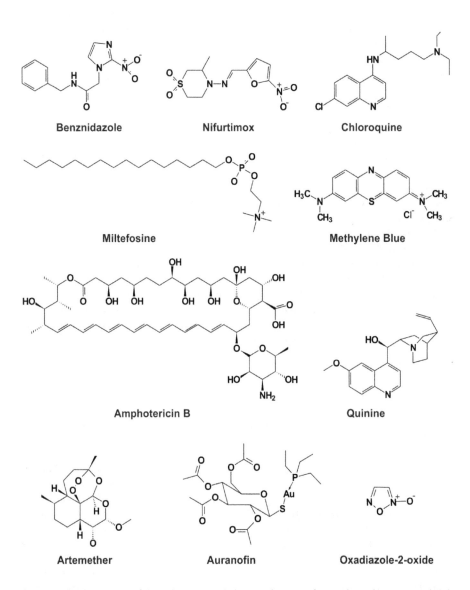

Figure 2. Molecular structures of chemotherapeutics which are used to treat infectious disease by generating directly or indirectly high levels reactive oxygen species.

Reliance on a single drug for mass treatment is risky. Therefore, anti-schistosomiasis drug development is on the way to identify new compounds with different modes of action. Recently it was demonstrated that artemisinin-based compounds (e.g. artemether, figure 2) are active against immature stages of schistosomes. Although a number of potential drug targets have been proposed, the mode of action remains ambiguous (O'Neill et al., 2010). It is thought that the primary activator of the drug is an iron source. Therefore, interaction with heme in the worm gut has been suggested, leading to the formation of an unstable species that generates ROS and thus kills the worm (Utzinger et al., 2001). Since artemisinins are critically important for malaria chemotherapy, they are not available for MDA.

Schistosomes seem to be poorly adapted to cope with oxidative stress. This is surprising, since they have to deal with host-immune and self-generated ROS and, furthermore, with ROS generated during the consumption of host haemoglobin (Huang et al., 2012).The highly restricted antioxidant network has been widely accepted as an excellent drug target for schistosomes and other platyhelminths, since it is unique and differs significantly from the human host. Interestingly, the parasites have merged the Trx- and GSH-system using a hybrid enzyme, the thioredoxin-glutathione reductase (TGR) (Salinas et al., 2004, Huang et al., 2012). Using RNA interference, the TGR was found to be essential for parasite survival (Kuntz et al., 2007). TGR was indicated to be the main target of schistosomicidal drugs used in the past (antimonyl potassium tartrate and oltipraz) and of the anti-arthritic drug auranofin (Fig. 2), with a significant worm reduction observed in infected mice (Kuntz et al., 2007; Angelucci et al., 2009). A quantitative high-throughput screen identified highly potent lead compounds against the Schistosoma TGR (Simeonov et al., 2008), with low inhibitory constants being found with derivatives of phosphinic amides, isoxazolones and the oxadiazole-2-oxide chemotype (Furoxan) (Fig. 2) (Huang et al., 2012).

Preventive chemotherapy is the mainstay in the control of human soil-transmitted helminthiasis (STH). STH is primarily caused by the nematodes *Ancylostoma duodenale* and *Necator americanus* (hookworms), *Ascaris lumbricoides* (roundworm) and *Trichuris trichiura* (whipworm) that parasitize the human gastrointestinal tract. Four anthelminthics that exhibit a broad spectrum of activity are currently recommended by the World Health Organization: The benzimidazoles albendazole and mebendazole, the synthetic phenylimidazolthiazole levamisole and the pyrimidine derivative pyrantel pamoate. While benzimidazoles bind to free β-tubulin, leading to tubule capping and degradation (Beech et al., 2011), the cholinergic agonist levamisole activates ligand-gated acetylcholine receptors (Lewis et al., 1980) and the pyrimidine derivative pyrantel pamoate induces persistent activation of nicotinic acetylcholine receptors (Utzinger and Keiser, 2004). The GABA agonist piperazine, the nicotinic acetylcholine receptor agonist tribendimidine are further drugs used in STH. Currently neither drug class used to control or treat STH, has been implicated as influencing the redox biology of parasites. Instead, most of the currently used or proposed drugs (Olliaro et al., 2011) of gastro-intestinal nematodes affect ion channel function of the neuromuscular synapses. These neuroactive drugs cause paralysis of the worm and result in its rapid expulsion or killing.

Filarial parasites are classified according to the habitat of the adult worms in the vertebral host, with the cutaneous (*Loa loa* and *Onchocerca volvulus*) and lymphatic (*Wuchereria bancrofti, Brugia malayi* and *Brugia timori*) groups being the most clinically significant. Chemotherapeutic approaches to control parasite transmission and to treat onchocerciasis rely on the macrocyclic lactone ivermectin, an effective and safe microfilaricide (Basáñez et al., 2008). Ivermectin is an agonist of ligand-gated Cl⁻ channels, with particular activity against gluta-mate-gated Cl⁻ channels of invertebrates (Martin et al., 1997). While ivermectin is less effec-tive against adult worms, it causes reproductive quiescence and disappearance of microfilaria from skin or blood. Interestingly, cultured microfilariae are unaffected by iver-mectin at concentrations found in treated patients (Bennett et al., 1993), making interference of the drug with protective mechanisms employed against the human immune response fea-sible (Geary et al., 2010). The development of ivermectin-resistant strains of *Caenorhabditis elegans* has shown that resistance to low levels of ivermectin is associated with an increased expression of drug efflux pumps and an increase in GSH-synthesis and -conjugation is ob-served. Since the overall levels of glutathione decrease, increased drug conjugation and re-moval from the cells is suggested (James and Davey, 2009). In a recent study, ivermectin has been identified as a cytotoxic agent to leukemia cells and a previously unknown indirect in-fluence of ivermectin on the intracellular redox balance was demonstrated. Mechanistically, ivermectin induced chloride influx, membrane hyperpolarization, and generated ROS, the latter being functionally important for ivermectin-induced cell death (Shrameen et al., 2010).

Diethylcarbamazine (DEC) is still the mainstay for the treatment of lymphatic filariasis and first choice of therapy of loiasis. Surprisingly, its molecular mechanism of action is still not completely understood. Since pharmacologically relevant concentrations of DEC do not have an effect on microfilariae in culture, its mode of action must involve both the worm and its host. A possible involvement of host arachidonate- and NO-dependent pathways was observed (McGarry et al., 2005). Currently no verification of an influence on the redox biology of helminths is available.

It has been postulated that antioxidant enzymes, that defend against host-generated ROS, are of particular importance for long-lived tissue-dwelling parasites that are involved in chronic infections. Here, surface or secreted antioxidant enzymes are of great importance since they can directly neutralize ROS that pose real danger, thereby protecting surface membranes against peroxides. Secreted filarial antioxidant enzymes include SOD, GPx and Prx (Henkle-Dührsen and Kampkötter, 2001). Additionally to their antioxidant role, the Prx have recently been shown to contribute to the development of Th2-responses by altering the function of macrophages (Donnelly et al., 2008). Interestingly, GSH-dependent proteins have been observed that are capable of modifying the local environment via modulation of the immune response. Here the secretory GSTs from *O. volvulus* combine several features that make them excellent drug target: they are accessible since they are located directly at the parasite–host interface, they detoxify and/or transport various electrophilic compounds and secondary products of lipid peroxidation and they are involved in the synthesis of po-tential immunmodulators. Significant structural differences to the host homologues are ob-served in the xenobiotic binding site; this may support the structure-based design of specific inhibitors (Sommer et al., 2003; Perbandt et al., 2008; Liebau et al., 2008).

As outlined above, GSH-dependent detoxification pathways defend against current drugs and also play a role in mediating resistance to anthelmintics. The antioxidant pathways also provide the parasite with a means to protect against ROS-attack by its host and/or vector. In the model nematode *C. elegans*, GSH-synthesis and a large variety of primary and secondary antioxidant enzymes and GSH-dependent detoxification enzymes are tightly regulated by the sole NF-E2-related (Nrf) transcription factor SKN-1 (An and Blackwell, 2003). Inhibiton of SKN-1 would thus target the expression of a multitude of enzymatic antioxidants and detoxification enzymes rather than affecting only one single protein or protein class, resulting in the downregulation of xenobiotic detoxification and in an enormous increase of oxidative stress. Since SKN-1 is also essential for embryonic development, this would be an additional bonus. Nematode-specific structural differences are observed that make SKN-1 an excellent candidate for the development of specific nematocidal drugs (Choe et al., 2012).

11. Conclusion

The current bottle-neck for the treatment of parasitic diseases with chemotherapeutics is the increasing drug resistance which forces the continuous discovery and development of new antiparasitic drugs. There is an urgent need for novel chemotherapeutic targets. New drugs should be generated to specifically target the parasite with minimal (or no) toxicity to the human host. Therefore, good drug targets should be distinctly different from processes in the host, or ideally be absent in the latter. Targeting the peculiarities - which are absent in the host - is proposed as such a strategy. In this sense, the parasite-specific biosyntheses represent ideal drug targets; similar to the already exploited antifolate interference with the parasite's dihydrofolate (vitamin B9) biosynthesis. There are a variety of reports about reactive compounds that have antiparasitic activity; however, not all of these are therapeutically viable drug-like molecules due to various limitations such as toxicity, low bioavailability, rapid inactivation under *in vivo* conditions and development of resistance. Recently studies on drug synergism raised special attention, which can open new avenues to improve the efficacy of antiparasitic drugs in combination with others. Since parasites such as *Plasmodium*, *Trypanosoma* or helminths are highly susceptible to oxidative stress - as outlined within this chapter - the identification of new lead compounds that target the parasite's redox systems by inducing oxidative stress, will be an efficient approach to discover novel drugs.

In this chapter we have tried to give an outline of the present situation of redox-active antiparasitic molecules that target human infectious diseases. In future the mechanisms, evolutionarily developed by the parasite to circumvent the crucial presence of ROS, will open new avenues for the development of novel antiparasitic drugs that combat resistant human pathogens effectively.

Acknowledgement

The authors would like to thank FAPESP (Fundação de Amparo à Pesquisa do Estado de São Paulo) for financial support (Project No. 2009/54325-2 to CW). The support of the DFG (Deutsche Forschungsgemeinschaft, grant LI 793/5-0 to EL) is acknowledged.

Author details

Carsten Wrenger[1], Isolmar Schettert[2] and Eva Liebau[3*]

*Address all correspondence to: cwrenger@icb.usp.br or liebaue@uni-muenster.de

1 Department of Parasitology, Institute of Biomedical Science, University of São Paulo, Av. Prof. Lineu Prestes, São Paulo-SP, Brazil

2 Laboratory of Genetics and Molecular Cardiology, Heart Institute InCor, Av. Dr. Eneas de Carvalho Aguiar, São Paulo-SP, Brazil

3 Department of Molecular Physiology, University of Münster, Hindenburgplatz, Münster, Germany

References

[1] Ahmad R, Srivastava AK, Tripathi RP, Batra S, Walter RD. (2007) Synthesis and bio-logical evaluation of potential modulators of malarial glutathione-S-transferase(s). J Enzym Inhib Med Chem. 22:327-342

[2] Akoachere M, Buchholz K, Fischer E, Burhenne J, Haefeli WE, Schirmer RH, Becker K. (2005) In vitro assessment of methylene blue on chloroquine-sensitive and -resist-ant *Plasmodium falciparum* strains reveals synergistic action with artemisinins. Anti-microb Agents Chemother. 49:4592-4597

[3] Amato VS, Tuon FF, Bacha HA, Neto VA, Nicodemo AC. (2008) Mucosal leishmania-sis: current scenario and prospects for treatment. Acta Trop. 105:1-9

[4] An JH, Blackwell TK. (2003) SKN-1 links C. elegans mesendodermal specification to a conserved oxidative stress response. Genes Dev. 17:1882-93

[5] Angelucci F, Basso A, Bellelli A, Brunori M, Pica Mattoccia L, Valle C. (2007) The an-ti-schistosomal drug praziquantel is an adenosine antagonist. Parasitology 134:1215-1221

[6] Angelucci F, Sayed AA, Williams DL, Boumis G, Brunori M, Dimastrogiovanni D, Miele AE, Pauly F, Bellelli A. (2009) Inhibition of *Schistosoma mansoni* thioredoxin-glutathione reductase by auranofin: structural and kinetic aspects. J Biol Chem. 284:28977-28985

[7] Andreyev AY, Kushnareva YE, Starkov AA. (2005) Mitochondrial metabolism of re-active oxygen species. Biochemistry (Moscow) 70:200-214

[8] Aragon AD, Imani RA, Blackburn VR, Cupit PM, Melman SD, Goronga T, Webb T, Loker ES, Cunningham C. (2009) Towards an understanding of the mechanism of ac-tion of praziquantel. Mol Biochem Parasitol. 164:57-65

[9] Atamna H, Ginsburg H. (1995) Heme degradation in the presence of glutathione. A proposed mechanism to account for the high levels of non-heme iron found in the membranes of hemoglobinopathic red blood cells. J Biol Chem. 270:24876-24883

[10] Balana-Fouce R, Reguera RM, Cubria JC, Ordonez D. (1998) The pharmacology of leishmaniasis. Gen Pharmacol. 30:435-443

[11] Bandyopadhyay U, Dey S. (2011) Antimalarial drugs and molecules inhibiting hemozoin formation. In: Apicomplexan Parasites: Molecular Approaches Toward Targeted Drug Development, edited by Becker K. Weinheim, Germany: Wiley-VCH Verlag & Co. KGaA, 205-234.

[12] Banerjee AK, Arora N, Murty US. (2009) Structural model of the *Plasmodium falciparum* thioredoxin reductase: a novel target for antimalarial drugs. J Vector Borne Dis. 46:171-183

[13] Becker K, Kanzok SM, Iozef R, Fischer M, Schirmer RH, Rahlfs S. (2003) Plasmoredoxin, a novel redox-active protein unique for malarial parasites. Eur J Biochem. 270:1057-1064

[14] Beech RN, Skuce P, Bartley DJ, Martin RJ, Prichard RK, Gilleard JS (2011) Anthelmintic resistance: markers for resistance, or susceptibility? Parasitology. 138:160–174

[15] Bennett JL, Williams JF, Dave V (1993) Pharmacology of ivermectin. Parasitol Today 4:226-228

[16] Biot C, Bauer H, Schirmer RH, Davioud-Charvet E. (2004) 5-substituted tetrazoles as bioisosteres of carboxylic acids. Bioisosterism and mechanistic studies on glutathione reductase inhibitors as antimalarials. J Med Chem. 47:5972-5983

[17] Boucher IW, Brzozowski AM, Brannigan JA, Schnick C, Smith DJ, Kyes SA, Wilkinson AJ. (2006) The crystal structure of superoxide dismutase from *Plasmodium falciparum*. BMC Struct Biol. 6:20

[18] Buchholz K, Schirmer RH, Eubel JK, Akoachere MB, Dandekar T, Becker K, Gromer S. (2008) Interactions of methylene blue with human disulfide reductases and their orthologues from *Plasmodium falciparum*. Antimicrob Agents Chemother. 52:183-191

[19] Butzloff S, Groves MR, Wrenger C, Müller IB. (2012) Cytometric quantification of singlet oxygen in the human malaria parasite *Plasmodium falciparum*. Cytometry A. 81:698-703

[20] Chatelain E, Ioset JR. (2011) Drug discovery and development for neglected diseases: the DNDi model. Drug Des Devel Ther. 5:175-181.

[21] Chibale K, Haupt H, Kendrick H, Yardley V, Saravanamuthu A, Fairlamb AH, Croft SL. (2001) Antiprotozoal and cytotoxicity evaluation of sulfonamide and urea analogues of quinacrine. Bioorg Med Chem Lett 11: 2655-2657

[22] Choe KP, Leung CK, Miyamoto MM. (2012) Unique structure and regulation of the nematode detoxification gene regulator, SKN-1: implications to understanding and controlling drug resistance. Drug Metab Rev. 44:209-23

[23] Cirimotich CM, Dong Y, Clayton AM, Sandiford SL, Souza-Neto JA, Mulenga M, Dimopoulos G (2011) Natural microbe-mediated refractoriness to Plasmodium infection in *Anopheles gambiae*. Science, 332:855-858

[24] Croft SL, Sundar S, Fairlamb AH. (2006) Drug resistance in leishmaniasis. Clin. Microbiol. Rev. 19:111-126

[25] Davioud-Charvet E, McLeish MJ, Veine DM, Giegel D, Arscott LD, Andricopulo AD, Becker K, Müller S, Schirmer RH, Williams CH, Jr., Kenyon GL. (2003) Mechanism-based inactivation of thioredoxin reductase from *Plasmodium falciparum* by Mannich bases. Implication for cytotoxicity. Biochemistry 42:13319-13330

[26] Dedet JP, Pratlong F. (2009) Protozoa infection in G. Cook, A. Zumla (Eds.), Manson's Tropical Diseases, Saunders, Philadelphia 1341-1367

[27] Díaz de Toranzo EG, Castro JA, Franke de Cazzulo BM, Cazzulo JJ. (1988) Interaction of benznidazole reactive metabolites with nuclear and kinetoplastic DNA, proteins and lipids from *Trypanosoma cruzi*. Experientia, 44:880-881

[28] Docampo R. (1990) Sensitivity of parasites to free radical damage by antiparasitic drugs. Chem Biol Interact. 73:1-27

[29] Donnelly S, Stack CM, O'Neill SM, Sayed AA, Williams DL, Dalton JP. (2008) Helminth 2-Cys peroxiredoxin drives Th2 responses through a mechanism involving alternatively activated macrophages. FASEB J 22:4022–4032

[30] Ehrenshaft M, Chung KR, Jenns AE, Daub ME. (1999) Functional characterization of SOR1, a gene required for resistance to photosensitizing toxins in the fungus *Cercospora nicotianae*. Curr Genet. 34:478-485

[31] Egan TJ, Hunter R, Kaschula CH, Marques HM, Misplon A, Walden J. (2000) Structure-function relationships in aminoquinolines: effect of amino and chloro groups on quinoline-hematin complex formation, inhibition of beta-hematin formation, and antiplasmodial activity. J Med Chem. 43:283-291

[32] Fairlamb AH, Blackburn P, Ulrich P, Chait BT, Cerami A. (1985) Trypanothione: a novel bis(glutathionyl)spermidine cofactor for glutathione reductase in trypanosomatids. Science 227:1485-1487

[33] Fernandes AP, Holmgren A (2004) Glutaredoxins: Glutathione-dependent redox enzymes with functions far beyond a simple thioredoxin backup system. Antioxid Redox Signal. 6:63-74

[34] Filardi LS, Brener Z. (1987) Susceptibility and natural resistance of *Trypanosoma cruzi* strains to drugs used clinically in Chagas disease. Trans R Soc Trop Med. Hyg. 81:755-759

[35] Forman HJ, Maiorino M, Ursini F (2010) Signaling functions of reactive oxygen species. Biochemistry 49:835-842

[36] Frey PA. (1997) Radicals in enzymatic reactions. Curr Opin Chem Biol. 1:347-356

[37] Freinbichler W, Colivicchi MA, Stefanini C, Bianchi L, Ballini C, Misini B, Weinberger P, Linert W, Varešlija D, Tipton KF, Della Corte L. (2011). Highly reactive oxygen species: detection, formation, and possible functions. Cell Mol Life Sci. 68:2067-2079

[38] Friebolin W, Jannack B, Wenzel N, Furrer J, Oeser T, Sanchez CP, Lanzer M, Yardley V, Becker K, Davioud-Charvet E. (2008) Antimalarial dual drugs based on potent inhibitors of glutathione reductase from *Plasmodium falciparum*. J Med Chem. 51:1260-1277

[39] Francis SE, Sullivan DJ, Daniel E. (1997) Hemoglobin metabolism in the malaria parasite *Plasmodium falciparum*. Annu. Rev. Microbiol. 51:97-123

[40] Fyfe PK, Westrop GD, Silva AM, Coombs GH, Hunter WN. (2012) Leishmania TDR1 structure, a unique trimeric glutathione transferase capable of deglutathionylation and antimonial prodrug activation. Proc Natl Acad Sci U S A. 109:11693-11698

[41] Geary TG, Woo K, McCarthy JS, Mackenzie CD, Horton J, Prichard RK, de Silva NR, Olliaro PL, Lazdins-Helds JK, Engels DA, Bundy DA. (2010) Unresolved issues in anthelmintic pharmacology for helminthiases of humans. Int J Parasitol. 40:1-13

[42] Gallo V, Schwarzer E, Rahlfs S, Schirmer RH, van Zwieten R, Roos D, Arese P, Becker K. (2009) Inherited glutathione reductase deficiency and *Plasmodium falciparum* malaria—a case study. PLoS One 4:e7303

[43] Garavito G, Bertani S, Rincon J, Maurel S, Monje MC, Landau I, Valentin A, Deharo E. (2007) Blood schizontocidal activity of methylene blue in combination with antimalarials against *Plasmodium falciparum*. Parasite. 14:135-140

[44] Gradoni L, Soteriadou K, Louzir H, Dakkak A, Toz SO, Jaffe C et al. (2008) Drug regimens for visceral leishmaniasis in Mediterranean countries. Trop Med Int Health 13:1272-1276

[45] Gratepanche S, Menage S, Touati D, Wintjens R, Delplace P, Fontecave M, Masset A, Camus D, Dive D. (2002) Biochemical and electron paramagnetic resonance study of the iron superoxide dismutase from *Plasmodium falciparum*. Mol Biochem Parasitol. 120:237-246

[46] Grellier P, Maroziene A, Nivinskas H, Sarlauskas J, Aliverti A, Cenas N. (2010) Antiplasmodial activity of quinones: roles of aziridinyl substituents and the inhibition of *Plasmodium falciparum* glutathione reductase. Arch Biochem Biophys. 494:32-39

[47] Halliwell B (1999) Antioxidant defense mechanisms: from the beginning to the end (of the beginning) Free Radic Res. 31:261-272.

[48] Henkle-Dührsen K, Kampkötter A (2001) Antioxidant enzyme families in parasitic nematodes. Mol Biochem Parasitol. 114:129-142.

[49] Herwaldt, BL (1999). "Leishmaniasis." Lancet 354 (9185): 1191-1199

[50] Holzmuller P, Sereno D, Lemesre JL. (2005) Lower nitric oxide susceptibility of trivalent antimony-resistant amastigotes of *Leishmania infantum*. Antimicrob Agents Chemother. 49:4406-4409

[51] Hotez PJ, Brindley PJ, Bethony JM, King CH, Pearce EJ, Jacobson J (2008) Helminth infections: the great neglected tropical diseases. J Clin Invest. 118:1311-1321

[52] Huang HH, Rigouin C, Willams DL (2012) The redox biology of schistosome parasites and application for drug development. Curr Pharm Des. 18:3595-3611

[53] Ignatushchenko MV, Winter RW, Bachinger HP, Hinrichs DJ, Riscoe MK. (1997) Xanthones as antimalarial agents; studies of a possible mode of action. FEBS Lett. 409:67-73

[54] James CE, Davey MW. (2009) Increased expression of ABC transport proteins is associated with ivermectin resistance in the model nematode *Caenorhabditis elegans*. Int J Parasitol. 39:213-20

[55] Jeziorski MC, Greenberg RM. (2006) Voltage-gated calcium channel subunits from platyhelminths: potential role in praziquantel action. Int J Parasitol 36:625–632

[56] Jones DP, Go YM. (2010) Redox compartmentalization and cellular stress. Diabetes, Obes. Metab. 12:116–125.

[57] Kanzok SM, Rahlfs S, Becker K, and Schirmer RH. (2002) Thioredoxin, thioredoxin reductase, and thioredoxin peroxidase of malaria parasite *Plasmodium falciparum*. Methods Enzymol. 347:370-381

[58] Kanzok SM, Schirmer RH, Turbachova I, Iozef R, Becker K. (2000) The thioredoxin system of the malaria parasite *Plasmodium falciparum*. Glutathione reduction revisited. J Biol Chem. 275:40180-40186

[59] Kawazu S, Komaki K, Tsuji N, Kawai S, Ikenoue N, Hatabu T, Ishikawa H, Matsumoto Y, Himeno K, Kano S. (2001) Molecular characterization of a 2-Cys peroxiredoxin from the human malaria parasite *Plasmodium falciparum*. Mol Biochem Parasitol. 116:73-79

[60] Kehr S, Jortzik E, Delahunty C, Yates JR, Rahlfs S, Becker K. (2011) Protein s-glutathionylation in malaria parasites. Antioxid Redox Signal. 15:2855-2865

[61] Khan AU, Kasha M. (1994) Singlet molecular oxygen in the Haber-Weiss reaction. Proc Natl Acad Sci USA. 91:12365-12367

[62] Khaw M, Panosian CB. (1995) Human antiprotozoal therapy: past, present, and future. Clin Microbiol Rev. 8:427-439.

[63] Kirchhoff LV. (2000) American trypanosomiasis (Chagas' disease) in R.E. Rakel (Ed.), Conn's Current Therapy, W. B. Saunders, New York: 101-102

[64] Knöckel J, Müller IB, Butzloff S, Bergmann B, Walter RD, Wrenger C. (2012) The anti-oxidative effect of *de novo* generated vitamin B6 in *Plasmodium falciparum* validated by protein interference. Biochem J. 443:397-405

[65] Koenderink JB, Kavishe RA, Rijpma SR, Russel FG. (2010) The ABCs of multidrug resistance in malaria. Trends Parasitol. 26:440-446

[66] Kotecka BM, Barlin GB, Edstein MD, Rieckmann KH. (1997) New quinoline di-Mannich base compounds with greater antimalarial activity than chloroquine, amodiaquine, or pyronaridine. Antimicrob Agents Chemother. 41:1369-1374

[67] Krauth-Siegel RL, Bauer H, Schirmer RH. (2005) Dithiol proteins as guardians of the intracellular redox milieu in parasites: old and new drug targets in trypanosomes and malaria-causing plasmodia. Angew Chem Int Ed Engl. 44:690-715

[68] Krauth-Siegel RL, Comini MA. (2008) Redox control in trypanosomatids, parasitic protozoa with trypanothione-based thiol metabolism. Biochim. Biophys. Acta 1780:1236-1248

[69] Krnajski Z, Gilberger TW, Walter RD, Cowman AF, Müller S. (2002) Thioredoxin reductase is essential for the survival of *Plasmodium falciparum* erythrocytic stages. J Biol Chem. 277:25970-25975

[70] Krnajski Z, Walter RD, Müller S. (2001) Isolation and functional analysis of two thioredoxin peroxidases (peroxiredoxins) from *Plasmodium falciparum*. Mol Biochem Parasitol. 113:303-308

[71] Kumar S, Christophides GK, Cantera R, Charles B, Han YS, Meister S, Dimopoulos G, Kafatos FC, Barillas-Mury C. (2003) The role of reactive oxygen species on Plasmodium melanotic encapsulation in *Anopheles gambiae*. Proc Natl Acad Sci USA. 100:14139-14144

[72] Kumar S, Das SK, Dey S, Maity P, Guha M, Choubey V, Panda G, Bandyopadhyay U. (2008) Antiplasmodial activity of [(aryl)arylsulfanylmethyl]Pyridine. Antimicrob Agents Chemother. 52:705-715

[73] Kuntz AN, Davioud-Charvet E, Sayed AA, Califf LL, Dessolin J, Arnér ES, Williams DL. (2007) Thioredoxin glutathione reductase from *Schistosoma mansoni*: an essential parasite enzyme and a key drug target. PLoS Med. 4:e206

[74] Lewis JA, Wu CH, Berg H, Levine JH (1980) The genetics of levamisole resistance in the nematode *Caenorhabditis elegans*. Genetics 95:905–928

[75] Li R, Kenyon GL, Cohen FE, Chen X, Gong B, Dominguez JN, Davidson E, Kurzban G, Miller RE, Nuzum EO, et al. (1995) In vitro antimalarial activity of chalcones and their derivatives. J Med Chem. 38:5031–5037

[76] Liebau E, Bergmann B, Campbell AM, Teesdale-Spittle P, Brophy PM, Luersen K, Walter RD. (2002) The glutathione S-transferase from *Plasmodium falciparum*. Mol Biochem Parasitol. 124:85-90

[77] Liebau E, De Maria F, Burmeister C, Perbandt M, Turella P, Antonini G, Federici G, Giansanti F, Stella L, Lo Bello M, Caccuri AM, Ricci G. (2005) Cooperativity and pseudo-cooperativity in the glutathione S-transferase from *Plasmodium falciparum*. J Biol Chem. 280:26121-26128.

[78] Liebau E, Höppner J, Mühlmeister M, Burmeister C, Lüersen K, Perbandt M, Schmetz C, Büttner D, Brattig N. (2008) The secretory omega-class glutathione transferase OvGST3 from the human pathogenic parasite *Onchocerca volvulus*. FEBS J. 275:3438-3453.

[79] Liebau E, Dawood KF, Fabrini R, Fischer-Riepe L, Perbandt M, Stella L, Pedersen JZ, Bocedi A, Petrarca P, Federici G, Ricci G.(2009) Tetramerization and cooperativity in *Plasmodium falciparum* glutathione S-transferase are mediated by atypic loop 113-119. J Biol Chem. 284:22133-22139.

[80] Maltezou HC. (2010) Drug resistance in visceral leishmaniasis. J. Biomed. Biotechnol. 617521

[81] Martin RJ, Robertson AP, Bjorn H (1997) Target sites of anthelmintics. Parasitology 114:111–124

[82] Massimine KM, McIntosh MT, Doan LT, Atreya CE, Gromer S, Sirawaraporn W, Elliott DA, Joiner KA, Schirmer RH, Anderson KS. (2006) Eosin B as a novel antimalarial agent for drug-resistant *Plasmodium falciparum*. Antimicrob Agents Chemother. 50:3132-3141

[83] Mason RP, Holtzman JL. (1975) The role of catalytic superoxide formation in the O2 inhibition of nitroreductase. Biochem Biophys Res Commun. 67:1267-1274

[84] Maya JD, Rodríguez A, Pino L, Pabon A, Ferreira J, Pavani M, Repetto Y, Morello A. (2004) Effects of buthionine sulfoximine nifurtimox and benznidazole upon trypanothione and metallothionein proteins in *Trypanosoma cruzi*. Biol Res. 37:61-69

[85] Maya JD, Cassels BK, Iturriaga-Vásquez P, Ferreira J, Faúndez M, Galanti N, Ferreira A, Morello A. (2007) Mode of action of natural and synthetic drugs against *Trypanosoma cruzi* and their interaction with the mammalian host. Comp Biochem Physiol A Mol Integr Physiol. 146:601-620

[86] McGarry HF, Plant LD, Taylor MJ (2005) Diethylcarbamazine activity against *Brugia malayi* microfilariae is dependent on inducible nitric-oxide synthase and the cyclooxygenase pathway. Filaria J. 4:4

[87] Monostori P, Wittmann G, Karg E, Turi S. (2009) Determination of glutathione and glutathione disulfide in biological samples: an in-depth review. J. Chromatogr. B Analyt Technol Biomed Life Sci 877:3331-3346

[88] Moreno SN, Docampo R, Mason RP, León W, Stoppani AO. (1982) Different behaviors of benznidazole as free radical generator with mammalian and *Trypanosoma cruzi* microsomal preparations. Arch Biochem Biophys. 218:585-591

[89] Mukherjee AK, Gupta G, Bhattacharjee S, Guha SK, Majumder S, Adhikari A et al. (2010) Amphotericin B regulates the host immune response in visceral leishmaniasis: reciprocal regulation of protein kinase C isoforms. J Infect. 61:173–184

[90] Meunier B, Robert A. (2010) Heme as trigger and target for trioxane-containing anti-malarial drugs. Acc Chem Res 43: 1444-1451

[91] Müller S, Liebau E, Walter RD, Krauth-Siegel RL. (2003) Thiol-based redox metabolism of protozoan parasites. Trends Parasitol. 19:320-328

[92] Müller S. (2003) Thioredoxin reductase and glutathione synthesis in *Plasmodium falciparum*. Redox Rep. 8:251-255

[93] Muller T, Johann L, Jannack B, Bruckner M, Lanfranchi DA, Bauer H, Sanchez C, Yardley V, Deregnaucourt C, Schrevel J, Lanzer M, Schirmer RH, Davioud-Charvet E. (2011) A glutathione reductase-catalyzed cascade of redox reactions to bioactivate potent antimalarial 1,4-naphthoquinones-a new strategy to combat malarial parasites. J Am Chem Soc. 133:11557-11571

[94] O'Neill PM, Mukhtar A, Stocks PA, Randle LE, Hindley S, Ward SA, Storr RC, Bickley JF, O'Neil IA, Maggs JL, Hughes RH, Winstanley PA, Bray PG, Park BK. (2003) Isoquine and related amodiaquine analogues: a new generation of improved 4-aminoquinoline antimalarials. J Med Chem. 46:4933-4945

[95] O'Neill PM, Barton VE, Ward SA. (2010) The molecular mechanism of action of artemisinin--the debate continues. Molecules. 15:1705-1721

[96] Olliaro P, Seiler J, Kuesel A, Horton J, Clark JN, Don R, Keiser J. (2011) Potential drug development candidates for human soil-transmitted helminthiases. PLoS Negl Trop Dis. 5:e1138

[97] Pal C, Bandyopadhyay U. (2012) Redox-active antiparasitic drugs. Antioxid Redox Signal. 17:555-582

[98] Perbandt M, Höppner J, Burmeister C, Lüersen K, Betzel C, Liebau E. (2008) Structure of the extracellular glutathione S-transferase OvGST1 from the human pathogenic parasite *Onchocerca volvulus*. J Mol Biol. 377:501-511.

[99] Prata A. (2001) Clinical and epidemiological aspects of Chagas disease. Lancet, Infect. Dis. 1:92-100

[100] Prichard RK, Basáñez MG, Boatin BA, McCarthy JS, García HH, Yang GJ, Sripa B, Lustigman S. (2012) A research agenda for helminth diseases of humans: intervention for control and elimination. PLoS Negl Trop Dis. 6:e1549.

[101] Rakotomanga M, Loiseau PM, Saint-Pierre-Chazalet M. (2004) Hexadecylphospho-choline interaction with lipid monolayers. Biochim Biophys Acta. 1661:212-218

[102] Renslo AR, McKerrow JH. (2006) Drug discovery and development for neglected parasitic diseases. Nat Chem Biol. 2:701-710

[103] Ribeiro F, Coelho PM, Vieira LQ, Watson DG, Kusel JR. (1998) The effect of prazi-quantel treatment on glutathione concentration in *Schistosoma mansoni*. Parasitology. 116:229-236

[104] Roberts, MT. (2006). Current understandings on the immunology of leishmaniasis and recent developments in prevention and treatment. Br Med Bull 75-76:115-130

[105] Rodriques Coura J, de Castro SL. (2002) A critical review on Chagas disease chemo-therapy. Mem. Inst. Oswaldo Cruz. 97:3-24

[106] Saint-Pierre-Chazalet M, Ben BM, Le ML, Bories C, Rakotomanga M, Loiseau PM. (2009) Membrane sterol depletion impairs miltefosine action in wild-type and milte-fosine-resistant *Leishmania donovani* promastigotes. J Antimicrob Chemother. 64:993-1001

[107] Salinas G, Selkirk ME, Chalar C, Maizels RM, Fernández C. (2004) Linked thioredox-in-glutathione systems in platyhelminths. Trends Parasitol. 20:340-346

[108] Sarma GN, Savvides SN, Becker K, Schirmer M, Schirmer RH, Karplus PA. (2003) Glutathione reductase of the malarial parasite *Plasmodium falciparum*: crystal struc-ture and inhibitor development. J Mol Biol. 328:893-907

[109] Sau A, Pellizzari Tregno F, Valentino F, Federici G, Caccuri AM. (2010) Glutathione transferases and development of new principles to overcome drug resistance. Arch Biochem Biophys. 500:116-122.

[110] Seeber F, Aliverti A, Zanetti G. (2005) The plant-type ferredoxin-NADP+reductase/ferredoxin redox system as a possible drug target against apicomplexan human para-sites. Curr Pharm Des. 11:3159-3172

[111] Seifert K, Perez-Victoria FJ, Stettler M, Sanchez-Canete MP, Castanys S, Gamarro F et al. (2007) Inactivation of the miltefosine transporter, LdMT, causes miltefosine resist-ance that is conferred to the amastigote stage of *Leishmania donovani* and persists *in vivo*. Int J Antimicrob Agents. 30:229-235

[112] Sharma U, Singh S. (2008) Insect vectors of Leishmania: distribution, physiology and their control. J Vector Borne Dis. 45:255-272

[113] Sharmeen S, Skrtic M, Sukhai MA, Hurren R, Gronda M, Wang X, Fonseca SB, Sun H, Wood TE, Ward R, Minden MD, Batey RA, Datti A, Wrana J, Kelley SO, Schimmer AD. (2010) The antiparasitic agent ivermectin induces chloride-dependent membrane hyperpolarization and cell death in leukemia cells. Blood 116:3593-603.

[114] Sherman IW. (1977) Amino acid metabolism and protein synthesis in malarial para-sites. Bull World Health Organ. 55:265-276

[115] Sies H (1999) Glutathione and its role in cellular functions. Free Radic Biol Med. 27:916-921.

[116] Simeonov A, Jadhav A, Sayed AA, Wang Y, Nelson ME, Thomas CJ, Inglese J, Williams DL, Austin CP. (2008) Quantitative high-throughput screen identifies inhibitors of the *Schistosoma mansoni* redox cascade. PLoS Negl Trop Dis. 2:e127

[117] Singh C, Srivastav NC, Puri SK. (2002) *In vivo* active antimalarial isonitriles. Bioorg Med Chem Lett. 12:2277-2279

[118] Sommer A, Rickert R, Fischer P, Steinhart H, Walter RD, Liebau E. (2003) A dominant role for extracellular glutathione S-transferase from *Onchocerca volvulus* is the production of prostaglandin D2. Infect Immun. 71:3603-3606

[119] Soulere L, Delplace P, Davioud-Charvet E, Py S, Sergheraert C, Perie J, Ricard I, Hoffmann P, Dive D. (2003) Screening of *Plasmodium falciparum* iron superoxide dismutase inhibitors and accuracy of the SOD-assays. Bioorg Med Chem. 11:4941-4944

[120] Souza AS, Giudice A, Pereira JM, Guimaraes LH, de Jesus AR, de Moura TR et al. (2010) Resistance of *Leishmania (Viannia) braziliensis* to nitric oxide: correlation with antimony therapy and TNF-alpha production. BMC Infect Dis 10:209

[121] Sturm N, Hu Y, Zimmermann H, Fritz-Wolf K, Wittlin S, Rahlfs S, Becker K. (2009) Compounds structurally related to ellagic acid show improved antiplasmodial activity. Antimicrob Agents Chemother. 53:622-630

[122] Sundar S, Rai M. (2002) Advances in the treatment of leishmaniasis. Curr Opin Infect Dis 15:593–598

[123] Tambasco-Studart M, Titiz O, Raschle T, Forster G, Amrhein N, Fitzpatrick TB. (2005) Vitamin B6 biosynthesis in higher plants. Proc Natl Acad Sci USA. 102:13687-13692

[124] Temperton NJ, Wilkinson SR, Meyer DJ, Kelly JM. (1998) Overexpression of superoxide dismutase in *Trypanosoma cruzi* results in increased sensitivity to the trypanocidal agents gentian violet and benznidazole. Mol Biochem Parasitol. 96:167-176

[125] Trachootham D, Weiqin L, Ogasawara MA, Valle NRD, Huang P. (2008) Redox Regulation of Cell Survival. Antioxid Redox Signal. 10:1343-1374

[126] Turrens JF, Watts Jr BP, Zhong L, Docampo R. (1996) Inhibition of *Trypanosoma cruzi* and *T. brucei* NADH fumarate reductase by benznidazole and anthelmintic imidazole derivatives. Mol Biochem Parasitol. 82:125-129

[127] Utzinger J, Xiao S, N'Goran EK, Bergquist R, Tanner M. (2001) The potential of artemether for the control of schistosomiasis. Int J Parasitol 31:1549-1562.

[128] Utzinger J, Keiser J. (2004) Schistosomiasis and soil-transmitted helmintiasis: common drugs for treatment and control. Expert Opin. Pharmacother. 5:263-285.

[129] Vanaerschot M, Maes I, Ouakad M, Adaui V, Maes L, De DS et al. (2010) Linking in vitro and in vivo survival of clinical *Leishmania donovani* strains. PLoS One 5:e12211

[130] Van Assche T, Deschacht M, da Luz RA, Maes L, Cos P. (2007) Leishmania-macrophage interactions: insights into the redox biology. Free Radic Biol Med. 51:337-351

[131] Vennerstrom JL, Ellis WY, Ager AL, Jr., Andersen SL, Gerena L, Milhous WK. (1992) Bisquinolines. N,N-bis(7-chloroquinolin-4-yl)alkanediamines with potential against chloroquine-resistant malaria. J Med Chem. 35:2129-2134

[132] Vercruysse J, Albonico M, Behnke J, Kotze A, Prichard R, et al.(2011) Is anthelmintic resistance a concern for the control of human soil-transmitted helminths? Int J Parasitol: Drugs Drug Res. 1:14–27

[133] Wang X, Quinn PJ. (1999). Vitamin E and its function in membranes. Prog Lipid Res. 38:309-336

[134] Wangroongsarb P, Satimai W, Khamsiriwatchara A, Thwing J, Eliades JM, Kaewkungwal J, Delacollette C. (2011) Respondent-driven sampling on the Thailand-Cambodia border. II. Knowledge, perception, practice and treatment-seeking behaviour of migrants in malaria endemic zones. Malar J. 10:117

[135] Wrenger C, Eschbach ML, Müller IB, Warnecke D, Walter RD. (2005) Analysis of the vitamin B6 biosynthesis pathway in the human malaria parasite *Plasmodium falciparum*. J Biol Chem. 280:5242-5248

[136] Wright AD, Wang H, Gurrath M, Konig GM, Kocak G, Neumann G, Loria P, Foley M, Tilley L. (2001) Inhibition of heme detoxification processes underlies the antimalarial activity of terpene isonitrile compounds from marine sponges. J Med Chem. 44:873-885

[137] Xu Kelly J, Winter R, Riscoe M, Peyton DH. (2001) A spectroscopic investigation of the binding interactions between 4,5-dihydroxyxanthone and heme. J Inorg Biochem. 86:617-625

[138] Zahoor A, Lafleur MV, Knight RC, Loman H, Edwards DI. (1987) DNA damage induced by reduced nitroimidazole drugs. Biochem Pharmacol. 36:3299–3304

Chapter 8

Practical Considerations of Liquid Handling Devices in Drug Discovery

Sergio C. Chai, Asli N. Goktug, Jimmy Cui,
Jonathan Low and Taosheng Chen

Additional information is available at the end of the chapter

1. Introduction

Automated liquid handling has become an indispensable tool in drug discovery, particularly in screening campaigns ranging millions of compounds. Intense innovations of these devices go hand in hand with the progression towards assay miniaturization, accelerating dramatically the discovery of drug candidates and chemical probes for querying biological systems. The advancement in this technology is driven in large part by much impetus in cost reduction and efficiency. In addition to increased throughput, streamlining screening operations using automated fluid devices ensures consistency and reliability while avoiding human error.

In this chapter, we provide a general overview of existing liquid handlers, with emphasis on their strengths and limitations. Notably, we discuss practical considerations in the implementation of these devices, methods to discern performance quality and potential sources of error.

2. Types of liquid handling devices

A whole array of liquid handlers has been developed for every aspect of drug discovery. These instruments encompass different technologies for distinct purposes. In terms of application, they are broadly classified as bulk liquid dispensers, transfer devices and plate washers (Rudnicki and Johnston 2009).

Based on the way the reagent is being transferred, these instruments can follow two dispensing modes: contact or non-contact (Kong et al. 2012). Contact-based devices allow the fluid to be transferred to touch the surface of the destination container or solution, offering a simple and dependable alternative to sub-microliter fluid handling. Non-contact devices utilize additional force other than gravity to eject liquids, as minute volumes cannot be dispensed efficiently with gravity alone (Kong et al. 2012). The process is faster than using permanent tips or pins (Fig.1), because there is no washing step between delivery, while reducing cross-contamination and evaporation (Dunn and Feygin 2000).

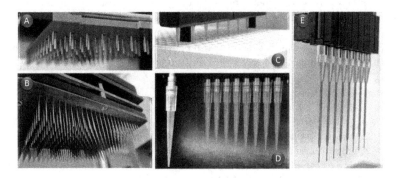

Figure 1. Various types of liquid handling tips, pins and heads from A) washer B) pintool C) peristaltic pump-based bulk dispenser D) liquid handler with single and 8-channel pipettors E) pipettor with 8-independent channels.

2.1. Peristaltic-based devices

The peristaltic pump is used for bulk reagent dispensing in conjunction with a nozzle head (Fig.1C) and a flexible tubing cartridge. The tubings stretch around a set of rollers connected to a motor. With the rotating motion of the motor, the rollers compress the tubings creating a continuous fluid motion due to positive displacement.

Typically, this type of dispenser is capable of handling volumes as low as 5 µL, offering a fast dispensing option for 96-/384-/1536-well plate formats. The disposable tubing cartridge is pre-sterilized, and the entire liquid path can be autoclaved. Additionally, these devices are normally equipped with programing capabilities that allow discrete column-wise dispensing, variable rolling speed settings and adjustable dispensing volume. The pump can roll both forward and backwards to execute priming and emptying functions, respectively. A major limitation is the lack of capabilities to dispense into individual wells.

2.2. Fixed-tip transfer devices

Fluid handlers that utilize fixed-tips (Fig.1E) are usually efficient at transferring relatively small volumes (100 µL or above) and have been largely used for compound pipetting ("cherry picking") and serial dilutions. They incorporate 2-/ 4-/ 8-channel expandable liquid handling arms in addition to 96- and 384-channel heads. This type of liquid handling device functions based on air displacement mechanism. The dilutor or syringe plunger pulls system liquid from the pipette tubing to aspirate the sample, with an air gap separating both fluids. The plunger speed, syringe size and resolution are factors that affect pipetting flow rate.

2.3. Changeable-tip transfer devices

The use of disposable tips (Fig.1D) is a simple alternative to avoid washing steps required for fixed-tip based systems, while eliminating completely the risk of cross-contamination. These instruments employ a conventional air displacement mechanism. A wide array of commercially-available tip sizes, materials and molding qualities offers the scientist great flexibility. There are even specialized tips with nanoliter-scale transfer capabilities that can be used in any conventional pipettor (Murthy et al. 2011; Ramírez et al. 2008).

2.4. Pintool transfer devices

Pintool is a contact-based dispensing method widely used for handling volumes at the nanoliter scale (Cleveland and Koutz 2005). It consists of a set of stainless steel pins (Fig. 1B) carefully crafted for consistent dimensions. The bottom end of the pins can be solid, grooved or slotted, with the option of having a hydrophobic coating to prevent non-specific binding (Dunn and Feygin 2000; Rudnicki and Johnston 2009). Solutions are transferred through a combination of capillary action and surface tension, with the volume being highly dependent on the contact surfaces and solution properties (Dunn and Feygin 2000). The pin array is normally assembled in a floating pin cassette to ensure soaking of all the pins amid uneven surfaces, which also minimizes pin damage. After liquid transfer, the pins have to cycle through washing steps to prevent cross-contamination.

2.5. Piezoelectric devices

The piezoelectric dispenser is a non-contact technology, where solutions are delivered as multiple tiny drops of defined size (Niles and Coassin 2005). This technology has been utilized in contemporary inject printers and refined to be implemented in the biological sciences. Various biochemical solutions (DNA, RNA, proteins) and bacterial suspensions have been tested with no negative effects (Schober et al. 1993). The system is composed of a capillary tube made of quartz or steel, with one end connected to the reagent reservoir and the other end ending in an orifice from which droplets are ejected (Niles and Coassin 2005). A piezoelectric crystal collar is bound to the capillary, which is filled with solution. Upon voltage application, the piezoelectric element contracts causing pressure on the capillary to generate fine drops. The ejection is at high acceleration with minimal wetting of the nozzle (Schober et al. 1993). Several thousand drops can be dispensed per second, with attainable drop sizes spanning the picoliter and nanoliter range (Schober et al. 1993). Droplet volume depends on several factors, including bore diameter, solution viscosity and the voltage pulse amplitude and frequency (James and Papen 1998; Kong et al. 2012).

2.6. Solenoid-based devices

Solenoid-based devices are non-contact dispensers that use a positive displacement mechanism (Bateman et al. 1999). The flow of pressurized liquid is occluded by a solenoid valve, which is actuated by electric current to allow for liquid to pass through the valve. The dispensed volume is regulated by the fluid pressure, duration of the valve in the open position, solution properties and orifice diameter (Bateman et al. 1999; Niles and Coassin 2005). Depending on the time the valve stays in the open position, the device can eject droplets or a continuous stream (Niles and Coassin 2005).

2.7. Acoustic devices

Acoustic droplet ejection (ADE) is a recent touch-less technology that surges in popularity in recent years. It adopts acoustic energy to propel droplets from various types of solutions with good precision (Ellson et al. 2003; Harris et al. 2008; Rudnicki and Johnston 2009; Shieh et al. 2006). The source plate remains stationary as the transducer and destination plate shuffle to allow for solution transfer from any well in the source plate to any well in the destination plate, the latter one lying in an inverted position (Olechno et al. 2006). This system does not require any additional consumable other than microplates (Olechno et al. 2006), and it speeds up the process by avoiding washing steps and having the capability to prepare assay-ready plates (Turmel et al. 2010)

2.8. Microplate washers

Microplate washers are laboratory instruments designed to automate and expedite assay applications, where a washing step is essential. They play an important role in areas such as high-content screening and enzyme-linked immunosorbent assays (ELISA). In 1990, Stobbs developed the first multiple plate washer using readily available materials as a low cost alternative to the commercially available plate washers of the era (Stobbs 1990). Over the years, fully programmable plate washers have been developed with numerous features. The development of automated plate washers has decreased the time required for laborious washing steps involved in many screening assays and improved reproducibility through standardized plate handling across multiple wash cycles (defined as a single dispense and aspirate step per cycle).

The two most critical components of a plate washer are a plate carrier and a manifold containing a number of fixed stainless steel needle probes for solution dispensing (Fig.1A). This manifold (or a separate manifold depending on the design) aspirates the liquid from the wells after an optional soaking period, leaving a pre-defined residual volume in the wells. A third component is the vacuum/pump assembly, which supplies the necessary pressure differential to drive efficient aspiration. Sunghou Lee first developed an additional vacuum filtration system integrated with a conventional plate washer to speed up the wash process for applications involving filter plates (Lee 2006). Some plate washers have a built-in magnet or a vacuum filtration module for handling bead-based assays.

Microplate washers can be categorized into two types: strip washers, which wash a single column or row of a plate at a time, and full plate washers (Rudnicki and Johnston 2009). The availability of 8-/12-/16-channel manifolds for strip washers provides both single strip washing and full-plate washing capability in the same device, but at the cost of increased wash time for full plates. On the other hand, full plate washers with either a 96- or 384-channel manifold may be preferred for time-efficient wash operations (from a few seconds to a few minutes), but lack the flexibility of the 8-/12-/16-channel units.

The combination of plate washing and bulk dispensing features within the same device may be favored for a space-efficient solution. They are designed to dispense reliably low volumes and reduce prime volume (Rudnicki and Johnston 2009). A major advantage of the washer-dispenser combination comes into play with assay protocols that require the direct addition of fluid after or between the washing steps, such as cell fixation or microplate surface coating reagents.

3. Considerations for using liquid handling devices

3.1. Determination of quality assessment descriptors

Assessment of instrument performance has become important in order to minimize false-positive and false-negative rates in high-throughput screening (Taylor et al. 2002). One of the most important figures of merit in evaluating the performance of liquid handlers is accuracy, which is commonly reported as %bias (Rose 1999):

$$\%bias = 100 \times \left(\frac{V_M - V_T}{V_T} \right) \qquad (1)$$

where V_M is the measured volume and V_T is the theoretical volume (desired). %bias represents the deviation from the desired volume, with a value of 0% indicating no deviation from the true value.

The precision, a measure of reproducibility, is calculated from the mean and standard deviation (SD) of a set of measurements, and it is reported as percent coefficient of variation (%CV) or relative standard deviation (RSD), as shown in Eq. 2. For most cases, it is adequate to have a bias value below 5% and a CV below 10% (Rose 1999).

$$\%CV = 100 \times \frac{SD}{mean} \qquad (2)$$

There have been several approaches for volume verification, which typically consist of gravimetric or photometric methods. Gravimetric measurements utilize the mass and the density (ϱ) of the dispensed solution to determine the volume. It has been used extensively to calibrate and verify the accuracy of liquid dispensers (Bergsdorf et al. 2006; Rhode et al. 2004; Taylor et al. 2002). Typically, the solution is dispensed across a pre-weighed microtiter plate, which is weighed immediately after dispensing to prevent evaporation. %bias can be calculated based on the total weight of the dispensed solution (W_{total}) and the number of dispensed wells (n):

$$\%bias \text{ per well (gravimetric)} = 100 \times \frac{\left(\frac{W_{total}}{n \times \varrho}\right) - V_T}{V_T} \tag{3}$$

Environmental conditions (e.g. temperature and humidity) have major effects on the reliability of gravimetric methods, which facilitates evaporation and water uptake for hygroscopic solvents such as dimethyl sulfoxide (DMSO). These factors of variation can be minimized by placing gasketed lids on the microtiter plates immediately following dispense (Taylor et al. 2002).

Absorbance and fluorescence are the most common photometric methods utilized to test the accuracy and precision of the transferred volumes of a liquid handling device. In a study comparing the performance of the two methods on determining the precision in 96-/384-/1536-well plates, no significant difference was observed between the 96- and 384-well plates (Petersen and Nguyen 2005). However, to achieve similar results for both fluorescence and absorbance measurements in the 1536-well plate, a centrifugation step was required because of the irregular meniscus shape enhanced by the small well geometry. In another study performed on liquid handlers with two different mechanisms, absorbance was found to be a more reliable method as long as the pH stability of the dye-buffer solution is maintained (Rhode et al. 2004).

Fluorescence signal is also known to be susceptible to photobleaching, which can be prevented by shorter excitation times, suitable buffer solutions and adequate concentration of fluorophore (Diaspro et al. 2006; Harris and Mutz 2006). To overcome the problems encountered due to signal quenching in DMSO, sulforhodamine 101 was presented as an alternative fluorescence dye (Walling 2011). Fluorescein was found to be a suitable probe to use in liquid handling performance quantification as long as the DMSO concentration in the buffer solution does not exceed 1% and the stock solutions are stored in 70-100% DMSO in a dark environment (Harris and Mutz 2006). While photobleaching is not an issue in absorbance, the method is limited by high background levels and lower sensitivity compared to fluorescence (Bradshaw et al. 2007). Based on the physical characteristics of a transferred sample and the material of the consumables, unforeseen interactions may be observed influencing the assay results. Especially, DMSO-containing samples are highly affected by the hygroscopic properties of the solvent, which inflates sample volume (Berg et al. 2001).

3.2. Considerations for using bulk reagent dispensers: Peristaltic-based devices

A single screening experiment can be costly, requiring valuable compounds and biological reagents. Routine evaluation of liquid handlers, in particularly prior to each run, is a necessary mean for preventing disastrous outcomes. Simple procedures can be integrated to identify problems in a relatively short period of time, which in many instances, can be easily corrected. Routine analysis should be performed with the actual reagents, because there are several factors that affect the dispensed volumes, including viscosity, density, and temperature (McGown and Hafeman 1998). General considerations to prevent undesirable dispensing performance and common sources of variations include:

3.2.1. Uneven dispensing

Tubings tend to stretch after certain period of use, affecting the intended volume to be delivered. When not in use, the cartridges should be placed in the "rest" position. In addition, autoclaving the cassettes should be minimized. Dispensing speed and the height of the tips in relation to the plate have to be optimized for the intended reagent, as viscous solutions could miss the targeted well at low dispensing speed and large spacing between the tips and microtiter plate. When working with cells, uneven dispensing can be reduced by increasing the prime volume, constant mixing/stirring the cell suspension source and minimizing cell clumps. Solutions should be dispensed in the center of the well, and plates have to be centrifuged when dispensing low volumes to force droplets at the walls to the bottom of the well. Cassettes should be calibrated regularly as recommended by the supplier and checked for tip clogging.

3.2.2. Protein binding

Protein binding to dispensing components is an important point to consider in the implementation of biochemical assays, particularly at low protein concentrations. In some instances, enzymes appear to be inactivated over time when dispensing multiple plates using a liquid handler, when in reality the enzymes have been depleted from the solution due to non-specific binding to plastic, silicone and other polymer-based surfaces. This effect is amplified when dispensing sizeable number of plates, as there is larger exposure time of the assay components to the surfaces of reagent reservoirs and dispensing cassette elements. In order to circumvent this problem, blocking reagents can be added to the buffer, plastic surfaces can be coated, or a combination of both. The two major types of blocking reagents are detergents and proteins. It is preferable to use non-ionic detergents such as Tween-20, Triton X-100 or Nonidet-P40. Among the most widely-used protein blockers are bovine serum albumin (BSA) and casein. Protein blockers are better suited for coating surfaces, as detergents can be easily washed away. Typical working concentrations for detergents range from 0.01 to 0.1%, while protein blockers are used between 0.1 to 3 %. The selection of the appropriate type of blocking reagent and concentration is central to a robust assay. Other less common blocking reagents include polyethylene glycol (PEG), polyvinyl alcohol (PVA) and polyvinyl pyrrolidone (PVP). Additionally, the use of glass reagent reservoirs is recommended.

3.2.3. Clogging

Particles can obstruct the flow of a dispensing cassette mainly by blocking the tips. Complete clogging is fairly easy to recognize, as the lack of fluid coming out of the tips can be visibly noticed. Depending on the degree of obstruction, partial clogging may not be easily perceived by the naked eye, and it is detected only by photometric or gravimetric testing. However, there are certain indications of partial clogging, such as slanted fluid spray or drop formation at the tip. To prevent clogging, the tubing should be primed with deionized water shortly after use, especially prior to priming with alcohol, as salts in the buffer may precipitate and biological reagents may clump. When working with cells, it is recommended to wet the tubing with buffer or media before dispensing cells, and if possible, not to allow the cells to settle in the tubing by emptying the contents back to the reservoir immediate after dispensing (prime/empty cycle).

3.2.4. Foaming

Solutions with high protein content can cause frothing, including media containing serum and biochemical buffers with high percentage of BSA (used as blocking protein). To minimize frothing, it is recommended not to empty the tubing between dispensing (as ordinarily performed in fully automated platforms for large screenings). If tubing emptying is unavoidable, it is advisable to empty a volume smaller than the dead volume. Other means to reduce frothing involve decreasing dispensing speed and applying grease to the cassette tips. Torn or cracked tubing can pull air generating bubbles.

3.2.5. Reservoir container

The reservoir container is an important component of a liquid dispenser that is often neglected in troubleshooting. The material of the container can have a detrimental effect on the assay robustness, such as sticking of proteins to plastic surfaces. For peristaltic pump-based dispensers, we suggest using a jacketed glass flask connected to a water chiller (waterbath with adjustable temperature). Careful monitoring of the temperature in the flask using a thermometer is recommended, as the temperature set in the chiller is not always reflected in the container. Suspensions of cells, beads or nanoparticles have to be constantly stirred to prevent settling, which could result in uneven dispensing or clogging. The stirring speed needs to be optimized, as fast stirring can create bubbles and disturb biological components (cells). When working with large reagent volumes at the start of dispensing, the stirring may have to be reduced as the volume decreases to prevent foaming or bubble formation.

3.2.6. Tubing extension

Extensions can be implemented when the dispensing tubings cannot be immersed in the reservoir container because of its large dimensions. Some commercially available extensions allow for the 8 tubings of a standard cartridge to be coupled into single elongated tubing through metallic cannulas sticking out of a joint casing. For viscous solutions, these types of elongations can introduce bubbles due to the joint design, particularly during prime/empty cycles. The metallic cannulas can easily tear the tubing during fitting, which is ameliorated by using glycerol or alcohol to smoothen the surfaces. A better alternative is to build home-made extensions by attaching each of the new tubings to separate discarded tubings through connectors, which can be made by cutting the end of a pipette tip.

3.2.7. Routine quality assessment

During assay development and validation, factors affecting liquid dispenser performance are identified and corrected. However, setbacks can occur randomly regardless of detailed preparations ahead of the screens. For instance, torn tubing, tip blockage or incorrect cartridge setup cannot be prevented a priori. Therefore, it is recommended to rapidly monitor dispensing variations at the start of a screen, where problems encountered at this stage can be usually corrected fairly quickly.

We normally dispense a solution of fluorescein isothiocyanate (FITC) in PBS into a couple of 384-well plates. Fluorescence intensities are analyzed for signal variations corresponding to each cassette channel, as described by %CV and %bias' (Fig.2). Determination of %CV for the entire plate is frequently performed in many laboratories, but this approach cannot distinguish issues with individual channels. In addition, a flawed channel does not necessarily change drastically the %CV of the whole plate, as illustrated by Fig. 2A. The types of problems commonly associated to high %CV include improper cassette mounting, tubing stretching and damage.

There are instances when the tip is partially obstructed, leading to reduced volume delivered. Even when a channel displays low fluorescence counts, the signal can still have small %CV values (Fig. 2B). We have adapted the concept of %bias to detect significant deviations in signal intensity for each row (S_R) compared to that of the whole plate (S_T), resulting in %bias' (Eq. 4). Values lower than 10 %CV and 10 %bias' are acceptable.

$$\% \text{ bias }' = 100 \times \left(\frac{S_R \text{-} S_T}{S_T} \right) \tag{4}$$

3.3. Considerations for using transfer devices: Pintool

The pintool has become a mature technology for transferring nanoliter to sub-microliter volumes. Even though the system is regarded as fairly simple and robust, there are a number of points to consider for a consistent and reliable performance:

3.3.1. Volume variation

The volume delivered by a pin can change due to a number of factors. To minimize volume variations, there should be consistency in immersion depth (Dunn and Feygin 2000). There is a minimum volume required in the source plate, and the destination plate should not be dry (Rudnicki and Johnston 2009). The dwell time that pins spend in the fluid and withdrawal speed from the liquid surface should be optimized for solutions of very different properties (e.g. viscosity).

The slot of a pin can be tainted by compound precipitation or formation of suspension deposits (Fig. 3B). Sufficient and robust washing and drying steps are effective in preventing deposition and being critical to avoid carry-over and cross-contamination. The pins can be physically damaged by dipping in highly uneven surfaces, particularly when using slotted pins (Fig. 3C). Coated pins should avoid harsh washing procedures, such as going through powerful sonication washes.

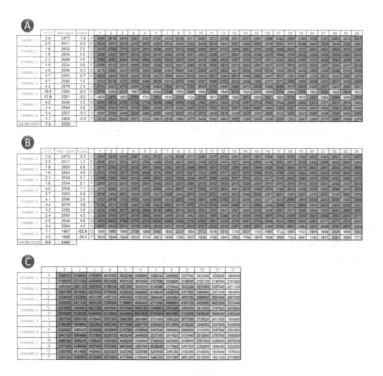

Figure 2. A-B) Delivery variation by a bulk reagent dispenser distributing a FITC solution into 384-well plates. Certain dispensing cassette channels display either higher %CV or %bias' values than the anticipated cut-off of 10%. C) Cell settling in the reagent reservoir when transferring to a microtiter plate using an automated pipetting system with an 8-channel head, with 1 min delay between transfers to each column. Cell settling is uneven due to the v-shaped bottom of the reservoir, causing the intensity pattern observed in the plate. The cells (HEK293T) were incubated with Cell-Titer-Glo® for 20 min prior to luminescence reading.

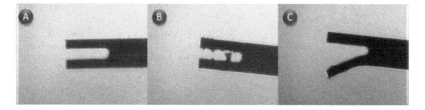

Figure 3. Magnified view of FP1NS50H pins (V&P Scientific, Inc.) with A) clean slot B) dirty slot C) damaged slot.

3.3.2. Carry-over

After transferring compounds from one plate to another, the pins are washed in DMSO, alcohol, water or a combination of these solutions. The pintool protocol involves dipping the pins in each solution bath certain number of times, at a particular speed and soaking time. The pins are then dried on lint-free blotting paper. Protocols of pintool devices used on robotic platforms are optimized for effectiveness in removing previous transfers while spending the minimum time between wash cycles. In many cases, the drugging (i.e., addition of compound to assay well) step using pintool becomes the bottleneck in a screening campaign, and the washing step accounts for most of the time consumed. However, certain assays can be very sensitive to compound carry-over, particularly if the compounds are very potent modulators and bind avidly to the pin surface. In such cases, increasing the number of dips and soaking time can improve cleanliness, albeit at the cost of increasing total transfer time.

Fig. 4 illustrates the effect of four different wash protocols in a kinase assay using staurosporine as the inhibitor. After compound transfer by pintool to the first assay plate, the pins are immersed in DMSO and isopropanol reservoirs, followed by drying on blotting paper. Subsequently, the pins are dipped in a second assay plate containing the kinase system. Residual staurosporine in the pins increases the signal variation as determined by %CV of a set of multiple wells. Protocol 1 has the least number of dips and soaking time per bath, resulting in the most dramatic signal variation due to carry-over. This general approach is recommended for detecting carry-over and selecting the appropriate pintool wash.

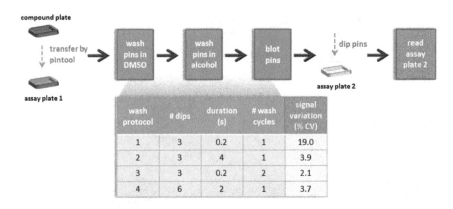

wash protocol	# dips	duration (s)	# wash cycles	signal variation (% CV)
1	3	0.2	1	19.0
2	3	4	1	3.9
3	3	0.2	2	2.1
4	6	2	1	3.7

Figure 4. General approach to detect compound carry-over and optimize pintool washing. A single wash cycle consists of dipping the pins in DMSO and isopropanol baths, followed by blotting on lint-free paper.

3.3.3. Routine quality assessment

Regular pintool calibration and quality assessment can considerably improve data quality. In screening runs at a single compound concentration, well-maintained pins can lead to a reduction of false negative hits, as damaged or dirty pins would usually deliver lower volumes than anticipated. In dose-response analysis, the quality of the curve fit is highly dependent on the variability of the data points.

A good quality control procedure should provide the transferred volume and the variation associated with the pin set. We implemented a relatively quick and simple procedure using a fluorescent dye (FITC). Prior to the test, the pins are washed as described above. A calibration curve is generated of fluorescence intensity as a function of FITC concentration. Using the pintool, FITC in DMSO is transferred from a source plate to several destination plates containing PBS (the use of 4 plates was shown to be sufficient). The average transferred volume per pin is calculated using the fluorescence signal of the destination plates and the calibration curve. Volume variation across the microtiter plate can be readily appreciated by plotting volume against well position (Fig. 5, top charts). The pink and green solid lines represent the upper and lower boundaries within 10% CV of the average volume, where outliers can be clearly identified. The frequency chart (Fig. 5, bottom chart) displays outliers present in 1, 2, 3 or all of the 4 destination plates, and it can be used to identify pins that consistently provide volumes outside a specified range. In the example shown in Fig. 5, pins corresponding to positions A13, B21, D8, F13, K1, N14 and P20 will have to be replaced. Depending on the need, stringency can be adjusted by changing the boundaries as specified by %CV. It is highly recommended to utilize the same freshly prepared fluorescent dye and buffer solutions in all aspects of the protocol. A template for data analysis can be easily created in conventional software such as MS-Excel.

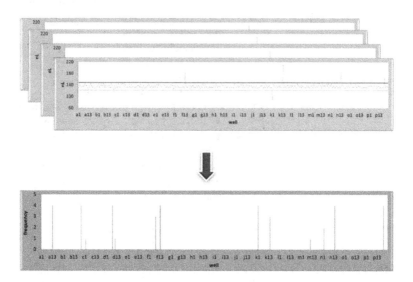

Figure 5. A simple and comprehensive approach to analyze pintool performance. Individual pins can be selected for replacement based on consistent variation across multiple transfers.

3.4. Considerations for using transfer devices: Pipettors

3.4.1. Pipette stations

The automation station is an integral part of any high throughput pipettor, regardless of the type of tips (fixed or disposable) it employs. It typically consists of ANSI/SBS standard compliant single or multiple deck positions on a stationary or moving platform to hold the labware, with a moving arm situated above the platform containing the single- or multi-channel pipette head. A major advantage of automated pipettor devices over manual or electronic multichannel hand-held pipettes is the elimination of inconsistency in the transfer process by minimizing human intervention, which also enables high throughput applications that are not otherwise feasible. The three major tasks that can be performed with suitable hardware settings are liquid transfer, cherry-picking and serial-dilution.

For plate-to-plate liquid transfers, 96- or 384-well pipette heads are preferred to work with 96-/384-/1536-well microplates to speed up the process and increase the throughput. While 4-/8-/12-/16-pipette heads can also be used for direct transfer applications, they are primarily used to perform serial-dilutions. On the other hand, a single channel pipette tip is an essential component to accomplish cherry-picking tasks.

The speed of an automated pipettor is important for time-sensitive experiments. Especially when performing small volume transfers into microplates, the amount of time spent to transfer liquids in a column-by-column or row-by-row manner may be problematic due to quick evaporation. If the speed of transfer is too slow, some evaporation in the first column or row may be observed before dispensing to the last column or row, causing inconsistent volume across the plate. To avoid evaporation issues during liquid transfers, deck size, pipettor speed, head type and the transfer volume should be considered.

3.4.2. Tip contamination

Sample carry-over is a common problem in liquid handling tasks requiring sequential dipping steps into various sample reservoirs. With fixed-tips, an adequate cleaning step is essential between two transfer operations to prevent sample carry-over. An on-deck cleaning protocol often consists of immersion in a bath (DMSO, alcohol and/or water) with optional sonication step. The tips should be allowed sufficient drying time to prevent sample dilution in the following transfer phase. Appropriate wash solutions should be selected and the optimum length of washing time should be determined during the assay development stage. Although fixed-tips may have the risk of carry-over, they enable more accurate and precise transfers in smaller volume ranges (Felton 2003).

Contamination can also be associated with disposable tips, especially when sterile and nuclease-free assay conditions are required. The speed at which the pipette tips are removed from a sample fluid was found to correlate to the amount of macroscopic droplets stuck to the outer surface of the polypropylene tips, which contributed to cross-contamination (Berg et al. 2001). It was also reported that to decrease this form of cross-contamination, which is influenced by the tip shape and the sample-polypropylene interactions, the removal speed should be slow enough to diminish droplet generation.

Impurities can also leach out of the disposable tips when in contact with solvents such as DMSO. Studies have shown that bioactive compounds released from plastic labware may interfere with assay readouts causing misleading experimental results (McDonald et al. 2008; Niles and Coassin 2008; Watson et al. 2009). Consumable materials, especially polypropylene tips, tend to adsorb certain compounds, leading to unreliable concentrations in the destination plates (Harris et al. 2010). Therefore, it is recommended to test and validate the influence of consumables on an assay during assay development and whenever there is a change in labware.

3.4.3. Foaming

Pipetting viscous and "sticky" samples is challenging due to bubble formation. Among the most important parameters to consider in avoiding these issues are the speed that the tips exit the sample fluid and the aspirate/dispense rates; they should be slow enough to avoid residuals at the inside and outside of the tips. Pre- and post-air pipetting options should be avoided.

3.4.4. Pipette behavior affecting dispensing variation

Most pipettor systems provide pre- and post-air aspiration functions to ensure accurate liquid transfers. Introduction of air into the tips before or after the aspiration of the sample liquid is recommended to improve volume accuracy by forcing all the liquid out of the tips. In a study performed to optimize the automated parameters to achieve a 10 µL transfer volume in a sequential transfer experiment, introduction of a 5 µL pre-air gap significantly reduced the relative volume inaccuracy along with the CV of the final transferred volume in a 96-well plate (Albert et al. 2007). While this method may help to achieve more precise results especially with small volume transfers, bubble formation in the destination wells may be inevitable unless proceeded by a shaking or centrifugation step. Post-air aspiration may also be applied to create an air gap between liquids, preventing unsought contamination in the source reservoirs when multiple samples are picked up sequentially into a single tip before the delivery into the destination reservoir.

When small and repetitive volume transfers into multiple destinations are needed, it is a common practice to pick up a single large volume and deliver smaller amounts in a sequential mode. However, with this method, it is hard to achieve accurate delivery in each step. In a study of multi-sequential dispense accuracy, it was shown that the first and last dispense steps led to relatively higher and lower transferred volumes, respectively, in addition to increased relative inaccuracy (Albert et al. 2007). Therefore, it is recommended to dispense the first and last steps into the source reservoir to enhance the precision in the destination plate. Delivery performance of the dry versus pre-wetted tips may also exhibit differences in variability depending on the sample characteristics.

Droplet formation at the end of the pipette tips after a dispense action remains an issue for liquids with high viscosity or low densities. Besides the selection of the optimum dispense speed, a "tip touch" function is a useful feature offered in some automated pipettors, where the tips contact the well wall at the end of a dispense step to force the release of the droplet. The path of the moving pipetting arm across the deck should be carefully determined to reduce the chance of contaminating other labware by hanging droplets.

Proper mixing of solutions in the source reservoir before aspiration and in the destination reservoir after dispensing may greatly affect the final assay quality due to the necessity of uniform sample concentrations. To avoid the formation of concentration gradient in wells, mixing can be performed by repetitive pipetting cycles. Mixing of the well contents by pipetting up and down is proven to be a quicker and more efficient method compared to free diffusion or shaking, which are not as successful due to the correlations between well size, content volume and the exerted capillary forces (Berg et al. 2001; Shieh et al. 2010; Travis et al. 2010). Mixing is necessary when dealing with suspensions (cells, beads, etc.). For instance, cell settling creates uneven cell density in the source reservoir, which would lead to aspiration of decreasing number of cells over time (Fig. 2C)

3.4.5. Routine quality assessment

Verification of transferred volumes and routine quality control (QC) are the most important and inevitable processes when working with liquid handling devices. While the verification method should be reliable enough to quantify the pipettor performance, it should also be easy and fast to be applied routinely. The performance assessment described for bulk liquid dispensers (section 3.2.7.) can also be applied to pipettors as long as the same volume is distributed throughout the plate for %CV and %bias' calculations.

As mentioned previously, liquid handlers are heavily used to perform serial dilutions, and suitable QC techniques should be employed to validate dilution performance, particularly when accurate compound potency is directly dependent on concentration accuracy. Dilution ratio, accuracy, precision and outlier distribution constitute the four major criteria that should be evaluated (Popa-Burke et al. 2009). Artel developed an approach to determine dilution and transferred volume accuracy by using dual-wavelength photometry, where two absorbance dyes with baseline resolved spectra are mixed at various ratios using a liquid handler (Albert 2007; Dong et al. 2007). This dual-dye ratiometric method can be applied by using a multichannel verification system (MVS) equipped with the necessary instrumentation and analysis (Bradshaw et al. 2005). Dual-dye photometry is also proven to be suitable to measure the efficiency of different mixing methods (Spaulding et al. 2006) and when pipetting non-aqueous solutions (Bradshaw et al. 2007).

3.5. Considerations for using microplate washers

3.5.1. General considerations

One of the major concerns with any high throughput microplate handler device is its compatibility with plates of various types and sizes. While most high throughput instruments are designed to accommodate labware with dimensions conforming to ANSI/SBS standards, an ideal plate washer is also able to support flat, v-shaped and round-bottom plates.

Both the vacuum assembly and the bottle setup are also important aspects of the plate washer. Although most washers operate through changes in vacuum pressure, pump-based vacuum-free and pressure-free systems are also offered.

Plate washers functioning by positive displacement principle are also available, enabling non-contact washing with no residual volume (Rudnicki and Johnston 2009). For assays where more than one wash buffer may need to be used, plate washers with multiple dispense channels and automatic buffer switching capability are preferred to minimize both operation time and contamination. Examples of other optional features for safe instrument operation include waste liquid level sensors and plate detection sensors to avoid unwanted overflows and jams. For BSL2 or higher level experiments, a washer with aerosol cover should be chosen to prevent spread of the contagious material.

3.5.2. Washer performance

Although compatibility and control properties are important, plate washers are predominantly evaluated by their wash performance. Plate washers provide a range of user-defined dispense/aspirate heights, flow rates, and needle probe positioning in reference to the well walls. By adjusting these parameters for each step of the wash cycle, optimal wash performance can be ensured. On the other hand, an adequate wash quality needs to be reached to diminish extensive background signal and high signal variations amongst wells. This can be primarily achieved by minimizing the amount of liquid left inside each well at the end of the aspiration step. Besides their effects on wash power, the above-mentioned parameters also have an impact on the residual volume and need to be fine-tuned in conjunction with the vacuum/pump settings. Some plate washers may also provide multipoint, secondary, crosswise or delayed aspiration modes aiming to deliver the best results. The number of wash cycles and the length of soaking time are other settings that can be modified to reduce background noise levels.

3.5.3. Washer maintenance

Since plate washers consist of tubing and needles which transport buffer solutions or waste liquid to or from the device, they require special cleaning processes as they are prone to be clogged by chemical residues such as salt and proteins from the wash liquids. Depending on the frequency of use, the fluid path may need to be rinsed daily to prevent blockage and contamination, especially if different buffers are being delivered through the same tubing. An efficient cleaning method alternates deionized water and a detergent such as Terg-a-Zyme®, which is highly recommended by plate washer manufacturers. Plate washers which provide an automatic cleaning feature or integrated ultrasonic washing technology are often easier to maintain. Models which do not contain built-in cleaning functionality are generally supplied with removable dispense/aspiration manifolds to ease the maintenance tasks.

Cleaning of the other detachable or fixed plate washer components should also be performed periodically.

3.5.4. Troubleshooting

Plate washers serve as an excellent alternative to time consuming manual wash procedures for many applications. Since all the wash parameters should be optimized for each specific application during the assay development stage, a tedious troubleshooting process may be inevitable while setting up wash protocols to meet specific assay needs. Table 1 presents a summary of wash parameters/components and their contributions to the wash performance along with various troubleshooting tips. Different assay types may require distinct considerations. With biochemical assays, minimizing the background signal and well-to-well variations are the most important tasks in the optimization process. Low background signal levels can be achieved by reducing the leftover liquid volume in each well. Decreasing the aspiration height and lowering the aspiration rate can greatly affect the residual volume leading to minimal liquid amounts in the wells. In order to prevent high standard deviations in the assay readouts, equal residual volumes should be attempted by optimizing the aspiration/dispense heights and rates. Depending on the viscosity of the wash buffer, high aspiration rates or low dispense rates may lead to unequal volumes. Inadequate priming volumes, unadjusted dispense or aspiration heights, clogged tubing, and physical misalignments between the manifolds and plate carrier should also be avoided to prevent high signal variations. The effect of the aspiration height on the final residual volume is presented in Fig. 6 for both 96- and 384-well black plates with clear bottom. The volume of the residual liquid (water) per well was measured with the gravimetric technique at several selected aspiration heights on a Biotek EL405 microplate washer, while all the other wash parameters were kept constant. A rising trend is observed in the final volume as the aspiration height is increased.

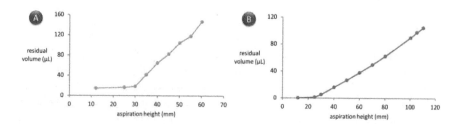

Figure 6. Effects of aspiration height on residual volume. Residual volume was measured in a) 96-well and B) 384-well plates at various aspiration heights. Residual volume was increased as the aspiration height from the bottom of the well was increased.

In cell-based assays, gentle cell washing is one of the most critical factors to produce reproducible assay results, and it can be controlled by several settings such as aspiration and dispense rates, heights and horizontal positions. For loosely-adherent cells, the cell layer attached to the bottom of the well may be easily disrupted by rigorous wash cycles, and the aspiration and dispense rates should be set low enough to prevent turbulence inside the wells. For the same purpose, wash fluid should be dispensed at a distance from the well bottom and may be even be aimed at the well walls when possible. To observe the consequences of inadequate washing and dispensing parameters on the cell layer endurance, a 3-cycle wash experiment was performed on HEK 293T cells, which are known for their low adherence and propensity to be frequently washed away in cell-based assays. The fixing solution was dispensed at medium speed, and the cells were washed before and after fixation. Representative images from wells containing an intact or damaged cell layer are presented in Fig. 7. When dealing with adherent cells, each step of the assay protocol should be optimized, including those involving other liquid handling devices such as bulk dispensers, pintools and pipettors.

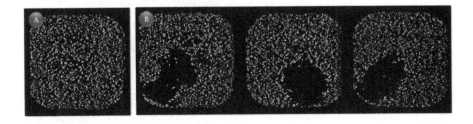

Figure 7. Effects of non-optimized dispensing and washing on low-adherent cells. HEK293T cells were fixed, stained with Hoechst 33258 and imaged with Acumen eX3 in a 384-well black clear bottom plates. The fixing solution was dispensed by a Thermo Scientific Matrix® Wellmate®. Representative images (shown here in false color green) of A) an intact cell layer and B) disrupted cell layers indicated cell loss due to harsh dispense and wash settings.

As with most high throughput instrument operations, it is a common practice to perform a periodic quality check on plate washers to assure a satisfactory wash performance at each use. It is important to perform these assessments with a wash buffer that has a similar viscosity to the buffers used in most of the applications. For evaluations on the residual volume, one can perform a mock wash with a dummy plate and measure the leftover liquid volume inside the wells with a single or multichannel manual pipettor. For more accurate results, gravimetric or colorimetric techniques can be used to calculate the average volume per well. This way, one can also test if dispensing/aspiration is consistent in all the probes, and if there is any physical failure with any of the device components.

parameter/component	effect	troubleshooting tips
prime	dispense performance	• prevent air bubble formation or no/uneven dispensing with adequate priming
aspiration rate	residual volume, gentle/rigorous washing	• higher residual volume if too fast • perturbed cell layer if too fast • uneven aspiration if too fast
aspiration height	residual volume, gentle/rigorous washing	• higher residual volume if too high • uneven aspiration if too low or too high • perturbed cell layer if aspiration probes touch the well bottom • undisturbed cell layer if high enough
horizontal aspirate position	gentle/rigorous washing	• prevent bead loss by offsetting the aspirate position (for magnetic bead assays)
dispense flow rate	dispense volume, gentle/rigorous washing	• uneven dispensing if too slow • fluid overflow if too slow or too fast • perturbed cell layer if too fast • air bubble formation if too slow
dispense height	dispense volume, gentle/rigorous washing	• uneven dispensing if too low or too high • fluid overflow if too high
horizontal dispense position	gentle/rigorous washing	• undisturbed cell layer if dispense position is offset to aim the well walls
assay buffer properties	residual volume, aspiration/dispense performance	• optimize for viscous/non-viscous buffer solutions • add surfactant to the buffer solution to reduce surface tension
vacuum/pump assembly	aspiration/dispense performance	• no/uneven aspiration with insufficient vacuum supply • no/uneven aspiration or leakage if tubing is defective, bent or clogged
plate carrier	aspiration/dispense performance	• uneven aspiration/dispense if plate carrier is not leveled or movement is blocked • plate is placed on the carrier with A1 in the correct position • enough plate clearance to prevent jams • higher throughput with lower plate clearance

Table 1. Wash parameters and troubleshooting advices

4. Conclusion

In order to fulfill the need for higher throughput options, the technology behind liquid handling devices is in constant progression, with systems capable of delivering smaller volumes at a faster rate with accuracy and precision. These developments should consider cost reduction by minimizing reagent and solvent expenditure, as well as reducing consumables.

The main concerns and limitations that liquid handling systems face are reproducibility and reliability. The devices should be robust to execute extensive experiments in a daily basis with minimal downtime and maintenance. However, as a single screen can generate thousands of data points, the user is required to ensure all the devices are functioning up to standards by implementing routine quality assessments. Regardless of the technological innovations and advancements, scientists are compelled to spend significant amount of time optimizing the liquid handling parameters to suit specific assay conditions. A thorough understanding of the principles, strengths and limitations of the instruments is advantageous in preventing undesirable results and facilitating troubleshooting.

Acknowledgements

This work was supported by the American Lebanese Syrian Associated Charities (ALSAC), St. Jude Children's Research Hospital, and National Cancer Institute grant P30CA027165.

Author details

Sergio C. Chai, Asli N. Goktug, Jimmy Cui, Jonathan Low and Taosheng Chen

High Throughput Screening Center, Department of Chemical Biology and Therapeutics, St. Jude Children's Research Hospital, USA

References

[1] Albert, KJ, Bradshaw, JT, Knaide, TR & Rogers, AL (2006). Verifying liquid-handler performance for complex or nonaqueous reagents: a new approach. *Journal of the Association for Laboratory Automation*, Vol. 11(4): pp. 172-80

[2] Bateman, TA, Ayers, RA & Greenway, RB (1999). An engineering evaluation of four fluid transfer devices for automated 384-well high throughput screening. *Laboratory Robotics and Automation*, Vol. 11(5): pp. 250-59

[3] Berg, M, Undisz, K, Thiericke, R, Zimmermann, P, Moore, T & Posten, C (2001). Evaluation of liquid handling conditions in microplates. *Journal of Biomolecular Screening*, Vol. 6(1): pp. 47-56

[4] Bergsdorf, C, Gewiese, N, Stolz, A, Mann, R, Parczyk, K & Bomer, U (2006). A cost-effective solution to reduce dead volume of a standard dispenser system by a factor of 5. *Journal of Biomolecular Screening*, Vol. 11(4): pp. 407-12

[5] Bradshaw, JT, Curtis, RH, Knaide, TR & Spaulding, BW (2007). Determining dilution accuracy in microtiter plate assays using a quantitative dual-wavelength absorbance method. *Journal of the Association for Laboratory Automation*, Vol. 12(5): pp. 260-66

[6] Bradshaw, JT, Knaide, T, Rogers, A & Curtis, R (2005). Multichannel Verification System (MVS): a dual-dye ratiometric photometry system for performance verification of multichannel liquid delivery devices. *Journal of the Association for Laboratory Automation*, Vol. 10(1): pp. 35-42

[7] Cleveland, PH & Koutz, PJ (2005). Nanoliter dispensing for uHTS using pin tools. *Assay and Drug Development Technologies*, Vol. 3(2): pp. 213-25

[8] Diaspro, A, Chirico, G, Usai, C, Ramoino, P & Dobrucki, J (2006). Photobleaching. In: *Handbook of Biological Confocal Microscopy*. J. B. Pawley. pp 690-702, Springer Science +Business Media, LLC, New York

[9] Dong, H, Ouyang, Z, Liu, J & Jemal, M (2006). The use of a dual dye photometric calibration method to identify possible sample dilution from an automated multichannel liquid-handling system. *Journal of the Association for Laboratory Automation*, Vol. 11(2): pp. 60-64

[10] Dunn, DA & Feygin, I (2000). Challenges and solutions to ultra-high-throughput screening assay miniaturization: submicroliter fluid handling. *Drug Discovery Today*, Vol. 5(12): pp. S84-S91

[11] Ellson, R, Mutz, M, Browning, B, Lee, L, Miller, MF & Papen, R (2003). Transfer of low nanoliter volumes between microplates using focused acoustics—automation considerations. *Journal of the Association for Laboratory Automation*, Vol. 8(5): pp. 29-34

[12] Felton, MJ (2003). Liquid handling: dispensing reliability. *Analytical Chemistry*, Vol. 75(17): pp. 397a-99a

[13] Harris, D, Mutz, M, Sonntag, M, Stearns, R, Shieh, J, Pickett, S, Ellson, R & Olechno, J (2008). Low nanoliter acoustic transfer of aqueous fluids with high precision and accuracy of volume transfer and positional placement. *Journal of the Association for Laboratory Automation*, Vol. 13(2): pp. 97-102

[14] Harris, D, Olechno, J, Datwani, S & Ellson, R (2010). Gradient, contact-free volume transfers minimize compound loss in dose-response experiments. *Journal of Biomolecular Screening*, Vol. 15(1): pp. 86-94

[15] Harris, DL & Mutz, M (2006). Debunking the myth: validation of fluorescein for testing and precision of nanoliter dispensing. *Journal of the Association for Laboratory Automation*, Vol.11(4): pp. 233-39

[16] James, P & Papen, R (1998). Nanolitre dispensing - a new innovation in robotic liquid handling. *Drug Discovery Today*, Vol. 3(9): pp. 429-30

[17] Kong, F, Yuan, L, Zheng, YF & Chen, W (2012). Automatic liquid handling for life science: a critical review of the current state of the art. *Journal of Laboratory Automation*, Vol. 17(3): pp. 169-85

[18] Lee, S (2006). Development of a vacuum filtration system for the conventional microplate washer. *Journal of Pharmacologicaland Toxicololgical Methods*, Vol. 53(3): pp. 272-6

[19] McDonald, GR, Hudson, AL, Dunn, SMJ, You, HT, Baker, GB, Whittal, RM, Martin, JW, Jha, A, Edmondson, DE & Holt, A (2008). Bioactive contaminants leach from disposable laboratory plasticware. *Science*, Vol. 322(5903): pp. 917-17

[20] McGown, EL & Hafeman, DG (1998). Multichannel pipettor performance verified by measuring pathlength of reagent dispensed into a microplate. *Analytical Biochemistry*, Vol. 258(1): pp. 155-57

[21] Murthy, TV, Kroncke, D & Bonin, PD (2011). Adding precise nanoliter volume capabilities to liquid-handling automation for compound screening experimentation. *Journal of the Association for Laboratory Automation*, Vol. 16(3): pp. 221-28

[22] Niles, WD & Coassin, PJ (2005). Piezo- and solenoid valve-based liquid dispensing for miniaturized assays. *Assay and Drug Development Technologies*, Vol. 3(2): pp. 189-202

[23] Niles, WD & Coassin, PJ (2008). Cyclic olefin polymers: innovative materials for high-density multiwell plates. *Assay and Drug Development Technologies*, Vol. 6(4): pp. 577-90

[24] Olechno, J, Shieh, J & Ellson, R (2006). Improving IC50 results with acoustic droplet ejection. *Journal of the Association for Laboratory Automation*, Vol. 11: pp. 240-46

[25] Petersen, J & Nguyen, J (2005). Comparison of absorbance and fluorescence methods for determining liquid dispensing precision. *Journal of the Association for Laboratory Automation*, Vol. 10: pp. 82-87

[26] Popa-Burke, I, Lupotsky, B, Boyer, J, Gannon, W, Hughes, R, Kadwill, P, Lyerly, D, Nichols, J, Nixon, E, Rimmer, D, Saiz-Nicolas, I, Sanfiz-Pinto, B & Holland, S (2009). Establishing quality assurance criteria for serial dilution operations on liquid-handling equipment. *Journal of Biomolecular Screening*, Vol. 14(8): pp. 1017-30

[27] Ramírez, M, Tudela, C, Crespo, JB, Rubles, A, Jiménez, A, Tarazona, G, Fernández, L, Sánchez, P, Kroncke, D, Tabanera, N, Pérez, J, Sánchez, M, Tormo, JR & Peláez, F (2008). Automation of sample dispensing using pocket tips for evaluation of CYP2C9

isoenzyme reversible inhibition in an evolution precision pipetting platform. *Journal of the Association for Laboratory Automation*, Vol. 13: pp. 289-96

[28] Rhode, H, Schulze, M, Renard, S, Zimmerman, P, Moore, T, Cumme, GA & Horn, A (2004). An improved method for checking HTS/uHTS liquid-handling systems. *Journal of Biomolecular Screening*, Vol. 9(8): pp. 726-33

[29] Rose, D (1999). Microdispensing technologies in drug discovery. *Drug Discovery Today*, Vol. 4(9): pp. 411-19

[30] Rudnicki, S & Johnston, S (2009). Overview of liquid handling instrumentation for high-throughput applications. *Current Protocols in Chemical Biology*, Vol. 1(1): pp. 43-54

[31] Schober, A, Gunther, R, Schwienhorst, A, Doring, M & Lindemann, BF (1993). Accurate high-speed liquid handling of very small biological samples. *Biotechniques*, Vol. 15(2): pp. 324-29

[32] Shieh, J, Ellson, RN & Olechno, J (2006). The effects of small molecule and protein solutes on acoustic drop ejection. *Journal of the Association for Laboratory Automation*, Vol. 11(4): pp. 227-32

[33] Shieh, J, Jamieson, B & Vivek, V (2010). Evaluating five microplate mixing techniques: diffusion, centrifugation, shaking, pipetting and ultrasonic mixing. Poster presented at Society for Biomolecular Sciences, Phoenix, AZ

[34] Spaulding, BW, Bradshaw, JT & Rogers, AL (2006). A method to evaluate mixing efficiency in 384-well plates. Poster presented at Society for Biomolecular Sciences, Seattle, WA

[35] Stobbs, LW (1990). Construction of a simple, inexpensive multiple enzyme-linked immunosorbent assay microdilution plate washer. *Applied and Environmental Microbiology*, Vol. 56(6): pp. 1763-7

[36] Taylor, PB, Ashman, S, Baddeley, SM, Bartram, SL, Battle, CD, Bond, BC, Clements, YM, Gaul, NJ, McAllister, WE, Mostacero, JA, Ramon, F, Wilson, JM, Hertzberg, RP, Pope, AJ &Macarron, R (2002). A standard operating procedure for assessing liquid handler performance in high-throughput screening. *Journal of Biomolecular Screening*, Vol. 7(6): pp. 554-69

[37] Travis, M, Vivek, V, Jamieson, B, Shieh, J & Weaver, D (2010). Mixing effectiveness – amethodology and study of microplate mixing techniques including ultrasonic HEN-DRIX SM100. Poster presented at Association for Laboratory Automation, Palm Spring, CA

[38] Turmel, M, Itkin, Z, Liu, D & Nie, D (2010). An innovative way to create assay ready plates for concentration response testing using acoustic technology. *Journal of the Association for Laboratory Automation*, Vol. 15(4): pp. 297-305

[39] Walling, LA (2011). An inline QC method for determining serial dilution perform-
      ance of DMSO-based systems. *Journal of the Association for Laboratory Automation*, Vol.
      16(3): pp. 235-40

[40] Watson, J, Greenough, EB, Leet, JE, Ford, MJ, Drexler, DM, Belcastro, JV, Herbst, JJ,
      Chatterjee, M & Banks, M (2009). Extraction, identification, and functional characteri-
      zation of a bioactive substance from automated compound-handling plastic tips.
      Journal of Biomolecular Screening, Vol. 14(5): pp. 566-72

Permissions

The contributors of this book come from diverse backgrounds, making this book a truly international effort. This book will bring forth new frontiers with its revolutionizing research information and detailed analysis of the nascent developments around the world.

We would like to thank Hany El-Shemy, for lending his expertise to make the book truly unique. He has played a crucial role in the development of this book. Without his invaluable contribution this book wouldn't have been possible. He has made vital efforts to compile up to date information on the varied aspects of this subject to make this book a valuable addition to the collection of many professionals and students.

This book was conceptualized with the vision of imparting up-to-date information and advanced data in this field. To ensure the same, a matchless editorial board was set up. Every individual on the board went through rigorous rounds of assessment to prove their worth. After which they invested a large part of their time researching and compiling the most relevant data for our readers. Conferences and sessions were held from time to time between the editorial board and the contributing authors to present the data in the most comprehensible form. The editorial team has worked tirelessly to provide valuable and valid information to help people across the globe.

Every chapter published in this book has been scrutinized by our experts. Their significance has been extensively debated. The topics covered herein carry significant findings which will fuel the growth of the discipline. They may even be implemented as practical applications or may be referred to as a beginning point for another development. Chapters in this book were first published by InTech; hereby published with permission under the Creative Commons Attribution License or equivalent.

The editorial board has been involved in producing this book since its inception. They have spent rigorous hours researching and exploring the diverse topics which have resulted in the successful publishing of this book. They have passed on their knowledge of decades through this book. To expedite this challenging task, the publisher supported the team at every step. A small team of assistant editors was also appointed to further simplify the editing procedure and attain best results for the readers.

Our editorial team has been hand-picked from every corner of the world. Their multi-ethnicity adds dynamic inputs to the discussions which result in innovative outcomes. These outcomes are then further discussed with the researchers and contributors who give their valuable feedback and opinion regarding the same. The feedback is then collaborated with the researches and they are edited in a comprehensive manner to aid the understanding of the subject.

Apart from the editorial board, the designing team has also invested a significant amount of their time in understanding the subject and creating the most relevant covers. They scrutinized every image to scout for the most suitable representation of the subject and create an appropriate cover for the book.

The publishing team has been involved in this book since its early stages. They were actively engaged in every process, be it collecting the data, connecting with the contributors or procuring relevant information. The team has been an ardent support to the editorial, designing and production team. Their endless efforts to recruit the best for this project, has resulted in the accomplishment of this book. They are a veteran in the field of academics and their pool of knowledge is as vast as their experience in printing. Their expertise and guidance has proved useful at every step. Their uncompromising quality standards have made this book an exceptional effort. Their encouragement from time to time has been an inspiration for everyone.

The publisher and the editorial board hope that this book will prove to be a valuable piece of knowledge for researchers, students, practitioners and scholars across the globe.

List of Contributors

Gabriel Magoma
Department of Biochemistry, Jomo Kenyatta University of Agriculture and Technology, Nairobi, Kenya

Jolanta Natalia Latosińska and Magdalena Latosińska
Faculty of Physics, Adam Mickiewicz University, Poznań, Poland

Irina Piatkov, Trudi Jones and Mark McLean
University of Western Sydney, Blacktown Clinical School and Research Centre, Blacktown Hospital, Western Sydney Local Health District, Blacktown, Australia

Elizabeth Hong-Geller and Sofiya Micheva-Viteva
Bioscience Division, Los Alamos National Laboratory, Bioscience Division, Los Alamos, NM, USA

Lourdes Rodríguez-Fragoso and Jorge Reyes-Esparza
Universidad Autónoma del Estado de Morelos, Facultad de Farmacia, Cuernavaca, México

Melanie A. Jordan
Midwestern University, College of Pharmacy – Glendale, Glendale, AZ, USA

Carsten Wrenger
Department of Parasitology, Institute of Biomedical Science, University of São Paulo, Av. Prof. Lineu Prestes, São Paulo-SP, Brazil

Isolmar Schettert
Laboratory of Genetics and Molecular Cardiology, Heart Institute InCor, Av. Dr. Eneas de Carvalho Aguiar, São Paulo-SP, Brazil

Eva Liebau
Department of Molecular Physiology, University of Münster, Hindenburgplatz, Münster, Germany

Sergio C. Chai, Asli N. Goktug, Jimmy Cui, Jonathan Low and Taosheng Chen
High Throughput Screening Center, Department of Chemical Biology and Therapeutics, St. Jude Children's Research Hospital, USA